Urology

Editor

ROBERT E. BRANNIGAN

MEDICAL CLINICS
OF NORTH AMERICA

www.medical.theclinics.com

Consulting Editor
BIMAL H. ASHAR

March 2018 • Volume 102 • Number 2

ELSEVIER

1600 John F. Kennedy Boulevard • Suite 1800 • Philadelphia, Pennsylvania, 19103-2899

http://www.theclinics.com

MEDICAL CLINICS OF NORTH AMERICA Volume 102, Number 2
March 2018 ISSN 0025-7125, ISBN-13: 978-0-323-58160-8

Editor: Jessica McCool
Developmental Editor: Kristen Helm

Medical Clinics of North America (ISSN 0025-7125) is published bimonthly by Elsevier Inc., 360 Park Avenue South, New York, NY 10010-1710. Months of publication are January, March, May, July, September, and November. Business and editorial offices: 1600 John F. Kennedy Boulevard, Suite 1800, Philadelphia, PA 19103-2899. Periodicals postage paid at New York, NY, and additional mailing offices. Subscription prices are USD $273.00 per year (US individuals), $574.00 per year (US institutions), $100.00 per year (US Students), $336.00 per year (Canadian individuals), $746.00 per year (Canadian institutions), $200.00 per year (Canadian and foreign students), $402.00 per year (foreign individuals), and $746.00 per year (foreign institutions). To receive student/resident rate, orders must be accompanied by name of affiliated institution, date of term, and the signature of program/residency coordinator on institution letterhead. Orders will be billed at individual rate until proof of status is received. Foreign air speed delivery is included in all Clinics' subscription prices. All prices are subject to change without notice. **POSTMASTER:** Send address changes to *Medical Clinics of North America*, Elsevier Health Sciences Division, Subscription Customer Service, 3251 Riverport Lane, Maryland Heights, MO 63043. **Customer Service: Telephone: 1-800-654-2452** (U.S. and Canada); **1-314-447-8871** (outside U.S. and Canada). **Fax: 314-447-8029. E-mail: journalscustomerserviceusa@elsevier.com** (for print support); **journalsonlinesupport-usa@elsevier.com** (for online support).

Reprints. For copies of 100 or more of articles in this publication, please contact the Commercial Reprints Department, Elsevier Inc., 360 Park Avenue South, New York, NY 10010-1710. Tel.: 212-633-3874; Fax: 212-633-3820; E-mail: reprints@elsevier.com.

Medical Clinics of North America is also published in Spanish by McGraw-Hill Interamericana Editores S. A., P.O. Box 5-237, 06500 Mexico, D.F., Mexico.

Medical Clinics of North America is covered in *MEDLINE/PubMed (Index Medicus), Current Contents, ASCA, Excerpta Medica, Science Citation Index,* and *ISI/BIOMED.*

Printed in the United States of America.

PROGRAM OBJECTIVE

The goal of the *Medical Clinics of North America* is to keep practicing physicians up to date with current clinical practice by providing timely articles reviewing the state of the art in patient care.

TARGET AUDIENCE

All practicing physicians and other healthcare professionals.

LEARNING OBJECTIVES

Upon completion of this activity, participants will be able to:

1. Review prostate cancer screening and treatment.
2. Discuss urinary stone disease, urinary tract symptoms, and female voiding dysfunction and incontinence.
3. Recognize male infertility, sexual dysfunction, hypogonadism, and urological emergencies.

ACCREDITATION

The Elsevier Office of Continuing Medical Education (EOCME) is accredited by the Accreditation Council for Continuing Medical Education (ACCME) to provide continuing medical education for physicians.

The EOCME designates this enduring material for a maximum of 15 *AMA PRA Category 1 Credit*(s)™. Physicians should claim only the credit commensurate with the extent of their participation in the activity.

All other healthcare professionals requesting continuing education credit for this enduring material will be issued a certificate of participation.

DISCLOSURE OF CONFLICTS OF INTEREST

The EOCME assesses conflict of interest with its instructors, faculty, planners, and other individuals who are in a position to control the content of CME activities. All relevant conflicts of interest that are identified are thoroughly vetted by EOCME for fair balance, scientific objectivity, and patient care recommendations. EOCME is committed to providing its learners with CME activities that promote improvements or quality in healthcare and not a specific proprietary business or a commercial interest.

The planning committee, staff, authors and editors listed below have identified no financial relationships or relationships to products or devices they or their spouse/life partner have with commercial interest related to the content of this CME activity:

Omar Al Hussein Alawamlh, MD; Hans C. Arora, MD, PhD; Steven C. Campbell, MD, PhD; Nathan Chertack, BS; Scott E. Eggener, MD; Michele Fascelli, MD; Sarah Flury, MD; Matthew Gettman, MD; Christopher M. Gonzalez, MD, MBA; Ramy Goueli, MD; Joel Heidelbaugh, MD; Mark S. Hockenberry, MD; Matthias D. Hofer, MD, PhD; Sudhir Isharwal, MD; Jason Jameson, MD; Steven A. Kaplan, MD; Jonathan E. Kiechle, MD; Stephanie J. Kielb, MD; Edgar W. Kirby, MD; Shilajit D. Kundu, MD; Richard K. Lee, MD, MBA; Leah Logan, MBA; Wesley W. Ludwig, MD; Adarsh S. Manjunath, MD; Brian R. Matlaga, MD, MPH; Jessica McCool; Adam Miller, MD; Martin M. Miner, MD; Michael M. Pan, MD; Mark Paulos, MD; Eugene Rhee, MD, MBA; John T. Sigalos, BA; Zachary L. Smith, MD; Jeyanthi Surendrakumar; Amanda Vo, MD; Adam B. Weiner, MD; Ryan P. Werntz, MD; Emily Yura, MD; JJ H. Zhang, MD.

The planning committee, staff, authors and editors listed below have identified financial relationships or relationships to products or devices they or their spouse/life partner have with commercial interest related to the content of this CME activity:

Nelson Bennett Jr, MD, FACS is a consultant/advisor for Endo Pharmaceuticals Inc., Boston Scientific Corporation, and Coloplast Corp.

William J. Catalona, MD has research support from Beckman-Coulter Inc. and OHMX Corporation.

Mohit Khera, MD, MBA, MPH is a consultant/advisor for Endo Pharmaceuticals Inc., Boston Scientific Corporation, Aytu BioScience, Inc., Coloplast Corp, and AbbVie Inc.

Larry I. Lipshultz, MD is on the speakers' bureau for American Medical Systems and Endo Pharmaceuticals and is a consultant/advisor for AbbVie Inc., Aytu BioScience, Inc., Lipocine Inc., and Endo Pharmaceuticals.

Alexander W. Pastuszak, MD, PhD is on the speakers' bureau and consultant/advisor for Endo Pharmaceuticals and received research support from Boston Scientific Corporation.

Allen D. Seftel, MD has employment affiliation with the Journal of Urology.

Aaron Spitz, MD is on the speakers' bureau for AbbVie Inc., and Endo Pharmaceuticals.

UNAPPROVED/OFF-LABEL USE DISCLOSURE

The EOCME requires CME faculty to disclose to the participants:

1. When products or procedures being discussed are off-label, unlabelled, experimental, and/or investigational (not US Food and Drug Administration [FDA] approved); and
2. Any limitations on the information presented, such as data that are preliminary or that represent ongoing research, interim analyses, and/or unsupported opinions. Faculty may discuss information about pharmaceutical agents that is outside of FDA-approved labelling. This information is intended solely for CME and is not intended to promote off-label use of these medications. If you have any questions, contact the medical affairs department of the manufacturer for the most recent prescribing information.

TO ENROLL

To enroll in the *Medical Clinics of North America* Continuing Medical Education program, call customer service at 1-800-654-2452 or sign up online at http://www.theclinics.com/home/cme. The CME program is available to subscribers for an additional annual fee of USD $300.90.

METHOD OF PARTICIPATION

In order to claim credit, participants must complete the following:

1. Complete enrolment as indicated above.
2. Read the activity.
3. Complete the CME Test and Evaluation. Participants must achieve a score of 70% on the test. All CME Tests and Evaluations must be completed online.

CME INQUIRIES/SPECIAL NEEDS

For all CME inquiries or special needs, please contact elsevierCME@elsevier.com.

MEDICAL CLINICS OF NORTH AMERICA

Contributors

CONSULTING EDITOR

BIMAL H. ASHAR, MD, MBA, FACP
Associate Professor of Medicine, Division of General Internal Medicine, The Johns
Hopkins University School of Medicine, Baltimore, Maryland

EDITOR

ROBERT E. BRANNIGAN, MD
Professor, Department of Urology, Director, Andrology Fellowship, Northwestern
University Feinberg School of Medicine, Chicago, Illinois

AUTHORS

OMAR AL HUSSEIN ALAWAMLH, MD
Department of Urology, Weill Cornell Medical College, Cornell University, James
Buchanan Brady Foundation, New York, New York

HANS C. ARORA, MD, PhD
Resident Physician, Department of Urology, Glickman Urological & Kidney Institute,
Cleveland Clinic, Cleveland, Ohio

NELSON BENNETT Jr, MD, FACS
Associate Professor, Department of Urology, Northwestern University Feinberg School of
Medicine, Chicago, Illinois

STEVEN C. CAMPBELL, MD, PhD
Professor of Surgery, Vice Chairman, Department of Urology, Center for Urologic
Oncology, Glickman Urological & Kidney Institute, Cleveland Clinic, Cleveland, Ohio

WILLIAM J. CATALONA, MD
Professor, Department of Urology, Northwestern University Feinberg School of Medicine,
Chicago, Illinois

NATHAN CHERTACK, BS
Case Western Reserve University School of Medicine, Cleveland, Ohio

SCOTT E. EGGENER, MD
Professor of Surgery and Radiology, Section of Urology, Department of Surgery,
The University of Chicago Medicine, Chicago, Illinois

MICHELE FASCELLI, MD
Resident Physician, Department of Urology, Glickman Urological & Kidney Institute,
Cleveland Clinic, Cleveland, Ohio

SARAH FLURY, MD
Assistant Professor, Department of Urology, Northwestern University Feinberg School of Medicine, Chicago, Illinois

MATTHEW GETTMAN, MD
Professor, Department of Urology, Mayo Clinic, Rochester, Minnesota

CHRISTOPHER M. GONZALEZ, MD, MBA
Chairman, Professor of Urology, Urology Institute, University Hospitals Cleveland Medical Center, Case Western Reserve University School of Medicine, Cleveland, Ohio

RAMY GOUELI, MD
Department of Urology, Weill Cornell Medical College, Cornell University, James Buchanan Brady Foundation, New York, New York

JOEL HEIDELBAUGH, MD
Clinical Professor, Departments of Family Medicine and Urology, University of Michigan Medical School, Ann Arbor, Michigan

MARK S. HOCKENBERRY, MD
Scott Department of Urology, Center for Reproductive Medicine and Surgery, Baylor College of Medicine, Houston, Texas

MATTHIAS D. HOFER, MD, PhD
Attending Physician, Department of Urology, Northwestern University Feinberg School of Medicine, Chicago, Illinois

SUDHIR ISHARWAL, MD
Fellow in Urologic Oncology, Department of Urology, Glickman Urological & Kidney Institute, Cleveland Clinic, Cleveland, Ohio

JASON JAMESON, MD
Division of Urology, Mayo Clinic, Scottsdale, Arizona

STEVEN A. KAPLAN, MD
Professor of Urology, Director, Benign Urologic Diseases and The Men's Health Program, Icahn School of Medicine at Mount Sinai, Mount Sinai Health System, New York, New York

MOHIT KHERA, MD, MBA, MPH
Scott Department of Urology, Baylor College of Medicine, Houston, Texas

JONATHAN E. KIECHLE, MD
Reconstructive Urology Fellow, Urology Institute, University Hospitals Cleveland Medical Center, Case Western Reserve University School of Medicine, Cleveland, Ohio

STEPHANIE J. KIELB, MD
Associate Professor, Departments of Urology, Medical Education, and Obstetrics and Gynecology, Northwestern University Feinberg School of Medicine, Chicago, Illinois

EDGAR W. KIRBY, MD
Scott Department of Urology, Center for Reproductive Medicine and Surgery, Baylor College of Medicine, Houston, Texas

SHILAJIT D. KUNDU, MD
Associate Professor, Department of Urology, Northwestern University Feinberg School of Medicine, Chicago, Illinois

RICHARD K. LEE, MD, MBA
Department of Urology, Weill Cornell Medical College, Cornell University, James Buchanan Brady Foundation, New York, New York

LARRY I. LIPSHULTZ, MD
Scott Department of Urology, Center for Reproductive Medicine and Surgery, Baylor College of Medicine, Houston, Texas

WESLEY W. LUDWIG, MD
Resident, Department of Urology, The James Buchanan Brady Urological Institute, The Johns Hopkins Hospital, The Johns Hopkins University School of Medicine, Baltimore, Maryland

ADARSH S. MANJUNATH, MD
Resident Physician, Department of Urology, Northwestern University Feinberg School of Medicine, Chicago, Illinois

BRIAN R. MATLAGA, MD, MPH
Professor, Department of Urology, The James Buchanan Brady Urological Institute, The Johns Hopkins Hospital, The Johns Hopkins University School of Medicine, Baltimore, Maryland

ADAM MILLER, MD
Resident, Department of Urology, Mayo Clinic, Rochester, Minnesota

MARTIN M. MINER, MD
Clinical Professor, Departments of Family Medicine and Urology, Co-Director, Men's Health Center, The Miriam Hospital, The Warren Alpert Medical School of Brown University, Providence, Rhode Island

MICHAEL M. PAN, MD
Scott Department of Urology, Baylor College of Medicine, Houston, Texas

ALEXANDER W. PASTUSZAK, MD, PhD
Center for Reproductive Medicine, Scott Department of Urology, Baylor College of Medicine, Houston, Texas

MARK PAULOS, MD
Clinical Assistant Professor of Medicine and Urology, Departments of Internal Medicine and Urology, Men's Health Center, The Miriam Hospital, The Warren Alpert Medical School of Brown University, Providence, Rhode Island

EUGENE RHEE, MD, MBA
Regional Coordinating Chief Kaiser Permanente Southern California, National Chair Interregional Urology Chiefs' Group, Assistant Area Medical Director, Department of Urology, Kaiser Permanente San Diego, San Diego, California

ALLEN D. SEFTEL, MD
Chief, Division of Urology, Cooper University Hospital, Professor of Urology, Cooper Medical School of Rowan University, Camden, New Jersey

JOHN T. SIGALOS, BA
Baylor College of Medicine, Houston, Texas

ZACHARY L. SMITH, MD
Urologic Oncology Fellow, Section of Urology, Department of Surgery, The University of Chicago Medicine, Chicago, Illinois

AARON SPITZ, MD
Assistant Clinical Professor, Department of Urology, University of California, Irvine, Partner, Orange County Urology Associates, Laguna Hills, California

AMANDA VO, MD
Resident, Department of Urology, Northwestern University Feinberg School of Medicine, Chicago, Illinois

ADAM B. WEINER, MD
Urology Resident, Department of Urology, Northwestern University Feinberg School of Medicine, Chicago, Illinois

RYAN P. WERNTZ, MD
Urologic Oncology Fellow, Section of Urology, Department of Surgery, The University of Chicago Medicine, Chicago, Illinois

EMILY YURA, MD
Urology Resident, Department of Urology, Northwestern University Feinberg School of Medicine, Chicago, Illinois

JJ.H. ZHANG, MD
Resident Physician, Department of Urology, Glickman Urological & Kidney Institute, Cleveland Clinic, Cleveland, Ohio

Contents

> During the prostate-specific antigen-based prostate cancer (PCa) screening era there has been a 53% decrease in the US PCa mortality rate. Concerns about overdiagnosis and overtreatment combined with misinterpretation of clinical trial data led to a recommendation against PCa screening, resulting in a subsequent reversion to more high-risk disease at diagnosis. Re-evaluation of trial data and increasing acceptance of active surveillance led to a new draft recommendation for shared decision making for men aged 55 to 69 years old. Further consideration is needed for more intensive screening in men with high-risk factors. PCa screening significantly reduces PCa morbidity and mortality.

> Given the high incidence of prostate cancer and the need for shared decision making before screening, it is imperative that primary care providers understand treatment options and treatment adverse effects. In this article, the treatment options for the localized and metastatic prostate cancer are discussed, including the different modalities and their indications, adverse effects, oncologic outcomes, posttreatment monitoring, and potential treatment options following cancer recurrence.

> Malignancies of the urinary tract (kidney, ureter, and bladder) are distinct clinical entities. Hematuria is a unifying common presenting symptom for these malignancies. Surgical management of localized disease continues to be the mainstay of treatment, and early detection is important in the prognosis of disease. Patients often require life-long follow-up and assessment for recurrence.

> There were an estimated 8720 new cases of testicular cancer (TC) in the United States in 2016. The cause of the disease is complex, with several

environmental and genetic risk factors. Although the disease is rare, the incidence has been steadily increasing. Fortunately, substantial advances in treatment have occurred over the last few decades, making TC one of the most curable malignancies. However, because TC typically occurs in younger men, considerations of the treatment impact on fertility, quality of life, and long-term toxicity are paramount; an individualized approach must be taken with patients based on their clinical and pathologic findings.

Clinical suspicion of urolithiasis should be evaluated with low-dose computed tomography as the first-line imaging modality for nonpregnant, adult patients. A period of observation may be appropriate for ureteral stones less than 10 mm, and medical expulsive therapy may be beneficial for facilitating passage of distal ureteral stones. Regardless of stone type, patients should adhere to a low-sodium diet and attempt to achieve a urine volume of more than 2.5 L daily. Individuals with calcium stones should maintain a normal calcium diet, and if stones persist, citrate therapy or thiazide diuretics in the setting of hypercalciuria may be indicated.

Individuals with cutaneous diseases of the external genitalia often initially present to their primary care provider. When present, these conditions may be associated with considerable physical symptoms and psychological distress. Dermatoses affecting the genitals may be of infectious, inflammatory, or neoplastic cause and can be processes confined to the genitalia or a manifestation of a more widespread dermatologic condition. This article provides a guide to recognizing and managing common genital dermatoses and when to refer for specialist opinion.

Lower urinary tract symptoms (LUTS) consist of a common set of urologic symptoms that can affect the elderly. The prevalence of LUTS is expected to increase owing to the continued increase of numbers of the elderly. Although benign prostatic hyperplasia is considered a common cause of LUTS, the broader potential causes of LUTS are myriad. A wide range of diagnostic modalities and treatments are available to manage patients with LUTS, and their utilization should not be limited to the urologist.

Female voiding dysfunction and incontinence are common in the general population, and symptoms have been shown to have a significant negative impact on health-related quality of life. This article highlights the epidemiology, evaluation, diagnosis, pharmacologic therapies, and surgical treatment for overactive bladder, stress urinary incontinence, and urogenital fistulas.

to diagnosis, whereas imaging is increasingly used to confirm diagnoses. Acute urinary retention should be relieved with Foley placement. Penile emergencies include paraphimosis, which can be treated by foreskin reduction, whereas penile fracture and priapism require urologic intervention. Fournier gangrene and testicular torsion are scrotal emergencies requiring emergent surgery. Nephrolithiasis, although painful, is not an emergency unless there is concern for concomitant urinary tract infection, both ureters are obstructed by stones, or there is an obstructing stone in a solitary kidney.

Telemedicine use in urology is an evolving practice. In this article, the authors review the early experience of telemedicine specifically as it relates to urologic practice and discuss the future implications and the utility of telemedicine as it applies to other fields.

Men's mental health and how they think about their health are critical to the future of men's health. Poor health choice patterns are established under age 50 years, when men are twice more likely to die than women. As the future of medicine focuses on quality and value, a better understanding of the social determinants of men's health will identify areas for improvement. The presentation of a man with a sexual health complaint to a clinician's office presents an opportunity for more complete evaluation. The future of men's health will be well served by integrated men's health centers that focus on the entire man.

Foreword
Go with the Flow

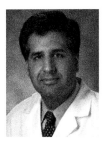

Bimal H. Ashar, MD, MBA, FACP
Consulting Editor

When I was a third-year medical student many years ago, my senior resident shared an old adage with me: "Urine and pus must come out." He actually used a different term for "urine" that made the saying a bit more memorable. The importance of proper functioning of the urinary system has been historically recognized. In 3000 BC, the ancient Egyptians developed the first urinary catheters that were made of bronze, reed, straw, or curled-up palm leaves.[1] Later, rigid catheters made of silver or lead were developed, but trauma often ensued. The urinary catheter underwent a number of changes through the years, particularly with respect to materials used. In the 1930s, Frederic Foley first described the use of an indwelling catheter consisting of a longitudinal-grooved rubber tube with an inflatable balloon near the tip. This type of indwelling catheter is still used today.

Although the term "urology" is derived from the Greek words $o \check{v} \rho o \nu$ (ouron) and $-\lambda o \gamma i \alpha$ (-logia), which are literally translated as "the study of urine," the field of urology extends far beyond the excretion of water and organic compounds. Tumors of the genitourinary system, sexual dysfunction, urinary retention and incontinence, and infertility are just a few issues encompassed by this field. Every person will likely experience some urologic issue in their lifetime.

In this issue of the *Medical Clinics of North America*, Dr Brannigan has enlisted experts from around the country to assist internists in identifying, assessing, and (in some cases) treating common urologic problems. In addition, cutting-edge topics like the association between sexual dysfunction and cardiometabolic disease and the future

Med Clin N Am 102 (2018) xv–xvi
https://doi.org/10.1016/j.mcna.2017.12.002
0025-7125/18/© 2017 Published by Elsevier Inc.

utility of telemedicine are discussed. It is hoped that this issue will serve as a resource for general practitioners when faced with genitourinary complaints that require more than just making sure that urine is flowing.

Bimal H. Ashar, MD, MBA, FACP
Division of General Internal Medicine
Johns Hopkins University School of Medicine
601 North Caroline Street, #7143
Baltimore, MD 21287, USA

E-mail address:
Bashar1@jhmi.edu

REFERENCE

1. Nacey J, Delahunt B. The evolution and development of the urinary catheter. Aust N Z J Surg 1993;63(10):815–9.

Preface

Urology and Medicine

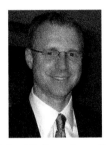

Robert E. Brannigan, MD
Editor

In this issue of *Medical Clinics of North America*, the multifaceted aspects of urology encountered by medical physicians are explored. Medical physicians are on the front-lines of health care, and urologic health concerns prompt large numbers of male and female patient visits annually. While some urologic conditions affect primarily aging individuals, large numbers of genitourinary health issues are prevalent across the lifespan. For these reasons, familiarity with the epidemiology, pathophysiology, diagnosis, management, and long-term treatment outcomes associated with urologic conditions is essential for the practicing medical physician.

Prostate cancer is the second most common cancer among American men, with 1 in 7 US men receiving this diagnosis in their lifetimes.[1] Prostate cancer has garnered substantial attention and controversy in recent years, with ongoing debate over how assertive clinicians should be in both diagnosing and treating this condition. Two articles in this issue thoughtfully address the complementary issues of prostate cancer screening (Catalona) and treatment (Weiner and Kundu) in the modern era. Arora and colleagues provide a highly informative and practical overview regarding the diagnosis and treatment of kidney, ureteral, and bladder cancers, conditions that can masquerade undiagnosed if the clinician is unfamiliar with their presenting signs and symptoms. Smith and colleagues round out this issue's genitourinary oncologic topics with a thoughtful consideration of testicular cancer, a condition for which the prognosis has evolved over the last several decades with marked improvements in treatment outcomes, particularly for patients with metastatic disease.[2]

Kidney stones affect nearly 1 in 11 Americans and can be the source of debilitating pain and life-threatening infections.[3] Kidney stone incidence is clearly on the rise, which many investigators attribute at least in part to rising rates of obesity and diabetes mellitus.[4] Ludwig and Matlaga provide an outstanding and practical review of urinary stone disease, including the optimal approaches for both diagnosis and treatment. Cutaneous lesions of the external genitalia can arise due to a number of infectious, inflammatory, and neoplastic conditions, and Yura and Flury have done an excellent job describing the

Med Clin N Am 102 (2018) xvii–xix
https://doi.org/10.1016/j.mcna.2017.12.001
0025-7125/18/© 2017 Published by Elsevier Inc.

diagnosis and management of cutaneous lesions involving the genitalia. Male and female voiding dysfunction is a highly prevalent medical condition that can develop due to a diverse array of underlying medical abnormalities. Voiding dysfunction can cause severe bother and adversely impact quality of life for affected patients. Hussein and colleagues provide a compelling overview of lower urinary tract symptoms and benign prostatic hypertrophy in men, and Vo and Kielb expertly address the problematic issues of female voiding dysfunction and urinary incontinence. These two articles serve as effective roadmaps to diagnose and treat patients impacted by these highly troubling conditions. Kiechle and colleagues provide an extremely well-written contribution regarding the growing field of penile and urethral reconstructive surgery. Urethral issues are often diagnosed in a delayed fashion, long after the onset of associated symptoms. For this reason, medical practitioners should be aware that urethral stricture disease is the root cause of urinary symptoms for large numbers of men. The symptoms associated with urethral strictures typically do not respond to medical therapy, given that the underlying problem is a fixed anatomical narrowing of the urinary tract.

Fifteen percent of couples will experience fertility issues, and half of these couples have a male factor cause involved. Pan and colleagues have authored an outstanding article that comprehensively addresses the diagnosis and treatment of male infertility in the era of in vitro fertilization. This is an important article, given that historically the burden for diagnostic and therapeutic procedures has largely been relegated to the female partner, bypassing opportunities to treat the male partner. Sexual dysfunction (Bennett) and hypogonadism (Sigalos and colleagues) are both expertly addressed in this issue, including the wide array of effective treatment options available for each of these bothersome conditions.

The genitourinary system is not immune to emergent pathology, and the medical practitioner is often on the "frontlines" of care for affected patients. Familiarity with the clinical signs and symptoms of urologic emergencies is thus imperative, and Manjunath and Hofer provide a very well-written piece detailing the wide breadth of urologic conditions that require emergent intervention. Telemedicine is a novel modality of patient engagement, and early studies show it has great potential for increasing patient access to care.[5] Miller and colleagues are experts in telemedicine who provide a thoughtful overview for clinicians who are considering application of this evolving approach to patient care. Finally, Miner and colleagues close this issue with an expertly written and highly informative article describing men's health, which sits at the intersection of medicine and urology.

In closing, this issue of *Medical Clinics of North America* is comprised of a wide breadth of incredibly well-written pieces that cover the full scope of adult urology. The authors are all highly respected experts who have worked hard to provide a state-of-the-art perspective for each topic. Collectively, these contributions will provide medical physicians with an invaluable roadmap as they treat male and female patients facing genitourinary conditions over the course of their lifetimes.

Robert E. Brannigan, MD
Department of Urology
Northwestern University
Feinberg School of Medicine
Galter Pavilion, Suite 20-150
675 North Saint Clair Street
Chicago, IL 60611, USA

E-mail address:
r-brannigan@northwestern.edu

REFERENCES

1. American Cancer Society. Cancer facts & figures 2017. Atlanta (GA): American Cancer Society; 2017.
2. Hanna NH, Einhorn LH. Testicular cancer—discoveries and updates. N Engl J Med 2014;371(21):2005–16.
3. Scales CD, Smith AC, Hanley JM, et al. Prevalence of kidney stones in the United States. Eur Urol 2012;62:160–5.
4. Shoag J, Tasian GE, Goldfarb DS, et al. The new epidemiology of nephrolithiasis. Adv Chronic Kidney Dis 2015;22:273–8.
5. Ellimoottil C, Skolarus T, Gettman M, et al. Telemedicine in urology: state of the art. Urology 2016;94:10–6.

Prostate Cancer Screening

William J. Catalona, MD

KEYWORDS

- Prostate • Prostate cancer • Prostate cancer screening
- Prostate cancer screening guidelines • Prostate-specific antigen • PSA
- History of prostate cancer screening • United States Preventive services Task Force

KEY POINTS

- Prostate cancer (PCa) screening is controversial. PSA-based screening has effected a dramatic stage shift from mostly incurable to mostly curable disease along with a greater than 53% reduction in the US PCa mortality rate; however, concerns have arisen about overdiagnosis and treatment of screen-detected indolent tumors.
- Randomized clinical trials of varying quality and much of their misinterpreted data have created confusion about the benefits versus harms of screening, leading to flawed recommendations in 2008 and 2012 against PSA screening by the US Preventive Services Task Force (USPSTF).
- In the aftermath of the USPSTF recommendations, the widespread rejection of screening by many primary care physicians has had far-reaching consequences, notably, a reversion to more PCa cases being high-grade and advanced at diagnosis.
- A 2017 statistical modeling reanalysis of the large European Randomized Study of Screening for Prostate Cancer (ERSPC) and the US Prostate, Lung, Colorectal, and Ovarian (PLCO) screening trials by the Cancer Intervention and Surveillance Modeling Network of the National Cancer Institute revealed that screening in ERSPC produced a 25% to 31% reduction in PCa mortality versus a 27% to 32% reduction in PLCO.
- The USPSTF has now issued a revised draft recommendation, suggesting shared decision making for screening healthy men 55 years to 69 years of age.
- Consequently, the USPSTF has dropped its total opposition to PCa screening, with a draft recommendation for shared decision making for patients ages 55 years to 69 years old. Further consideration is needed for more intensive screening in men with high-risk factors, such as African ancestry and/or a strong family history of PCa, as well as for healthy men aged greater than or equal to 70 years.
- Further consideration is needed for more intensive screening in men with high-risk factors, such as African ancestry and/or a strong family history of PCa, as well as for healthy men age greater than or equal to 70 years. When correctly interpreted, the data are clear: PSA screening significantly reduces suffering and death from PCa.

Disclosure Statement: The author has received research support from Beckman-Coulter Inc and OHMX, Inc, developers of prostate-specific antigen–based assays.
Department of Urology, Northwestern University Feinberg School of Medicine, 675 North Saint Clair Street, Suite 20-150, Chicago, IL 63110, USA
E-mail address: wcatalona@nm.org

INTRODUCTION

The US Preventive Services Task Force (USPSTF) has dropped its opposition to routine prostate cancer (PCa) screening in favor of a shared decision-making process between men aged 55 years to 69 years and their physicians. Screening for prostate cancer is controversial, but it should not be. In the United States, PCa is the third leading cause of cancer death in men, with an estimated 161,360 new cases diagnosed in 2017 and 26,730 projected cancer deaths.[1] PCa seldom produces symptoms until it is incurable, and currently available methods cannot accurately distinguish between tumors that progress so slowly that they do not produce symptoms and those that are likely to cause suffering or death. Therefore, with no known means of preventing PCa or for curing metastatic disease, the sole hope for reducing suffering and death from PCa is through early detection and appropriate and effective patient management.

THE PRE–PROSTATE-SPECIFIC ANTIGEN SCREENING ERA

In the 6 decades before the PSA screening era, PCa death rates progressively increased, because more men lived long enough to succumb to PCa,[1] and most PCa patients were diagnosed with incurable disease. For those who did not die of other causes within 15 years, many died from PCa.

Prostate-Specific Antigen as a First-Line Screening Test

Because of overlap in PSA levels in men with benign prostatic hyperplasia, prostatitis, and PCa, it was believed that PSA could not be not used for early detection of PCa. In 1991, Catalona and colleagues[2] showed that PSA could be used as a first-line screening test for PCa in men without suspicious digital rectal examination (DRE) findings. Subsequently, PSA testing was widely adopted, causing a spike in PCa incidence rates, because the inventory of previously undetectable PCa was unmasked. This led to the creation of a new clinical-stage classification (T1c), that is, PCa with a normal DRE that has become the most common stage in practice.[3]

Randomized Clinical Trials of Prostate-Specific Antigen Screening

Randomized clinical trials (RCTs) were launched to evaluate PSA screening. Of these, the Swedish Göteborg trial is the highest-quality study. It is population based, included younger men, used lower PSA cutoffs for biopsy, had the longest follow-up, and had the lowest rate of contamination. Göteborg initially reported a 41% lower rate of advanced-stage PCa at diagnosis in the screening arm (66% lower in men actually screened) and a 44% lower PCa mortality rate (56% lower in men actually screened), despite 33% of patients being managed with active surveillance. The trial subsequently contributed 59% of its data from men in the core age group of the multinational European Randomized Study of Screening for Prostate Cancer (ERSPC)[4] that reported a 21% lower PCa mortality rate in the screening arm (29% after adjustment for noncompliance with screening, and 38% for those with 10 to 11 years of follow-up).[4–6]

Among the other RCTs of PSA screening,[7,8] the US Prostate, Lung, Colorectal, and Ovarian (PLCO) trial that reported no overall PCa mortality benefit from screening was noninformative on the benefits of screening versus no screening, because nearly 90% of PLCO controls had PSA testing before or during the trial.[9–12] A recent statistical modeling reanalysis of ERSPC and PLCO by the Cancer Intervention and Surveillance Modeling Network (CISNET) of the National Cancer Institute estimated that screening in ERSPC produced a 25% to 31% reduction in PCa mortality versus a 27% to 32% reduction in PLCO.[13]

US Food and Drug Administration Approval of Prostate-Specific Antigen as an Aid to the Early Detection of Prostate-Specific Antigen–Based Prostate Cancer

In 1994, a pivotal study demonstrated that a 4.0 ng/mL PSA cutoff was effective in selecting patients for biopsy.[14] For every 100 men tested, approximately 85 had PSA less than 4.0 ng/mL; the remaining 15 could then undergo prostate biopsy, of whom 4 to 5 were found to have PCa. The FDA approved PSA testing as an aid to early PCa detection using this cutoff; however, subsequent studies showed that many clinically significant PCas are missed with a 4.0 PSA cutoff, especially in men with PSA levels in the 2.5 ng/mL to 4.0 ng/mL range,[15–17] in which cancers have more favorable features and progression-free survival rates.[18]

The probability of a PCa diagnosis increases with increasing serum PSA levels.[2,19,20] The Prostate Cancer Prevention Trial demonstrated that 15% of men with a PSA level of less than or equal to 4.0 ng/mL and a normal DRE had PCa diagnosed (>20% with PSA of 2–4 ng/mL).[16] Approximately 30% to 35% of men with PSA 4 to 10 ng/mL and greater than 67% of men with PSA levels greater than 10 ng/mL have PCa diagnosed.[21,22] PSA levels correlate with the rate of change of PSA, the proportion of patients with high-grade tumors, the progression-free survival rate, and PCa mortality.[23] A caveat is that some poorly differentiated and/or neuroendocrine PCas do not produce much PSA, which reduces the value of PSA as a biomarker for these types of tumors.[24]

THE PROSTATE-SPECIFIC ANTIGEN SCREENING ERA (1991–2008)

With the advent of PSA screening, there was a dramatic stage migration, with most patients being diagnosed with curable disease. Thus, patients could elect treatment or observation, or they could opt not to have PSA testing and run the risk of later being diagnosed with incurable PCa.

Epidemiologic Impact of Prostate-Specific Antigen Screening

Widespread PSA testing had a profound impact on the epidemiologic features of PCa.[1] In the United States, the age-adjusted PCa mortality rate decreased by greater than 53% during the PSA screening era[22] resulting from an 80% decrease in the proportion of patients with metastases at diagnosis.[1,25] CISNET estimated that 45% to 70% of this decrease was attributable directly to PSA screening.[26,27] Benefits of PSA screening also are reflected in RCTs in which patients with clinically localized PCa randomized to prompt prostatectomy fared better than those randomized to observation, including the ProtecT trial (Prostate Testing for Cancer and Treatment) that exclusively enrolled men with screen-detected PCa.[28–30]

Enhancements of Prostate-Specific Antigen Tests to Increase Specificity

Because elevated PSA levels can be caused by conditions other than PCa, enhancements have been sought to increase the specificity of PSA testing.

Prostate-specific antigen velocity

PSA velocity (PSAV) correlates with both PCa risk and aggressiveness[31–36] but is confounded by benign prostatic hyperplasia and by prostatitis, and its short-term utility is limited because of the time required to determine whether PSA increases persist.[37,38] In men without PCa, PSAV increases by approximately 0.15 ng/mL/y versus approximately 0.35 ng/mL/y to 0.40 ng/mL/y with PCa.[32,34–36,39–41] The natural history of PSAV in PCa patients is that PSA increases by 2% per year prior to a change point when increases accelerate. After this, PSA increases by 15% in patients presenting with localized disease and 63% in those presenting with metastases. Usually, the change point occurs at PSA levels below 4.0 ng/mL, and the median age at the change point is 57 years old, occurring in the 40s in many patients.[41] PSA velocities greater than 2.0 ng/mL/y not caused by prostatitis may reflect incurable PCa.[34,42]

Prostate-specific antigen velocity risk count
PSAV risk count quantifies the persistence of PSA increases over time, that is, the number of times the PSAV increases by a specific amount, such as 0.2 ng/mL/y or 0.4 ng/mL/y. Unless a long PSA history is available, PSAV risk count also is limited by the time required to obtain a valid result.[33,43]

Prostate-specific antigen density
PSA density (PSAD) (PSA ÷ prostate volume) measurements factor in the prostate size in relation to the serum PSA level, because an enlarged prostate produces higher serum PSA levels. PSAD is a valuable parameter to assess risk for clinically significant PCa. A PSAD greater than 0.10 ng/mL/cm^3 to 0.15 ng/mL/cm^3 indicates a high risk.

Age-specific median prostate-specific antigen values
Age-specific median PSA values help guide whether an individual's PSA value is elevated by comparing them to levels in his peer age group (**Table 1**). Baseline PSA levels in men in their 40s and 50s are the most powerful predictors of the risk for PCa metastases and death decades later[44,45]—even more powerful than family history or African American race.[46]

Median values are from the author's PSA studies from approximately 30,000 subjects; they are consistent with other reports.[39,47–51]

The risk for aggressive PCa is increased in men with PSA levels above the median for their age group, with more than half of PCa deaths occurring in men with PSA levels in the highest 25th percentile of their age-specific PSA reference range at age 40 to 55 years.[52–54]

Free-to-total prostate-specific antigen
Free PSA–to–total PSA percent: free PSA (free PSA ÷ total PSA × 100) correlates with the probability of PCa and the presence of aggressive disease. If the free PSA–to–total PSA ratio is less than 10%, there is greater than 50% probability that a biopsy would show PCa. In contrast, a ratio greater than 25% is associated with less than 10% probability of PCa diagnosis.[55]

Prostate health index
The Prostate Health Index (*phi*) FDA-approved blood test measures total PSA, free PSA, and [−2]proPSA.[56,57] These values are used in a mathematical model,

Table 1
Median prostate-specific antigen by age

Age (y)	Prostate-Specific Antigen (ng/mL)
30–39	0.5
40–49	0.7
50–59	0.9
60–69	1.3
70–79	1.7
80–89	2.1

phi = ([−2] proPSA/free PSA) × ($\sqrt{}$total PSA). The output of the phi test is the probability that a biopsy would show PCa and also clinically significant disease. A multivariable model including phi also has been developed to improve risk prediction.[58]

The 4KScore

The 4KScore blood test incorporates measurements of total PSA, free PSA, human kallikrein 2, and intact PSA into a clinical model that combines these measurements with information about DRE and patient age to give statistical probabilities that a patient will have a high-grade tumor. 4KScore is commercially available but not FDA approved.[59,60]

Concerns About Prostate-Specific Antigen Screening

Screening for PCa has been challenged because of concerns about the risk of triggering unnecessary biopsies and the overdiagnosis and overtreatment of screen-detected, indolent tumors with possible untoward side effects.[61]

Politics of Prostate-Specific Antigen Testing: The US Preventive Services Task Force

Policymakers consider screening at the population level, whereas clinicians are trained to view PSA testing at the individual-patient level.[62] Most physicians have little knowledge of the USPSTF, of the processes under which it operates, or that reform of the process continues to be a legislative priority.[63,64]

The USPSTF was created in 1984, as an advisory committee to Medicare. It consists of 16 volunteers serving 4-year terms and is funded from the Agency for Health Research and Quality. Its mission is to evaluate the benefits and harms of health services and make recommendations for primary care physicians. The USPSTF panel is composed of internists, pediatricians, family physicians, obstetricians, gynecologists, and nurses but no urologists, radiation oncologists, or medical oncologists.[61] It is allowed to select the studies it deems most relevant to review and typically weighs RCTs most heavily.[62]

Functionally, the USPSTF reviews the specialty care literature and translates it into the context of primary care practice, scoring the services in terms of merit as either A, B, C, D, or I (incomplete information). A D score means there is a moderate-to-high certainty that the intervention has no net benefit or that harms outweigh benefits. Under its charter, the USPSTF initially functioned solely as an advisory panel to physicians and patients and deliberately excluded any specialty stakeholders. Thus, physicians and patients were free to evaluate USPSTF recommendations and decide how best to incorporate them into clinical practice.

The USPSTF's authority was broadened under the 2008 Medicare Improvements for Patients and Providers Act (MIPPA) that changed the way Medicare conducted business. MIPPA created a National Coverage Determination process that was still under Medicare's control but was significantly influenced by the USPSTF. Under MIPPA, a USPSTF recommendation of A or B permitted Medicare to expand its coverage of a service without the action of Congress, based on the advisory capacity of the USPSTF. This was a pivotal change, because all other entities that advise other government agencies are governed by a completely different set of rules.

The USPSTF's role was further expanded under the Affordable Care Act (ACA) that transformed the role of the USPSTF from an advisory capacity to a funding mandate. Under the ACA, if the USPSTF issued an A or B recommendation, Medicare would have to cover it and would be permitted to deny coverage for services that had a D rating. Furthermore, if, the USPSTF simply opted not to review a service and did not issue a recommendation, the Secretary of Health and Human Services or

Medicare would be permitted to deny coverage. This transformed the USPSTF from an agency that merely advised physicians and patients to one that now advised Medicare and could set mandatory payment policy. This is problematic, because the USPSTF was not chartered as an agency that would advise the government; it is exempt from all of the important regulations that govern entities that do advise government agencies.

In 2008, the USPSTF issued a grade D recommendation against screening men greater than 75 years old[65] despite the fact that RCT data to support this recommendation was limited. One year later, after the first reports of the ERSPC and PLCO trials,[4,9] the USPSTF began a new evidence review, 1 year ahead of schedule.[62] Giving prostate cancer screening a grade C recommendation would have required physicians to counsel men. Instead, the USPSTF gave a grade D recommendation, concluding that the harms outweigh the benefits.[61] Grade D reduced access to PSA testing because, under the ACA, grades A and B get full coverage by Medicare with no copayment; whereas, grade D does not have to be covered and, if it is, beneficiaries must make copayment.[62]

2008 TO 2017: THE PROSTATE-SPECIFIC ANTIGEN PROHIBITION ERA

In the aftermath of the USPSTF's 2008 and 2012 grade D recommendations, PSA testing declined in the United States by 25% to 30%,[66] significantly reducing overall PCa incidence rates and precluding early PCa detection in many patients.[67–71] Beginning with the 2008 recommendation, in men over age 75, there has been a reversal of the favorable tumor stage migration, and since 2011, among men greater than or equal to 75 years old, there has been a significant increase in the proportion and the absolute number of men presenting with metastases at the time of diagnosis with a similar trend in younger men.[67] CISNET has projected that if screening had been completely phased out in 2012, as recommended by the USPSTF, the number of cases of distant-stage disease would return to the pre-PSA screening era levels by the year 2025 (Etzioni R, personal communication, 2016). Empirically, in the Göteborg screening trial, 9 years after the termination of PSA testing, the incidence of potentially lethal cancers was the same as that of nonscreened men.[72,73]

Criticisms of US Preventive Services Task Force Analysis

The USPSTF overstepped its mandate by superimposing the harms of treatment on those of testing and diagnosis.[74–79] The USPSTF placed screening in a context that would be applied across the population, which underestimates benefits and overestimates harms with reasonable use in appropriate candidates. It incorrectly assumed that every man with abnormal screening results would undergo biopsy and that all men diagnosed with PCa would undergo definitive treatment.

Overdiagnosis and overtreatment are inherent in all cancer screening. From statistical modeling studies, overdiagnosis of PCa with screening has been estimated to be 17% to 66%. The true extent cannot be determined for individual patients and can only be approximately estimated in populations using excess cases diagnosed in the screening arm of an RCT as a proxy measure.[80] Using incidence data from RCT, however, produces inflated results, because the excess incidence in the screened arm, the typical proxy for overdiagnosis, consists of a mixture of overdiagnosed cases and true life-threatening cases, but because it is not possible to distinguish between them, they all get counted as overdiagnosed cases. Thus, empirical results of RCT do not accurately inform about the benefits of screening versus no screening, overdiagnosis, or the number of PCas that must be detected to save

1 life,[81] and early trial data especially exaggerates overdiagnosis. It is likely that the current estimates based on incidence data from the PLCO and ERSPC trials are too high.

RCTs conducted over a short time period do not reveal accurate estimates of the absolute benefits of screening over a lifetime. There is a delay from the start of an RCT until a screening-induced mortality reduction can be attained, and early data underestimate benefits and exaggerates harms.[82]

Unlike mortality rates that are affected by both early detection and better treatment, the frequency of metastases at diagnosis is determined only by early detection.[83] The USPSTF 2012 analysis failed to consider preventing suffering and treatment of metastatic disease. Avoiding metastases shifts the balance of harms and benefits. Also, many men in the RCTs who died of PCa were diagnosed with metastases on their first screening visit. Better results are achieved over the long term with longitudinal screening. In ERSPC, the rate of metastases was lower across all sites.[84,85] In an intent-to-screen analysis, there was a 50% reduction in metastases at diagnosis and a 30% reduction of metastases during 12 years of follow-up (42% for men who were actually screened).[6,85] The initial incidence of metastases was 22% lower in the screening arm of PLCO; however, PLCO did not report on the cumulative incidence of metastases.[83]

The most important criticism of the USPSTF methodology is its heavy weighting of PLCO results in which it was only later revealed that nearly 90% of controls had PSA testing before or during the trial. In arriving at its grade D recommendation, the USPSTF relied on the incorrectly reported approximately 50% rate of PSA testing in the control arm in the 2009 PLCO report:

> ...approximately 50% of men in the control group received at least 1 PSA test during the study.[9]

In contrast, in a 2016 independent evaluation of the PLCO data, Shoag and colleagues[86] reported,

> ... the proportion of control participants who reported having undergone at least 1 PSA test before or during the trial was close to 90%.

PLCO coauthors published a re-evaluation of PSA testing in the control group in 2010 in a publication that received little public notice.[10,11] Their most recent report cites an 86% rate of PSA testing in the control arm versus 99% in the intervention arm and asserts that 46% of controls underwent yearly testing during the screening phase compared with 84% in the screening arm. They concede that PLCO is not informative on the benefits of screening versus no screening but maintain that it is a trial demonstrating no advantage of organized screening over opportunistic screening.[12]

Shoag and colleagues[86] responded that before their independent review of PLCO data, guideline panels had not recognized the high rate of contamination when formulating policy recommendations (eg, the 2010 PLCO article was not cited in the USPSTF's announcement of its grade D recommendation).[61]

Gulati and Albertsen[87] editorialized that the PLCO trial may have reached a saturation point for screening in both arms, beyond which more frequent screening could not produce more benefits. They suggested that certain methods of organized screening could, in fact, be superior to certain methods of opportunistic screening. In this regard, Arnsrud Godtman and colleagues[88] reported on opportunistic and organized screening in the Göteborg trial, in which organized screening produced a 42% reduction in PCa mortality over opportunistic screening.

Psychological Effects

Most quality-of-life studies of PSA screening have revealed significant early excess bother from urinary, sexual, and bowel dysfunction with active treatment and excess anxiety associated with conservative management; however, after longer-term follow-up, global quality of life and sense of well-being are not significantly different between screened and nonscreened men. These studies reflect substantial declines in sexual and urinary function in untreated men in their 60s to 80s.[28,89–93] The ERSPC's quality-of-life adjustment study reported the total benefit was 73 life-years gained per 1000 men screened (mean 8.4 years per death avoided). The net benefit had to be reduced by 23% due to risks and harms, but there were still 56 life-years gained per 1000 men screened.[89]

EPILOGUE: 2017 CANCER INTERVENTION AND SURVEILLANCE MODELING NETWORK REANALYSIS OF PROSTATE, LUNG, COLORECTAL, AND OVARIAN TRIAL AND EUROPEAN RANDOMIZED STUDY OF SCREENING FOR PROSTATE CANCER DATA

In 2017, CISNET published a statistical modeling study examining the conflicting ERSPC and PLCO results by focusing on differences in implementation of screening between the trials. In an intent-to-treat analyses, they calculated a continuous score reflecting how much earlier participants in the screening arm were diagnosed relative to a nonscreened population from the pre-PSA era, called the "mean lead time." They found the greater the mean lead time, the greater the reduction in mortality. They reported that screening produced a significant 25% to 31% reduction in PCa mortality in ERSPC and a 27% to 32% reduction in PLCO. Thus, correcting for the implementation of screening, both trials showed that PSA screening saves lives.[13]

2017—THE FUTURE: PROSTATE-SPECIFIC ANTIGEN SCREENING RENAISSANCE
US Preventive Services Task Force Backs Away from Total Ban on Prostate-Specific Antigen Testing

In May 2017, the USPSTF backed away from its grade D recommendation and issued a draft recommendation that clinicians inform men aged 55 years to 69 years about the potential benefits and harms of PSA screening. The new draft recommendation, however, maintains the grade D score for men younger than 55 and older than 69 years, even though PSA screening has not been adequately tested in RCTs in men less than 55 years or greater than or equal to 70 years. Therefore, there is insufficient evidence to recommend for or against early detection in men in these younger and older age groups. The limited evidence from the Göteborg trial that included screening of men at age 50 suggests that screening is beneficial in this age group. Thus, the new USPSTF draft recommendation excludes baseline screening in men in their 40s for assessment for future risk for metastatic or lethal PCa.

The USPSTF 2017 draft also lacks a recommendation for more intensive screening in high-risk men, such as men with a family history of PCa or for men of African ancestry, for whom there is compelling evidence of greater risk of PCa morbidity and mortality and thus potentially greater potential of screening benefits.[94,95] In the PLCO trial, men with a positive family history had a 56% higher PCa detection rate and a 51% higher PCa mortality rate. In the screening arm, there was a trend ($P = .06$) toward a 50% lower PCa mortality rate that was not statistically significant, owing to the small sample size.[96] Similarly, evidence suggests possible increased benefits from earlier and more frequent PSA testing in African American men.[94,97,98]

The USPSTF stated that although it is possible that screening may offer greater benefits for African American men, currently no direct evidence demonstrates whether this is true. It is well documented, however, that African American men present with more advanced disease and have shorter progression-free survival after treatment.[94,95,98] African American men are more likely to have longer time intervals between screenings; thus, more frequent screening may reduce their risk of advanced-stage disease.[94,97] A natural history modeling study reported that African American men have more preclinical and progressive PCa and are more likely to develop PCa at a younger age and more likely to progress to a metastases or higher stage or grade before clinical diagnosis. This suggests that African American men should consider beginning screening earlier and/or more frequently.[94]

The Burden of Prostate-Specific Antigen–Based Prostate Cancer in the Future

It has been estimated that, with changing age demographics, the number of PCa deaths in the United States will increase 3-fold in the mid-2000s.[99–101] PCa diagnosed in older men is more frequently aggressive, and nearly half of US PCa deaths occur in men diagnosed after the age of 74 years, despite men in this age group comprising only approximately one-fourth of PCa patients.[102] Thus, in the future, even with reinstitution of widespread PSA testing, more men will live long enough to succumb to PCa, and there will be more total PCa deaths. It is sobering to consider that without PSA testing, the death rate would be more than twice as high.[83]

Author's Recommendations for Prostate-Specific Antigen Testing

The controversy over PSA screening has not ended despite unequivocal evidence that it saves lives. Although the USPSTF's 2017 draft recommendation is a step in the right direction, there is more progress to be made with respect to

1. Baseline testing in men in their 40s to assess future risk for life-threatening disease
2. Earlier testing of high-risk men, such as African-Americans and men with a family history whose risk of metastatic and lethal PCa is greater
3. Testing healthy men greater than or equal to 70 who are also at higher risk for life-threatening PCa[103]

If a man asks his physician whether or not he should have a PSA test, the physician should encourage appropriate testing. Moreover, men in their 40s should be informed that baseline PSA testing in their 40s is the best way to assess their risk for subsequent life-threatening PCa, because those in the top 10% PSA levels for their age group account for almost half of all PCa deaths up to 30 years later, and those with levels above 1.0 ng/mL clearly warrant more careful monitoring. Healthy men in their 70s should not be discouraged from being tested if their life expectancy is greater than or equal to 10 years. Life expectancy at age 70 years in the United States is greater than 15 years; therefore, some older men will benefit from early detection and treatment of a potentially aggressive tumor.[104,105]

In interpreting PSA testing results, age-specific PSA cutoffs should be used to help determine whether an individual has an elevated PSA level, and testing intervals should not exceed 1 year to 2 years, because less frequent PSA testing limits the ability to detect aggressive cancers that have the shortest preclinical phases. Some investigators have recommended increasing the PSA trigger for recommending a biopsy of men greater than 69 years to 10 ng/mL. Higher thresholds for biopsy, however, are less likely to detect aggressive cancers that produce less PSA while they are in a curable stage. Deferring or discontinuing screening in men with a low baseline PSA also may critically delay the diagnosis of aggressive PCa.

Prostate Cancer Screening Renaissance

The USPSTF recommendation against all screening was patently wrong and has engendered cynicism about USPSTF procedures. Its recommendations have created a generation of primary care physicians who reject PSA testing. The release of the USPSTFs 2017 draft recommendation is a first step in acknowledging to the medical community that the benefits of PSA screening outweigh the harms, and physicians and patients should now accept the truth and the value of the practical application of PSA testing, which will reduce the suffering and death from PCa.

ACKNOWLEDGMENTS

The author gratefully acknowledges the assistance of Phillip Richard Cooper in preparing the article.

REFERENCES

1. Siegel RL, Miller KD, Jemal A. Cancer statistics, 2017. CA Cancer J Clin 2017; 67(1):7–30.
2. Catalona WJ, Smith DS, Ratliff TL, et al. Measurement of prostate-specific antigen in serum as a screening test for prostate cancer. N Engl J Med 1991; 324(17):1156–61.
3. Stormont TJ, Farrow GM, Myers RP, et al. Clinical Stage B0 or T1c prostate cancer: nonpalpable disease identified by elevated serum prostate-specific antigen concentration. Urology 1993;41(1):3–8.
4. Schroder FH, Hugosson J, Roobol MJ, et al. Screening and prostate-cancer mortality in a randomized European study. N Engl J Med 2009;360(13):1320–8.
5. Schroder FH, Hugosson J, Roobol MJ, et al. Screening and prostate cancer mortality: results of the European Randomised Study of Screening for Prostate Cancer (ERSPC) at 13 years of follow-up. Lancet 2014;384(9959):2027–35.
6. Schroder FH, Hugosson J, Roobol MJ, et al. Prostate-cancer mortality at 11 years of follow-up. N Engl J Med 2012;366(11):981–90.
7. Djulbegovic M, Beyth RJ, Neuberger MM, et al. Screening for prostate cancer: systematic review and meta-analysis of randomised controlled trials. BMJ 2010; 341:c4543.
8. Ilic D, O'Connor D, Green S, et al. Screening for prostate cancer: an updated cochrane systematic review. BJU Int 2011;107(6):882–91.
9. Andriole GL, Crawford ED, Grubb RL 3rd, et al. Mortality results from a randomized prostate-cancer screening trial. N Engl J Med 2009;360(13):1310–9.
10. Pinsky P, Prorok P. More on reevaluating PSA testing rates in the PLCO trial. N Engl J Med 2016;375(15):1500–1.
11. Pinsky PF, Blacka A, Kramer BS, et al. Assessing contamination and compliance in the prostate component of the prostate, lung, colorectal, and ovarian (PLCO) cancer screening trial. Clin Trials 2010;7(4):303–11.
12. Pinsky PF, Prorok PC, Yu K, et al. Extended mortality results for prostate cancer screening in the PLCO trial with median follow-up of 15 years. Cancer 2017; 123(4):592–9.
13. Tsodikov A, Gulati R, Heijnsdijk EAM, et al. Reconciling the effects of screening on prostate cancer mortality in the ERSPC and PLCO trials. Ann Intern Med 2017;167(7):449–55.

14. Catalona WJ, Hudson MA, Scardino PT, et al. Selection of optimal prostate specific antigen cutoffs for early detection of prostate cancer: receiver operating characteristic curves. J Urol 1994;152(6 Pt 1):2037–42.
15. Zhu H, Roehl KA, Antenor JA, et al. Biopsy of men with PSA level of 2.6 to 4.0 ng/mL associated with favorable pathologic features and PSA progression rate: a preliminary analysis. Urology 2005;66(3):547–51.
16. Thompson IM, Pauler DK, Goodman PJ, et al. Prevalence of prostate cancer among men with a prostate-specific antigen level < or =4.0 ng per milliliter. N Engl J Med 2004;350(22):2239–46.
17. Punglia RS, D'Amico AV, Catalona WJ, et al. Effect of verification bias on screening for prostate cancer by measurement of prostate-specific antigen. N Engl J Med 2003;349(4):335–42.
18. Antenor JA, Roehl KA, Eggener SE, et al. Preoperative PSA and progression-free survival after radical prostatectomy for Stage T1c disease. Urology 2005; 66(1):156–60.
19. Crawford ED, Leewansangtong S, Goktas S, et al. Efficiency of prostate-specific antigen and digital rectal examination in screening, using 4.0 ng/ml and age-specific reference range as a cutoff for abnormal values. Prostate 1999;38(4): 296–302.
20. Gore JL, Shariat SF, Miles BJ, et al. Optimal combinations of systematic sextant and laterally directed biopsies for the detection of prostate cancer. J Urol 2001; 165(5):1554–9.
21. Catalona WJ, Richie JP, deKernion JB, et al. Comparison of prostate specific antigen concentration versus prostate specific antigen density in the early detection of prostate cancer: receiver operating characteristic curves. J Urol 1994; 152(6 Pt 1):2031–6.
22. Smith DS, Catalona WJ. The nature of prostate cancer detected through prostate specific antigen based screening. J Urol 1994;152(5 Pt 2):1732–6.
23. D'Amico AV, Chen MH, Roehl KA, et al. Preoperative PSA velocity and the risk of death from prostate cancer after radical prostatectomy. N Engl J Med 2004; 351(2):125–35.
24. Okotie OT, Roehl KA, Han M, et al. Characteristics of prostate cancer detected by digital rectal examination only. Urology 2007;70(6):1117–20.
25. Boring CC, Squires TS, Tong T. Cancer statistics, 1992. CA Cancer J Clin 1992; 42(1):19–38.
26. Etzioni R, Tsodikov A, Mariotto A, et al. Quantifying the role of PSA screening in the US prostate cancer mortality decline. Cancer Causes Control 2008;19(2): 175–81.
27. Etzioni R, Gulati R, Tsodikov A, et al. The prostate cancer conundrum revisited: treatment changes and prostate cancer mortality declines. Cancer 2012; 118(23):5955–63.
28. Hamdy FC, Donovan JL, Lane JA, et al. 10-year outcomes after monitoring, surgery, or radiotherapy for localized prostate cancer. N Engl J Med 2016;375(15): 1415–24.
29. Bill-Axelson A, Holmberg L, Ruutu M, et al. Radical prostatectomy versus watchful waiting in early prostate cancer. N Engl J Med 2011;364(18):1708–17.
30. Wilt TJ, Brawer MK, Jones KM, et al. Radical prostatectomy versus observation for localized prostate cancer. N Engl J Med 2012;367(3):203–13.
31. Bill-Axelson A, Holmberg L, Ruutu M, et al. Radical prostatectomy versus watchful waiting in early prostate cancer. N Engl J Med 2005;352(19):1977–84.

32. Carter HB, Ferrucci L, Kettermann A, et al. Detection of life-threatening prostate cancer with prostate-specific antigen velocity during a window of curability. J Natl Cancer Inst 2006;98(21):1521–7.
33. Carter HB, Kettermann A, Ferrucci L, et al. Prostate-specific antigen velocity risk count assessment: a new concept for detection of life-threatening prostate cancer during window of curability. Urology 2007;70(4):685–90.
34. Carter HB, Pearson JD, Metter EJ, et al. Longitudinal evaluation of prostate-specific antigen levels in men with and without prostate disease. JAMA 1992; 267(16):2215–20.
35. Fang J, Metter EJ, Landis P, et al. PSA velocity for assessing prostate cancer risk in men with PSA levels between 2.0 and 4.0 ng/ml. Urology 2002;59(6): 889–93 [discussion: 893–4].
36. Smith DS, Catalona WJ. Rate of change in serum prostate specific antigen levels as a method for prostate cancer detection. J Urol 1994;152(4):1163–7.
37. Shoaibi A, Rao GA, Cai B, et al. Prostate specific antigen-growth curve model to predict high-risk prostate cancer. Prostate 2017;77(2):173–84.
38. Orsted DD, Bojesen SE, Kamstrup PR, et al. Long-term prostate-specific antigen velocity in improved classification of prostate cancer risk and mortality. Eur Urol 2013;64(3):384–93.
39. Loeb S, Nadler RB, Roehl KA, et al. Risk of prostate cancer for young men with a prostate specific antigen less than their age specific median. J Urol 2007; 177(5):1745–8.
40. Bent S, Kane C, Shinohara K, et al. Saw palmetto for benign prostatic hyperplasia. N Engl J Med 2006;354(6):557–66.
41. Inoue LY, Etzioni R, Slate EH, et al. Combining longitudinal studies of PSA. Biostatistics 2004;5(3):483–500.
42. Eggener SE, Yossepowitch O, Roehl KA, et al. Relationship of prostate-specific antigen velocity to histologic findings in a prostate cancer screening program. Urology 2008;71(6):1016–9.
43. Loeb S, Zhu X, Schroder FH, et al. Long-term radical prostatectomy outcomes among participants from the European Randomized Study of Screening for Prostate Cancer (ERSPC) Rotterdam. BJU Int 2012;110(11):1678–83.
44. Fang J, Metter EJ, Landis P, et al. Low levels of prostate-specific antigen predict long-term risk of prostate cancer: results from the Baltimore Longitudinal Study of Aging. Urology 2001;58(3):411–6.
45. Ulmert D, Cronin AM, Bjork T, et al. Prostate-specific antigen at or before age 50 as a predictor of advanced prostate cancer diagnosed up to 25 years later: a case-control study. BMC Med 2008;6:6.
46. Vertosick EA, Poon BY, Vickers AJ. Relative value of race, family history and prostate specific antigen as indications for early initiation of prostate cancer screening. J Urol 2014;192(3):724–8.
47. Smith DS, Humphrey PA, Catalona WJ. The early detection of prostate carcinoma with prostate specific antigen: the Washington University experience. Cancer 1997;80(9):1852–6.
48. Whittemore AS, Cirillo PM, Feldman D, et al. Prostate specific antigen levels in young adulthood predict prostate cancer risk: results from a cohort of Black and White Americans. J Urol 2005;174(3):872–6 [discussion: 876].
49. Morgan TO, Jacobsen SJ, McCarthy WF, et al. Age-specific reference ranges for serum prostate-specific antigen in black men. N Engl J Med 1996;335(5): 304–10.

50. Oesterling JE, Jacobsen SJ, Chute CG, et al. Serum prostate-specific antigen in a community-based population of healthy men. Establishment of age-specific reference ranges. JAMA 1993;270(7):860–4.
51. Loeb S, Roehl KA, Antenor JA, et al. Baseline prostate-specific antigen compared with median prostate-specific antigen for age group as predictor of prostate cancer risk in men younger than 60 years old. Urology 2006;67(2): 316–20.
52. Lilja H, Ulmert D, Bjork T, et al. Long-term prediction of prostate cancer up to 25 years before diagnosis of prostate cancer using prostate kallikreins measured at age 44 to 50 years. J Clin Oncol 2007;25(4):431–6.
53. Vickers AJ, Cronin AM, Bjork T, et al. Prostate specific antigen concentration at age 60 and death or metastasis from prostate cancer: case-control study. BMJ 2010;341:c4521.
54. Vickers AJ, Ulmert D, Sjoberg DD, et al. Strategy for detection of prostate cancer based on relation between prostate specific antigen at age 40-55 and long term risk of metastasis: case-control study. BMJ 2013;346:f2023.
55. Catalona WJ, Partin AW, Slawin KM, et al. Use of the percentage of free prostate-specific antigen to enhance differentiation of prostate cancer from benign prostatic disease: a prospective multicenter clinical trial. JAMA 1998; 279(19):1542–7.
56. Catalona WJ, Partin AW, Sanda MG, et al. A multicenter study of [-2]pro-prostate specific antigen combined with prostate specific antigen and free prostate specific antigen for prostate cancer detection in the 2.0 to 10.0 ng/ml prostate specific antigen range. J Urol 2011;185(5):1650–5.
57. Loeb S, Sanda MG, Broyles DL, et al. The prostate health index selectively identifies clinically significant prostate cancer. J Urol 2015;193(4):1163–9.
58. Loeb S, Shin SS, Broyles DL, et al. Prostate Health Index improves multivariable risk prediction of aggressive prostate cancer. BJU Int 2017;120(1):61–8.
59. Parekh DJ, Punnen S, Sjoberg DD, et al. A multi-institutional prospective trial in the USA confirms that the 4Kscore accurately identifies men with high-grade prostate cancer. Eur Urol 2015;68(3):464–70.
60. Bryant RJ, Sjoberg DD, Vickers AJ, et al. Predicting high-grade cancer at ten-core prostate biopsy using four kallikrein markers measured in blood in the ProtecT study. J Natl Cancer Inst 2015;107(7) [pii:djv095].
61. Moyer VA, U.S. Preventive Services Task Force. Screening for prostate cancer: U.S. Preventive Services Task Force recommendation statement. Ann Intern Med 2012;157(2):120–34.
62. Kaffenberger SD, Penson DF. The politics of prostate cancer screening. Urol Clin North Am 2014;41(2):249–55.
63. Kapoor D. Origins of The U.S. Preventive Services Task Force. Available at: https://www.urotoday.com/video-lectures/5-for-5-hot-topics-e-david-crawford/video/672-embedded-media2017-01-03-23-19-35.html?utm_source=bottom-links. Accessed June 19, 2017.
64. Kapoor DA. A history of the USPSTF; its expanding authority and need for reform. J Urol 2017 [pii:S0022-5347(17)77375-2].
65. U.S. Preventive Services Task Force. Screening for prostate cancer: U.S. Preventive Services Task Force recommendation statement. Ann Intern Med 2008;149(3):185–91.
66. Halpern JA, Shoag JE, Artis AS, et al. National trends in prostate biopsy and radical prostatectomy volumes following the US preventive services task

force guidelines against prostate-specific antigen screening. JAMA Surg 2017; 152(2):192–8.

67. Hu JC, Nguyen P, Mao J, et al. Increase in prostate cancer distant metastases at diagnosis in the United States. JAMA Oncol 2017;3(5):705–7.

68. Gaylis FD, Choi J, Kader AK. Trends in metastatic breast and prostate cancer. N Engl J Med 2016;374(6):594–5.

69. Jemal A, Fedewa SA, Ma J, et al. Prostate cancer incidence and PSA testing patterns in relation to USPSTF screening recommendations. JAMA 2015; 314(19):2054–61.

70. Aslani A, Minnillo BJ, Johnson B, et al. The impact of recent screening recommendations on prostate cancer screening in a large health care system. J Urol 2014;191(6):1737–42.

71. Cohn JA, Wang CE, Lakeman JC, et al. Primary care physician PSA screening practices before and after the final U.S. Preventive Services Task Force recommendation. Urol Oncol 2014;32(1):41.e23-30.

72. Grenabo Bergdahl A, Holmberg E, Moss S, et al. Incidence of prostate cancer after termination of screening in a population-based randomised screening trial. Eur Urol 2013;64(5):703–9.

73. Godtman RA, Carlsson S, Holmberg E, et al. The effect of start and stop age at screening on the risk of being diagnosed with prostate cancer. J Urol 2016; 195(5):1390–6.

74. Chou R, Croswell JM, Dana T, et al. Screening for prostate cancer: a review of the evidence for the U.S. Preventive Services Task Force. Ann Intern Med 2011; 155(11):762–71.

75. Catalona WJ, D'Amico AV, Fitzgibbons WF, et al. What the U.S. Preventive Services Task Force missed in its prostate cancer screening recommendation. Ann Intern Med 2012;157(2):137–8.

76. Allan GM, Chetner MP, Donnelly BJ, et al. Furthering the prostate cancer screening debate (prostate cancer specific mortality and associated risks). Can Urol Assoc J 2011;5(6):416–21.

77. McNaughton-Collins MF, Barry MJ. One man at a time–resolving the PSA controversy. N Engl J Med 2011;365(21):1951–3.

78. Sox HC. Quality of life and guidelines for PSA screening. N Engl J Med 2012; 367(7):669–71.

79. Hartzband P, Groopman J. There is more to life than death. N Engl J Med 2012; 367(11):987–9.

80. Etzioni R, Gulati R. Response: reading between the lines of cancer screening trials: using modeling to understand the evidence. Med Care 2013;51(4):304–6.

81. Etzioni RD, Thompson IM. What do the screening trials really tell us and where do we go from here? Urol Clin North Am 2014;41(2):223–8.

82. Gulati R, Mariotto AB, Chen S, et al. Long-term projections of the harm-benefit trade-off in prostate cancer screening are more favorable than previous short-term estimates. J Clin Epidemiol 2011;64(12):1412–7.

83. Scosyrev E, Wu G, Mohile S, et al. Prostate-specific antigen screening for prostate cancer and the risk of overt metastatic disease at presentation: analysis of trends over time. Cancer 2012;118(23):5768–76.

84. Buzzoni C, Auvinen A, Roobol MJ, et al. Metastatic prostate cancer incidence and prostate-specific antigen testing: new insights from the European randomized study of screening for prostate cancer. Eur Urol 2015;68(5):885–90.

85. Schroder FH, Hugosson J, Carlsson S, et al. Screening for prostate cancer decreases the risk of developing metastatic disease: findings from the European

Randomized Study of Screening for Prostate Cancer (ERSPC). Eur Urol 2012; 62(5):745–52.

86. Shoag JE, Mittal S, Hu JC. Reevaluating PSA testing rates in the PLCO trial. N Engl J Med 2016;374(18):1795–6.

87. Gulati R, Albertsen PC. Insights from the PLCO trial about prostate cancer screening. Cancer 2017;123(4):546–8.

88. Arnsrud Godtman R, Holmberg E, Lilja H, et al. Opportunistic testing versus organized prostate-specific antigen screening: outcome after 18 years in the Goteborg randomized population-based prostate cancer screening trial. Eur Urol 2015;68(3):354–60.

89. Heijnsdijk EA, Wever EM, Auvinen A, et al. Quality-of-life effects of prostate-specific antigen screening. N Engl J Med 2012;367(7):595–605.

90. Sanda MG, Dunn RL, Michalski J, et al. Quality of life and satisfaction with outcome among prostate-cancer survivors. N Engl J Med 2008;358(12): 1250–61.

91. Vasarainen H, Malmi H, Maattanen L, et al. Effects of prostate cancer screening on health-related quality of life: results of the finnish arm of the European randomized screening trial (ERSPC). Acta Oncol 2013;52(8):1615–21.

92. Korfage IJ, Essink-Bot ML, Borsboom GJ, et al. Five-year follow-up of health-related quality of life after primary treatment of localized prostate cancer. Int J Cancer 2005;116(2):291–6.

93. Krahn M, Ritvo P, Irvine J, et al. Patient and community preferences for outcomes in prostate cancer: implications for clinical policy. Med Care 2003; 41(1):153–64.

94. Tsodikov A, Gulati R, de Carvalho TM, et al. Is prostate cancer different in black men? Answers from 3 natural history models. Cancer 2017;123(12):2312–9.

95. Powell IJ. Epidemiology and pathophysiology of prostate cancer in African-American men. J Urol 2007;177(2):444–9.

96. Liss MA, Chen H, Hemal S, et al. Impact of family history on prostate cancer mortality in white men undergoing prostate specific antigen based screening. J Urol 2015;193(1):75–9.

97. Carpenter WR, Howard DL, Taylor YJ, et al. Racial differences in PSA screening interval and stage at diagnosis. Cancer Causes Control 2010; 21(7):1071–80.

98. Chornokur G, Dalton K, Borysova ME, et al. Disparities at presentation, diagnosis, treatment, and survival in African American men, affected by prostate cancer. Prostate 2011;71(9):985–97.

99. Weir HK, Thompson TD, Soman A, et al. The past, present, and future of cancer incidence in the United States: 1975 through 2020. Cancer 2015;121(11): 1827–37.

100. Chan JM, Jou RM, Carroll PR. The relative impact and future burden of prostate cancer in the United States. J Urol 2004;172(5 Pt 2):S13–6 [discussion: S17].

101. United States Census Bureau. 2014 National Population Projections. Available at: https://www.census.gov/population/projections/data/national/2014.html. Accessed May 24, 2017.

102. Scosyrev E, Messing EM, Mohile S, et al. Prostate cancer in the elderly: frequency of advanced disease at presentation and disease-specific mortality. Cancer 2012;118(12):3062–70.

103. Bechis SK, Carroll PR, Cooperberg MR. Impact of age at diagnosis on prostate cancer treatment and survival. J Clin Oncol 2011;29(2):235–41.

104. Wong YN, Mitra N, Hudes G, et al. Survival associated with treatment vs observation of localized prostate cancer in elderly men. JAMA 2006;296(22): 2683–93.
105. Litwin MS, Miller DC. Treating older men with prostate cancer: survival (or selection) of the fittest? JAMA 2006;296(22):2733–4.

Prostate Cancer

A Contemporary Approach to Treatment and Outcomes

Adam B. Weiner, MD, Shilajit D. Kundu, MD*

KEYWORDS

- Prostatic neoplasm • Therapeutics • Treatment outcomes • Surgical procedures
- Operative • Radiotherapy • Watchful waiting

KEY POINTS

- It is imperative for primary care providers to understand the different treatment options for prostate cancer given the high incidence and need for shared-decision making before screening.
- The mainstays of prostate cancer treatment include observation, surgery, and radiotherapy for localized diseased; and androgen deprivation therapy and chemotherapy for metastatic disease.
- Active surveillance for low-risk prostate cancer may minimize unnecessary treatment without compromising survival and is the preferred management approach.
- Radical prostatectomy and radiotherapy with or without androgen deprivation therapy, are used to treat localized prostate cancer and have similar cancer-specific outcomes but different adverse effects.
- Androgen deprivation therapy has a variety of adverse effects that require monitoring and preventive measures.

INTRODUCTION

Prostate cancer will be diagnosed in more than 160,000 men and claim the lives of more than 25,000 men in 2017.[1] Over the past decade, the diagnosis of prostate cancer using prostate-specific antigen (PSA)-directed screening has been scrutinized with concerns that it may lead to overtreatment of low-grade disease that may never have become symptomatic in a patient's lifetime or result in death from prostate cancer. In 2012, the US Preventive Services Task Force (USPSTF) recommended against routine prostate cancer screening, citing that the benefits of screening were outweighed by the potential harms associated with diagnosis and treatment.[2]

Disclosure Statement: None.
Department of Urology, Northwestern University, Feinberg School of Medicine, 303 East Chicago Avenue, 16-710, Chicago, IL 60611, USA
* Corresponding author.
E-mail address: Shilajit.Kundu@nm.org

Med Clin N Am 102 (2018) 215–229
https://doi.org/10.1016/j.mcna.2017.10.001

It is notable that recent trends in the approach to managing low-grade prostate cancer have moved more toward a risk-adaptive approach, including active surveillance, when appropriate, in the hopes of reducing overtreatment.[3,4] (See William J. Catalona's article, "Prostate Cancer Screening," in this issue.) In addition, data from large trials have supported that early screening and subsequent treatment may prevent progression to metastatic disease.[5] These trends have influenced the USPSTF to recently recommend screening for prostate cancer after discussion with a clinician about the potential harms and benefits of screening.[6] Therefore, it is imperative that, as the first point of contact, primary care providers are knowledgeable on the topic of prostate cancer management if they are going to advise patients about screening.

The traditional paradigm of treatment of adenocarcinoma of the prostate (which will henceforth be implied when referring to prostate cancer) includes observation, radical prostatectomy, and radiotherapy with or without androgen deprivation therapy (ADT) for localized, nonmetastatic prostate cancer. Systemic treatment alone, such as ADT and chemotherapy, are generally reserved for men with metastatic disease. Each of these management approaches has a unique combination of indications, advantages, disadvantages, adverse effects, and surveillance schedules.

The goal of this article is to serve as a reference for primary care providers who are counseling their patients on screening for and management of prostate cancer. It covers the standard approaches to the initial management of prostate cancer, posttreatment surveillance, and the adverse effects of each management approach. It also briefly reviews the management options following cancer recurrence and current areas of research interest.

OBSERVATION

Observation can be categorized into 2 subsets: watchful waiting and active surveillance. Both were developed as a means of reducing overtreatment in prostate cancer and have been increasingly implemented in recent years.[3,4]

Watchful Waiting: Treatment Only for Symptomatic Relief

Watchful waiting implies a passive monitoring of symptoms without treatment in the absence of clinical symptoms or extreme elevations in PSA (>100 ng/mL).[7] Development of symptoms associated with prostate cancer progression or extremely high PSA values (which may portend imminent symptoms) would trigger treatment intervention with intentions to palliate symptoms. Patients electing watchful waiting can expect possible blood tests and physical examinations no more frequently than every 6 months. Palliative measures may include ADT (see later discussion) or radiotherapy directed at painful bony metastases. In the largest randomized controlled trial comparing radical prostatectomy to watchful waiting, surgery was able to reduce the rate of developing metastatic disease for men aged 65 years and younger from 45% to 28%, but differences between the 2 treatment arms were minimal before 10 years of follow-up.[8] Thus, in general, patients who qualify as watchful waiting candidates have less than 5 years life expectancy or have low-risk or intermediate-risk disease according the National Comprehensive Cancer Network (NCCN) standards (**Table 1**) and a life expectancy of less than 10 years.[7]

The rationale to pursue watchful waiting is aimed at minimizing the adverse effects associated with treatment of patients who may derive minimal survival benefit from definitive local therapy, such as surgery or radiation. One important factor in enrolling a man into watchful waiting is his age, which serves as a surrogate for life expectancy.

Table 1
National Comprehensive Cancer Network prostate cancer risk groups

Risk Group	PSA (ng/mL)	Gleason Score	Clinical Tumor (T)-Stage	Clinical Node (N)-Stage or Metastasis (M)-Stage	Additional Information
Very low[a]	<10	≤6	T1	N0 and M0	Fewer than 3 biopsy cores with cancer, ≤50% cancer in each core, PSA density <0.15 ng/mL/g
Low	<10	≤6	T1–T2a	N0 and M0	—
Intermediate	10–20	3 + 4 = 7, 4 + 3 = 7	T2b–T2c	N0 and M0	—
High	>20	8–10	T3–T4	N0 and M0	—
Very High[b]	>20	8–10	T3–T4	N0 and M0	Primary Gleason pattern 5, >4 biopsy cores with Gleason score 8–10
Metastatic	Any	Any	Any	N1 or M1	—

Clinical T stages are defined as nonpalpable on digital rectal examination (T1), tumor involving less than one-half of 1 prostate lobe (T2a), tumor involving more than one-half of 1 prostate lobe (T2b), tumor involving both prostate lobes (T2c), tumor extending through the prostate capsule or seminal vesicles (T3), and tumor invading into adjacent organs, such as the bladder or pelvic side wall (T4).
 [a] Included in low-risk group.
 [b] Included in high-risk group.
 From National Comprehensive Cancer Network (NCCN). Prostate cancer, version 1.2017. Available at: https://www.nccn.org. Accessed April 17, 2017; with permission.

However, a patient's overall health must be taken into consideration when considering age with respect to life expectancy. The NCCN recommends beginning with a tool to help estimate life expectancy based on age, such as the Social Security Administration tools (https://www.ssa.gov/OACT/STATS/table4c6.html), and adding or subtracting 50% of the years if a patients is in the upper or lower quartile of health for his age, respectively.[7]

Active Surveillance: Disease Monitoring with Treatment on Progression or Patient Preference

Active surveillance, as its name implies, involves a more dynamic approach to observation than watchful waiting. Patients who enroll into active surveillance are candidates for definitive therapy with surgery or radiotherapy but choose to forego treatment due to low risk of progression to metastasis or death from prostate cancer. This may help to mitigate potential side effects associated with treatment. Ideal candidates for active surveillance have low-risk cancer, which includes low-grade (Gleason 3 + 3 = 6) with fewer than half of the total biopsy cores containing cancer. Some urologists will also consider surveillance for patients with favorable intermediate-risk disease. These patients will also have low volume of tumors as indicated by a low number of biopsy cores with cancer and tumor that is primarily composed of low-grade disease (Gleason 3 + 4 = 7 vs to Gleason 4 + 3 = 7).[9]

Although there is no single standardized approach to active surveillance, in general, patients can expect serial monitoring every 3 to 6 months with PSA measurements, digital rectal examinations at least annually, and prostate biopsies every 1 to 2 years. Over time, the surveillance intervals may increase.[7] A urologist may recommend a confirmatory prostate biopsy soon after the initial diagnostic biopsy before recommending active surveillance because as many as 20% of patients may demonstrate a higher grade disease on this second biopsy.[10] If available, an MRI–ultrasound fusion-guided prostate biopsy may improve the ability to detect higher grade disease on the confirmatory biopsy.[11]

Patients in whom there is evidence of cancer progression (PSA rise faster than normal or increase in Gleason grade) may discontinue surveillance and opt to undergo curative surgery or radiotherapy at that point.

To date, there are now several single-arm series assessing the safety of active surveillance[12–17] and 1 ongoing randomized controlled trial comparing surveillance to upfront surgery or radiotherapy.[18] Although these trials are heterogeneous in terms of who they deemed active surveillance candidates, surveillance schedules, and triggers for initiating surgery or radiotherapy, the general principles as previously outlined are relatively similar and results tend to be congruent.

The benefit of active surveillance is the potential to avoid or delay treatment-related adverse effect while monitoring for and treating any prostate cancer that progresses. The overall 5-year, 10-year, and 15-year treatment-free rates in reported studies are 60% to 81%, 60% to 64%, and 43% to 55%, respectively.[12–16] Over time, patients on active surveillance, including men who eventually receive curative treatment, are expected to maintain better urinary and sexual function compared with men who undergo initial radical prostatectomy, and better bowel function compared with men who undergo radiotherapy.[19,20]

Additionally, the risk of missing the window of opportunity for cure through surveillance is thought to be minimal. Metastasis-free and cancer-specific survival is very favorable with greater than 10 years of follow-up at 97.2% to 99.4%, and 98.5% to 99.7%, respectively.[12,15,18]

In summary, active surveillance is a safe management approach for select men with low-risk prostate cancer. Its use has the potential to reduce overtreatment without compromising cancer-specific survival, making it the preferred management approach for most men with low-risk prostate cancer.

RADICAL PROSTATECTOMY
Surgery and Oncologic Outcomes

Radical prostatectomy remains the cornerstone of curative treatment of prostate cancer and is deemed appropriate for men with localized prostate cancer with at least 10 years of life expectancy or any patient with high-risk prostate cancer (see **Table 1**).[7] Two large randomized controlled trials have compared radical prostatectomy to watchful waiting.[8,21] In general, data from the Scandinavian Prostate Cancer Group Study Number 4 (SPCG-4) study showed, with up to 23 years of follow-up, that surgery reduced prostate cancer–specific mortality by 11%, from 29% to 18%. The greatest mortality benefit was seen in men younger than 65 years of age and in those with intermediate-risk disease. A total of 8 men required surgery to save 1 from death due to prostate cancer. In men younger than 65 years of age the number needed to treat was reduced to 4 men. The accrual for SPCG-4 occurred largely before the widespread use of PSA screening and thus their cohort likely had worse cancer prognoses compared with that of the American Prostate Cancer Intervention versus Observation Trial (PIVOT).[21] In PIVOT, no difference in death due to prostate cancer was seen between the 2 treatment arms; however, in subgroup analyses, radical prostatectomy reduced cancer-specific death from 13% to 6% for men with PSA values greater than 10 ng/mL and from 18% to 9% for men with high-risk disease after a median of 10 years follow-up.

In general, one can infer from SPCG-4 and PIVOT that radical prostatectomy likely reduces prostate cancer–specific mortality for men with intermediate-risk and high-risk disease. Additionally, these trials support the use of some form of observation for men with low-risk disease, although active surveillance may currently be the optimal option for most of these men (see previous discussion). Importantly, both studies demonstrated that surgery led to significant reductions in the development of potentially morbid metastatic disease and SPCG-4 showed large reductions in the use of ADT for men who received surgery.[8,21]

In a recent randomized controlled trial comparing radical prostatectomy to active surveillance and radiotherapy, the Prostate Testing for Cancer and Treatment (ProtecT) trial showed no difference between the groups in terms of prostate cancer mortality after 10 years of follow-up.[18] However, prostate cancer–specific and overall mortality were significantly lower in ProtecT compared with PIVOT and SPCG-4, which likely reflects improvements in adjuvant treatment of prostate cancer progression (see later discussion) and overall health care. Importantly, from ProtecT, one can draw only limited conclusions on the mortality benefits of surgery for intermediate-risk and high-risk disease given that 77% of patients had a low-risk Gleason score 3 + 3 = 6 (77%). However, even within this relatively low-risk cohort, the development of metastatic disease was significantly reduced by surgery from 6% to 2% after 10 years compared with active surveillance.

The Adverse Effects of Surgery

From ProtecT and a dearth of other large series, one can predict the adverse effects of radical prostatectomy.[19,20,22–24] The 2 major adverse effects of surgery are impotence and urinary incontinence. In general, the major predictors of recovery of potency are younger patient age and use of nerve-sparing surgical technique.[23] The decision to spare the cavernous nerves, which control potency during radical prostatectomy either bilaterally or unilaterally, is largely determined by the surgeon, based on the location and aggressiveness of cancer within the prostate. Because of these factors, predicting the likelihood of recovering potency varies greatly by patient. Patients should see improvements in their impotence within 3 to 12 months following surgery, after which sexual function tends to plateau.[19,20,22,24] The use of erectile dysfunction medications in the early months following surgery, referred to as penile rehabilitation, may also improve long-term potency.[25] Long-term impotence tends to be worse among men who undergo radical prostatectomy compared with those who elect radiotherapy, especially among those with higher baseline erectile function.[19,20,22,24] However, in general, long-term bother from sexual dysfunction tends to be similar between patients who undergo surgery or radiotherapy.[19,24]

Lymph Node Dissection During Radical Prostatectomy

Studies investigating the use of a pelvic lymph node dissection during radical prostatectomy have demonstrated various effects on perioperative complications and conflicting reports on oncologic benefits.[26] Although this technique has not been tested in a randomized clinical trial, the NCCN does recommend it for men with greater than 2% risk of having nodal involvement based on any validated nomogram.[7]

Open Versus Robotic Radical Prostatectomy

The open retropubic approach to radical prostatectomy is still performed in the United States; however, more than 85% of all radical prostatectomies are performed with robotic assistance.[27] Only 1 phase 3 randomized controlled trial has been published that compared the 2 approaches; it showed no difference in postoperative complications or urinary, sexual, or bowel dysfunction 12 weeks following surgery.[28] There have been several retrospective series comparing open versus robotic surgery that have been thoroughly assessed in systematic reviews and metaanalyses. They have shown that the robot-assisted approach may improve urinary continence and potency at 12 months and may slightly reduce operative blood loss.[29–32] However, no differences in oncologic outcomes, such as cancer-specific mortality, have been shown yet.[31]

Disease Monitoring and Salvage Treatment Following Surgery

Following surgery, men generally undergo PSA measurements every 6 to 12 months for the first 5 years, then every 12 months thereafter. Annual monitoring may also include a digital rectal examination to detect local recurrences.

Although there is no standard approach to adjuvant and salvage therapies, there are some generally accepted principles. Adjuvant therapy usually refers to surgery followed by systemic therapy or radiotherapy to help decrease the risk of the cancer recurring. Adjuvant treatment with ADT is usually considered for men with cancer involving lymph nodes and other high-risk features.[33] External beam radiotherapy (EBRT), with or without ADT, is often considered for men with high-risk disease seen on final histologic assessment of the surgical specimen, including cancer with extraprostatic extension, seminal vesicles involvement, or extensive positive surgical margins.[34,35]

Salvage therapy, treatment following disease recurrence, also can involve the use radiotherapy and ADT. Patients who develop biochemical recurrent disease following surgery can be categorized into 2 groups. The first group includes those who reach a very low, but not undetectable level of PSA following surgery and see a very slow rise in PSA following surgery. These patients may have small amounts of benign tissue remaining and if they maintain low levels of PSA long term they may not require further treatment. The second group includes those men who reach an undetectable PSA level and subsequently experience a rise in PSA. It also includes those who never reach a low PSA, those who never nadir. These patients are thought to have remaining cancer. A failure for the PSA to decline following this treatment may indicate cancer has spread elsewhere in the body and, therefore, these men should receive metastatic evaluation, which may include a computed tomography scan and a bone scan. Radiotherapy directed at the prostatic fossa is often used for these patients, with or without ADT. Regardless of response in PSA, most men will receive ADT in this situation based on recent data suggesting radiotherapy with 24 months of ADT can reduce mortality from 13.4% to 5.8% compared with salvage radiotherapy alone.[36]

RADIOTHERAPY

Radiotherapy has been extensively studied to determine its efficacy and safety as a definitive treatment of localized prostate cancer. The 2 main categories of radiotherapy include EBRT and brachytherapy. Both have their distinct advantages and are considered safe and may be as effective as radical prostatectomy for nonmetastatic disease.[37,38] Radiotherapy is considered an option for men with low-risk prostate cancer and at least 10 years life expectancy. It is also considered an option for men with shorter life expectancies with intermediate-risk or high-risk prostate cancer, especially if those men are not considered surgical candidates. EBRT and brachytherapy are used as monotherapies for men with low-risk prostate cancer and are usually given with ADT for intermediate-risk and high-risk cancer.[7]

External Beam Radiotherapy

Standard EBRT takes place during several sessions over the course of 8 to 9 weeks or 4 to 6 weeks, depending on the type of technology used to deliver the radiation. In men with low-risk prostate cancer, EBRT alone will produce a disease-free survival rate of about 75% and a long-term cancer-specific survival rate of 99%.[39,40] The addition of ADT to the treatment of low-risk patients has not been shown to improve outcomes.[40] In studies largely composed of men with more advanced localized prostate cancer, the addition of androgen deprivation tended to improve progression-free and prostate cancer–specific survival.[41,42] The expected 10-year cancer-specific survival for men with high-risk disease who received both EBRT and androgen deprivation is about 84%.[42] Based on these results, ADT is recommended as adjunctive treatment of men with high-risk disease and should be considered for men with intermediate-risk disease.

The ProtecT trial is the only randomized controlled trial comparing radiotherapy directly to surgery and active surveillance.[18] As previously discussed, in this trial composed mostly of men with low-risk disease, the 3 treatment arms had similar rates of prostate cancer–specific survival, and both radiotherapy and surgery (2%–3%, respectively) did have significantly lower rates of developing metastatic disease compared with active surveillance (6%).

Proton therapy is another form of external radiotherapy that has been purported as having the theoretic benefit of reducing radiation toxicity to tissues adjacent to the prostate. Over the past decade, the number of facilities offering proton therapy have grown with minimal evidence about its benefits and increased costs to health care payers.[43] In general, there does not seem to be any added benefit to proton therapy compared with conventional EBRT.[44,45] Current NCCN recommendations state there is no clear benefit or decrement to the use of proton therapy compared with conventional EBRT.[7]

Brachytherapy

Brachytherapy is another potential curative treatment of localized prostate cancer. Similar to EBRT, it is often used as a monotherapy for low-risk prostate cancer and in addition to androgen deprivation for intermediate-risk and high-risk prostate cancer. The most important distinction for brachytherapy is between low-dose rate (LDR) and high-dose rate (HDR). LDR involves permanent irradiated seeds implanted transperineally, using transrectal ultrasound guidance. Different from EBRT, the brachytherapy seeds are delivered in a single session. Disadvantages include the need for general anesthesia for implantation. LDR alone tends to have similar disease-free survival compared with standard EBRT and surgery for low-risk prostate cancer.[46] LDR is often used with androgen deprivation and EBRT for intermediate-risk patients and is not usually used for high-risk patients.

HDR brachytherapy involves the insertion of temporary irradiated seeds that provide a boost dose to EBRT. The addition of HDR to EBRT has been shown to improve disease-free survival in patients with intermediate-risk and high-risk disease.[47] One large study demonstrated that prostate cancer–specific survival was only improved when both ADT and EBRT were added to HDR brachytherapy, and not just 1 or the other.[48] These data support the use of this trimodal therapy for patients with high-risk disease who are not surgical candidates.

Adverse Effects of Radiotherapy

The most common adverse effects of radiotherapy are irritative or obstructive voiding symptoms and bowel dysfunction. Compared with men undergoing surgery or active surveillance, men receiving radiotherapy report more bowel bother in the form bloody stools and bowel urgency.[19,20,24] One study demonstrated no difference in short-term bowel-related problems between brachytherapy and active surveillance, whereas EBRT was significantly worse than active surveillance at 3 months.[22] Overall, with long-term follow-up, 4% of men will report fecal incontinence at least once a week and 6% will report bloody stool about half of the time.[19]

Compared to patients who initially elect active surveillance, patients who undergo initial radiotherapy have similar rates of urinary incontinence but may experience worse short-term (6 months following treatment) urinary symptoms, such as nocturia, daytime frequency, and obstructive and irritative symptoms.[19] Importantly, by 1 year following treatment initiation, the rates of these irritative urinary symptoms may become similar to those of patients who initially elect active surveillance since some men on surveillance eventually undergo treatment. Compared to radical prostatectomy, patients undergoing radiotherapy are much less likely to experience urinary incontinence and bother from urinary incontinence in both the short and long terms.[19,20,24] Compared to LDR, HDR brachytherapy may be associated with lower rates of urinary frequency and urgency.[49] EBRT is generally considered to have fewer early and late urinary and bowel complications compared with LDR.[50]

Declines in erectile function following the initiation of radiotherapy may be worsened with concomitant use of ADT.[22] Compared with initial active surveillance, EBRT alone may not worsen sexual function significantly.[20] Compared with surgery, EBRT with androgen deprivation had lower rates of erectile dysfunction initially and then were about equivalent after 10 to 15 years of follow-up.[19,20] In the group of patients from the ProtecT trial who received both radiotherapy and androgen deprivation, baseline rates of erections adequate for intercourse were 68%. By 6 months this rate was 22% and by 3 years it recovered somewhat to 34%.[19]

Disease Monitoring and Salvage Treatment Following Radiotherapy

Following radiotherapy, disease monitoring is similar to that of radical prostatectomy. Patients can anticipate PSA measurements every 6 to 12 months for the first 5 years following treatment and annual measurements thereafter. PSA measurements may be more frequent for patients with high-risk disease (see **Table 1**). Annual digital rectal examinations can help detect local recurrences.[7] If patients have biochemical disease recurrence following radiotherapy, it is possible for them to undergo salvage radical prostatectomy if the recurrence is thought to be local. Salvage surgery can produce long-term cancer control; however, the risk of complications and injury to adjacent organs is much higher compared with upfront surgery.[51]

ANDROGEN DEPRIVATION THERAPY AND OTHER SYSTEMIC THERAPIES

Beginning in the 1940s, clinicians have been using the dependence of prostate tissue growth and differentiation on androgen to treat prostate cancer.[52] As previously mentioned, the indications for the use of ADT include adjunctive therapy with radiotherapy, and salvage treatment following surgery or radiotherapy. Additionally, ADT may be used in patients with metastatic disease at the time of diagnosis. ADT as a monotherapy for patients with localized prostate cancer is not considered to improve survival.[53]

The Basics of Androgen Deprivation Therapy

ADT comes in 3 general forms: bilateral orchiectomy, luteinizing hormone-releasing hormone (LHRH) agonist, or antagonist. These 3 forms of ADT are considered equally efficacious.[54] Administering an LHRH agonist may initially create an androgen flare, which may potentiate symptoms in patients with substantial metastatic disease, thus it is usually administered after initially blocking the systemic binding of testosterone to its receptor with an androgen antagonist.[55] Combining medical or surgical castration with an antiandrogen may also improve survival in patients with metastatic prostate cancer; however, the benefit is likely modest and should be balanced with potential added adverse effects.[56]

The Adverse Effects of Androgen Deprivation Therapy

The potential side-effect profile of ADT is significant, and urologists, oncologists, and primary care providers should be aware of signs and symptoms of ADT adverse effects. Androgen suppression greatly increases the risk of osteopenia and the risk for clinical fractures.[57] Baseline dual-energy X-ray absorptiometry (DEXA) scans may be useful at the initiation of ADT for men at an increased risk of fracture. Almost all men should receive supplement with 1200 mg calcium and 800 to 1000 IU vitamin D3. Additionally, men with established osteopenia or osteoporosis who continue on ADT should receive bisphosphonates to reduce fracture risk.[58] ADT has well-established links to increased rates of cardiovascular disease and type 2 diabetes mellitus,[59] and may increase rates of myocardial infarction, coronary artery disease, hyperlipidemia, acute kidney injury, and stroke.[60–62]

Additional adverse effects directly related to castrate levels of androgen include gynecomastia, decreased libido, hot flashes, and erectile dysfunction. Several studies have also linked the use of ADT with the development of psychiatric disorders such as Alzheimer disease, dementia, and depression.[63–65]

The use of surgical as compared with medical castration may be fewer associated osseous and cardiovascular adverse effects[61,66] in patients who are surgical candidates. ADT may also be dosed intermittently to reduce adverse effects.[67,68] For patients who either have biochemical recurrence following local therapy or are diagnosed with metastatic cancer, intermittent ADT usually begins with several weeks to months of induction ADT, followed by several months without ADT. ADT may be dosed again for another several months based on a regular cycle or if PSA measurements become elevated (typically >10 ng/mL).[67,68] Intermittent compared with continuous ADT may minimize adverse effects and theoretically delay the development of castration-resistant prostate cancer (CRPC; defined as biochemical disease progression with castrate levels of testosterone <50 ng/dL), although data are conflicting on the latter point.[69,70]

Second-Generation Androgen Deprivation Therapy

Some prostate cancers may develop castration resistance by increasing androgen levels within the prostate itself or through increased activity of the androgen receptor.[71–73] Second-generation ADT have been developed for patients with CRPC with the understanding that the androgen receptor may continue to play a role in the progression of some CRPC. Abiraterone acetate, an androgen synthesis inhibitor, and enzalutamide, an antiandrogen, are both available for advanced prostate cancer treatment, and both represent options that may improve survival in patients even after castration resistance develops.[74,75]

Chemotherapy for Prostate Cancer

The 2 most widely used chemotherapeutics for advanced prostate cancer are the taxanes docetaxel and cabazitaxel. Docetaxel has demonstrated benefits on overall survival for metastatic CRPC.[76,77] Recently, docetaxel has also established itself as a reasonable treatment of men with metastatic disease that is still sensitive to androgen deprivation. Two large randomized controlled trials showed an overall survival of 1.1 to 1.8 years among patients with androgen-sensitive metastatic disease who received docetaxel with ADT compared with ADT alone.[78,79] Additional survival benefits with docetaxel may also be seen in patients with high-risk nonmetastatic prostate cancer as with adjunctive therapy with EBRT and ADT.[80] The rates of significant adverse effects of treatments are largely similar among patients receiving ADT monotherapy and ADT with docetaxel.[78,79] Common adverse effects attributed to docetaxel include neutropenia in 16%, cardiovascular events in 15%, and nausea and vomiting in 20%.[77] Cabazitaxel is currently used for metastatic prostate cancer after docetaxel failure and may improve both survival and cancer-related pain.[81]

Immunotherapy for Prostate Cancer

The only currently accepted form of immunotherapy for prostate cancer is sipuleucel-T, a so-called cancer vaccine. The treatment consists of an autologous transfusion of antigen-presenting cells that are cultured ex vivo with a fusion protein that includes both a prostate-specific antigen and an immune-cell activator. Sipuleucel-T is administered by 3 infusion every 2 weeks. In a study of more than 500 subjects with CRPC and minimally symptomatic metastatic disease, sipuleucel-T administration was able to increase median overall survival from 21.7 to 25.8 months and 3-year survival from 23% to 32%.[82] This treatment has several attractive qualities, including the short-term duration of administration (4 weeks), it does not preclude subsequent chemotherapy use, and the minimal side effect profile, which are largely transient, minor, and related to infusion-related effects (chills in 51%, fever in 23%, fatigue in 16%, nausea in 14%, and headache in 11%).[82]

Bisphosphonates for Patients with Bone Metastases

In patients with bone metastases and CRPC, bisphosphonate therapy with denosumab or zoledronic acid has been shown to reduce skeletal-related events, such as pathologic fractures, need for skeletal-directed palliative radiotherapy, and spinal cord compression.[83,84] The most common adverse effects of bisphosphonate therapy compared with placebo include anemia (27% vs 18%), myalgia (25% vs 18%), and fever (20% vs 13%).[85] Patients may also experience hypocalcemia (6%–13%) and osteonecrosis of the jaw (1%–2%).[84]

FUTURE CONSIDERATIONS

There are several exciting ongoing areas of research for the treatment of prostate cancer that may potentially change practice.

For patients on active surveillance, a large, multiinstitutional trial is underway assessing the utility of biomarkers to indicate who is most likely to harbor more aggressive disease or progress to more advanced disease over time.[86] For patients undergoing radical prostatectomy, whole-genome analyses of their surgical specimens may help predict who will have recurrence and may benefit from earlier adjuvant radiation.[87,88]

REFERENCES

1. Siegel RL, Miller KD, Jemal A. Cancer statistics, 2017. CA Cancer J Clin 2017; 67(1):7–30.

2. Moyer VA, U.S. Preventive Services Task Force. Screening for prostate cancer: U.S. Preventive Services Task Force recommendation statement. Ann Intern Med 2012;157(2):120–34.
3. Cooperberg MR, Carroll PR. Trends in Management for Patients With Localized Prostate Cancer, 1990-2013. JAMA 2015;314(1):80–2.
4. Weiner AB, Patel SG, Etzioni R, et al. National trends in the management of low and intermediate risk prostate cancer in the United States. J Urol 2015;193(1): 95–102.
5. Schroder FH, Hugosson J, Carlsson S, et al. Screening for prostate cancer decreases the risk of developing metastatic disease: findings from the European Randomized Study of Screening for Prostate Cancer (ERSPC). Eur Urol 2012; 62(5):745–52.
6. Bibbins-Domingo K, Grossman DC, Curry SJ. The US Preventive Services Task Force 2017 draft recommendation statement on screening for prostate cancer: an invitation to review and comment. JAMA 2017;317(19):1949–50.
7. National Comprehensive Cancer Network. Prostate Cancer, Version 1.2017. 2017. Available at: https://http://www.nccn.org. Accessed April 17, 2017.
8. Bill-Axelson A, Holmberg L, Garmo H, et al. Radical prostatectomy or watchful waiting in early prostate cancer. N Engl J Med 2014;370(10):932–42.
9. Cooperberg MR, Cowan JE, Hilton JF, et al. Outcomes of active surveillance for men with intermediate-risk prostate cancer. J Clin Oncol 2011;29(2):228–34.
10. Porten SP, Whitson JM, Cowan JE, et al. Changes in prostate cancer grade on serial biopsy in men undergoing active surveillance. J Clin Oncol 2011;29(20): 2795–800.
11. Stamatakis L, Siddiqui MM, Nix JW, et al. Accuracy of multiparametric magnetic resonance imaging in confirming eligibility for active surveillance for men with prostate cancer. Cancer 2013;119(18):3359–66.
12. Klotz L, Vesprini D, Sethukavalan P, et al. Long-term follow-up of a large active surveillance cohort of patients with prostate cancer. J Clin Oncol 2015;33(3): 272–7.
13. Newcomb LF, Thompson IM Jr, Boyer HD, et al. Outcomes of active surveillance for clinically localized prostate cancer in the prospective, multi-institutional canary PASS cohort. J Urol 2016;195(2):313–20.
14. Selvadurai ED, Singhera M, Thomas K, et al. Medium-term outcomes of active surveillance for localised prostate cancer. Eur Urol 2013;64(6):981–7.
15. Tosoian JJ, Mamawala M, Epstein JI, et al. Intermediate and longer-term outcomes from a prospective active-surveillance program for favorable-risk prostate cancer. J Clin Oncol 2015;33(30):3379–85.
16. Welty CJ, Cowan JE, Nguyen H, et al. Extended followup and risk factors for disease reclassification in a large active surveillance cohort for localized prostate cancer. J Urol 2015;193(3):807–11.
17. Iremashvili V, Soloway MS, Rosenberg DL, et al. Clinical and demographic characteristics associated with prostate cancer progression in patients on active surveillance. J Urol 2012;187(5):1594–9.
18. Hamdy FC, Donovan JL, Lane JA, et al. 10-year outcomes after monitoring, surgery, or radiotherapy for localized prostate cancer. N Engl J Med 2016;375(15): 1415–24.
19. Donovan JL, Hamdy FC, Lane JA, et al. Patient-reported outcomes after monitoring, surgery, or radiotherapy for prostate cancer. N Engl J Med 2016; 375(15):1425–37.

20. Barocas DA, Alvarez J, Resnick MJ, et al. Association between radiation therapy, surgery, or observation for localized prostate cancer and patient-reported outcomes after 3 Years. JAMA 2017;317(11):1126–40.

21. Wilt TJ, Brawer MK, Jones KM, et al. Radical prostatectomy versus observation for localized prostate cancer. N Engl J Med 2012;367(3):203–13.

22. Chen RC, Basak R, Meyer AM, et al. Association between choice of radical prostatectomy, external beam radiotherapy, brachytherapy, or active surveillance and patient-reported quality of life among men with localized prostate cancer. JAMA 2017;317(11):1141–50.

23. Kundu SD, Roehl KA, Eggener SE, et al. Potency, continence and complications in 3,477 consecutive radical retropubic prostatectomies. J Urol 2004;172(6 Pt 1): 2227–31.

24. Resnick MJ, Koyama T, Fan KH, et al. Long-term functional outcomes after treatment for localized prostate cancer. N Engl J Med 2013;368(5):436–45.

25. Muller A, Parker M, Waters BW, et al. Penile rehabilitation following radical prostatectomy: predicting success. J Sex Med 2009;6(10):2806–12.

26. Fossati N, Willemse PM, Van den Broeck T, et al. The benefits and harms of different extents of lymph node dissection during radical prostatectomy for prostate cancer: a systematic review. Eur Urol 2017;72(1):84–109.

27. Oberlin DT, Flum AS, Lai JD, et al. The effect of minimally invasive prostatectomy on practice patterns of American urologists. Urol Oncol 2016;34(6):255.e1–5.

28. Yaxley JW, Coughlin GD, Chambers SK, et al. Robot-assisted laparoscopic prostatectomy versus open radical retropubic prostatectomy: early outcomes from a randomised controlled phase 3 study. Lancet 2016;388(10049):1057–66.

29. Ficarra V, Novara G, Ahlering TE, et al. Systematic review and meta-analysis of studies reporting potency rates after robot-assisted radical prostatectomy. Eur Urol 2012;62(3):418–30.

30. Ficarra V, Novara G, Rosen RC, et al. Systematic review and meta-analysis of studies reporting urinary continence recovery after robot-assisted radical prostatectomy. Eur Urol 2012;62(3):405–17.

31. Novara G, Ficarra V, Mocellin S, et al. Systematic review and meta-analysis of studies reporting oncologic outcome after robot-assisted radical prostatectomy. Eur Urol 2012;62(3):382–404.

32. Novara G, Ficarra V, Rosen RC, et al. Systematic review and meta-analysis of perioperative outcomes and complications after robot-assisted radical prostatectomy. Eur Urol 2012;62(3):431–52.

33. Messing EM, Manola J, Yao J, et al. Immediate versus deferred androgen deprivation treatment in patients with node-positive prostate cancer after radical prostatectomy and pelvic lymphadenectomy. Lancet Oncol 2006;7(6):472–9.

34. Van der Kwast TH, Bolla M, Van Poppel H, et al. Identification of patients with prostate cancer who benefit from immediate postoperative radiotherapy: EORTC 22911. J Clin Oncol 2007;25(27):4178–86.

35. Swanson GP, Goldman B, Tangen CM, et al. The prognostic impact of seminal vesicle involvement found at prostatectomy and the effects of adjuvant radiation: data from Southwest Oncology Group 8794. J Urol 2008;180(6):2453–7 [discussion: 2458].

36. Shipley WU, Seiferheld W, Lukka HR, et al. Radiation with or without antiandrogen therapy in recurrent prostate cancer. N Engl J Med 2017;376(5):417–28.

37. Wolff RF, Ryder S, Bossi A, et al. A systematic review of randomised controlled trials of radiotherapy for localised prostate cancer. Eur J Cancer 2015;51(16): 2345–67.

38. Hoskin PJ, Rojas AM, Bownes PJ, et al. Randomised trial of external beam radiotherapy alone or combined with high-dose-rate brachytherapy boost for localised prostate cancer. Radiother Oncol 2012;103(2):217–22.

39. Critz FA, Benton JB, Shrake P, et al. 25-Year disease-free survival rate after irradiation for prostate cancer calculated with the prostate specific antigen definition of recurrence used for radical prostatectomy. J Urol 2013;189(3):878–83.

40. Jones CU, Hunt D, McGowan DG, et al. Radiotherapy and short-term androgen deprivation for localized prostate cancer. N Engl J Med 2011;365(2):107–18.

41. Bolla M, Van Tienhoven G, Warde P, et al. External irradiation with or without long-term androgen suppression for prostate cancer with high metastatic risk: 10-year results of an EORTC randomised study. Lancet Oncol 2010;11(11):1066–73.

42. Pilepich MV, Winter K, Lawton CA, et al. Androgen suppression adjuvant to definitive radiotherapy in prostate carcinoma–long-term results of phase III RTOG 85-31. Int J Radiat Oncol Biol Phys 2005;61(5):1285–90.

43. Zietman AL. The Titanic and the Iceberg: prostate proton therapy and health care economics. J Clin Oncol 2007;25(24):3565–6.

44. Sheets NC, Goldin GH, Meyer AM, et al. Intensity-modulated radiation therapy, proton therapy, or conformal radiation therapy and morbidity and disease control in localized prostate cancer. JAMA 2012;307(15):1611–20.

45. Yu JB, Soulos PR, Herrin J, et al. Proton versus intensity-modulated radiotherapy for prostate cancer: patterns of care and early toxicity. J Natl Cancer Inst 2013;105(1):25–32.

46. Kupelian PA, Potters L, Khuntia D, et al. Radical prostatectomy, external beam radiotherapy <72 Gy, external beam radiotherapy > or =72 Gy, permanent seed implantation, or combined seeds/external beam radiotherapy for stage T1-T2 prostate cancer. Int J Radiat Oncol Biol Phys 2004;58(1):25–33.

47. Sathya JR, Davis IR, Julian JA, et al. Randomized trial comparing iridium implant plus external-beam radiation therapy with external-beam radiation therapy alone in node-negative locally advanced cancer of the prostate. J Clin Oncol 2005;23(6):1192–9.

48. D'Amico AV, Moran BJ, Braccioforte MH, et al. Risk of death from prostate cancer after brachytherapy alone or with radiation, androgen suppression therapy, or both in men with high-risk disease. J Clin Oncol 2009;27(24):3923–8.

49. Grills IS, Martinez AA, Hollander M, et al. High dose rate brachytherapy as prostate cancer monotherapy reduces toxicity compared to low dose rate palladium seeds. J Urol 2004;171(3):1098–104.

50. Eade TN, Horwitz EM, Ruth K, et al. A comparison of acute and chronic toxicity for men with low-risk prostate cancer treated with intensity-modulated radiation therapy or (125)I permanent implant. Int J Radiat Oncol Biol Phys 2008;71(2):338–45.

51. Chade DC, Eastham J, Graefen M, et al. Cancer control and functional outcomes of salvage radical prostatectomy for radiation-recurrent prostate cancer: a systematic review of the literature. Eur Urol 2012;61(5):961–71.

52. Huggins C, Hodges CV. Studies on prostatic cancer I. The effect of castration, of estrogen and of androgen injection on serum phosphatases in metastatic carcinoma of the prostate. Cancer Res 1941;293–7.

53. Lu-Yao GL, Albertsen PC, Moore DF, et al. Fifteen-year survival outcomes following primary androgen-deprivation therapy for localized prostate cancer. JAMA Intern Med 2014;174(9):1460–7.

54. Trachtenberg J, Gittleman M, Steidle C, et al. A phase 3, multicenter, open label, randomized study of abarelix versus leuprolide plus daily antiandrogen in men with prostate cancer. J Urol 2002;167(4):1670–4.

55. Schulze H, Senge T. Influence of different types of antiandrogens on luteinizing hormone-releasing hormone analogue-induced testosterone surge in patients with metastatic carcinoma of the prostate. J Urol 1990;144(4):934–41.

56. Samson DJ, Seidenfeld J, Schmitt B, et al. Systematic review and meta-analysis of monotherapy compared with combined androgen blockade for patients with advanced prostate carcinoma. Cancer 2002;95(2):361–76.

57. Shahinian VB, Kuo YF, Freeman JL, et al. Risk of fracture after androgen deprivation for prostate cancer. N Engl J Med 2005;352(2):154–64.

58. Smith MR, Egerdie B, Hernandez Toriz N, et al. Denosumab in men receiving androgen-deprivation therapy for prostate cancer. N Engl J Med 2009;361(8):745–55.

59. Keating NL, O'Malley A, Freedland SJ, et al. Diabetes and cardiovascular disease during androgen deprivation therapy: observational study of veterans with prostate cancer. J Natl Cancer Inst 2012;104(19):1518–23.

60. Eri LM, Urdal P, Bechensteen AG. Effects of the luteinizing hormone-releasing hormone agonist leuprolide on lipoproteins, fibrinogen and plasminogen activator inhibitor in patients with benign prostatic hyperplasia. J Urol 1995;154(1):100–4.

61. Jespersen CG, Norgaard M, Borre M. Androgen-deprivation therapy in treatment of prostate cancer and risk of myocardial infarction and stroke: a nationwide Danish population-based cohort study. Eur Urol 2014;65(4):704–9.

62. Lapi F, Azoulay L, Niazi MT, et al. Androgen deprivation therapy and risk of acute kidney injury in patients with prostate cancer. JAMA 2013;310(3):289–96.

63. Khosrow-Khavar F, Rej S, Yin H, et al. Androgen deprivation therapy and the risk of dementia in patients with prostate cancer. J Clin Oncol 2017;35(2):201–7.

64. Nead KT, Gaskin G, Chester C, et al. Androgen deprivation therapy and future Alzheimer's disease risk. J Clin Oncol 2016;34(6):566–71.

65. Dinh KT, Reznor G, Muralidhar V, et al. Association of androgen deprivation therapy with depression in localized prostate cancer. J Clin Oncol 2016;34(16):1905–12.

66. Sun M, Choueiri TK, Hamnvik OP, et al. Comparison of gonadotropin-releasing hormone agonists and orchiectomy: effects of androgen-deprivation therapy. JAMA Oncol 2016;2(4):500–7.

67. Crook JM, O'Callaghan CJ, Duncan G, et al. Intermittent androgen suppression for rising PSA level after radiotherapy. N Engl J Med 2012;367(10):895–903.

68. Hussain M, Tangen CM, Berry DL, et al. Intermittent versus continuous androgen deprivation in prostate cancer. N Engl J Med 2013;368(14):1314–25.

69. Hershman DL, Unger JM, Wright JD, et al. Adverse health events following intermittent and continuous androgen deprivation in patients with metastatic prostate cancer. JAMA Oncol 2016;2(4):453–61.

70. Magnan S, Zarychanski R, Pilote L, et al. Intermittent vs continuous androgen deprivation therapy for prostate cancer: a systematic review and meta-analysis. JAMA Oncol 2015;1(9):1261–9.

71. Scher HI, Sawyers CL. Biology of progressive, castration-resistant prostate cancer: directed therapies targeting the androgen-receptor signaling axis. J Clin Oncol 2005;23(32):8253–61.

72. Montgomery RB, Mostaghel EA, Vessella R, et al. Maintenance of intratumoral androgens in metastatic prostate cancer: a mechanism for castration-resistant tumor growth. Cancer Res 2008;68(11):4447–54.

73. Hu R, Dunn TA, Wei S, et al. Ligand-independent androgen receptor variants derived from splicing of cryptic exons signify hormone-refractory prostate cancer. Cancer Res 2009;69(1):16–22.

74. Ryan CJ, Molina A, Griffin T. Abiraterone in metastatic prostate cancer. N Engl J Med 2013;368(15):1458–9.
75. Fizazi K, Scher HI, Miller K, et al. Effect of enzalutamide on time to first skeletal-related event, pain, and quality of life in men with castration-resistant prostate cancer: results from the randomised, phase 3 AFFIRM trial. Lancet Oncol 2014; 15(10):1147–56.
76. Berthold DR, Pond GR, Soban F, et al. Docetaxel plus prednisone or mitoxantrone plus prednisone for advanced prostate cancer: updated survival in the TAX 327 study. J Clin Oncol 2008;26(2):242–5.
77. Petrylak DP, Tangen CM, Hussain MH, et al. Docetaxel and estramustine compared with mitoxantrone and prednisone for advanced refractory prostate cancer. N Engl J Med 2004;351(15):1513–20.
78. James ND, Sydes MR, Clarke NW, et al. Addition of docetaxel, zoledronic acid, or both to first-line long-term hormone therapy in prostate cancer (STAMPEDE): survival results from an adaptive, multiarm, multistage, platform randomised controlled trial. Lancet 2016;387(10024):1163–77.
79. Sweeney CJ, Chen YH, Carducci M, et al. Chemohormonal therapy in metastatic hormone-sensitive prostate cancer. N Engl J Med 2015;373(8):737–46.
80. Fizazi K, Faivre L, Lesaunier F, et al. Androgen deprivation therapy plus docetaxel and estramustine versus androgen deprivation therapy alone for high-risk localised prostate cancer (GETUG 12): a phase 3 randomised controlled trial. Lancet Oncol 2015;16(7):787–94.
81. Bahl A, Oudard S, Tombal B, et al. Impact of cabazitaxel on 2-year survival and palliation of tumour-related pain in men with metastatic castration-resistant prostate cancer treated in the TROPIC trial. Ann Oncol 2013;24(9):2402–8.
82. Kantoff PW, Higano CS, Shore ND, et al. Sipuleucel-T immunotherapy for castration-resistant prostate cancer. N Engl J Med 2010;363(5):411–22.
83. Saad F, Gleason DM, Murray R, et al. Long-term efficacy of zoledronic acid for the prevention of skeletal complications in patients with metastatic hormone-refractory prostate cancer. J Natl Cancer Inst 2004;96(11):879–82.
84. Fizazi K, Carducci M, Smith M, et al. Denosumab versus zoledronic acid for treatment of bone metastases in men with castration-resistant prostate cancer: a randomised, double-blind study. Lancet 2011;377(9768):813–22.
85. Saad F, Gleason DM, Murray R, et al. A randomized, placebo-controlled trial of zoledronic acid in patients with hormone-refractory metastatic prostate carcinoma. J Natl Cancer Inst 2002;94(19):1458–68.
86. Lin DW, Newcomb LF, Brown EC, et al. Urinary TMPRSS2:ERG and PCA3 in an active surveillance cohort: results from a baseline analysis in the Canary Prostate Active Surveillance Study. Clin Cancer Res 2013;19(9):2442–50.
87. Spratt DE, Yousefi K, Deheshi S, et al. Individual patient-level meta-analysis of the performance of the decipher genomic classifier in high-risk men after prostatectomy to predict development of metastatic disease. J Clin Oncol 2017;35(18): 1991–8.
88. Dalela D, Santiago-Jimenez M, Yousefi K, et al. Genomic classifier augments the role of pathological features in identifying optimal candidates for adjuvant radiation therapy in patients with prostate cancer: development and internal validation of a multivariable prognostic model. J Clin Oncol 2017;35(18):1982–90.

Kidney, Ureteral, and Bladder Cancer
A Primer for the Internist

Hans C. Arora, MD, PhD[a], Michele Fascelli, MD[a], JJ.H. Zhang, MD[a],
Sudhir Isharwal, MD[a], Steven C. Campbell, MD, PhD[b],*

KEYWORDS

- Kidney cancer • Bladder cancer • Ureteral cancer • Urothelial carcinoma
- Renal cell carcinoma • Evaluation • Surgery • Treatment

KEY POINTS

- Hematuria (gross or microscopic) is a common presenting symptom in kidney, bladder, and ureteral cancer.
- High-quality contrast-enhanced cross-sectional abdominal imaging, such as computed tomography urogram or magnetic resonance urogram, is the most sensitive radiological studies for evaluation of suspected renal or upper tract malignancy.
- Cystoscopy is an important component of the evaluation of any patient with gross or microscopic hematuria.
- Early recognition and referral to an urologist for further work-up and management is critical to optimize prognosis.

INTRODUCTION

Malignancies of the urinary tract (kidney, ureter, and bladder) differ in their cellular origins and thus represent distinct clinical entities. The overarching term kidney cancer most commonly refers to malignancies of the renal parenchyma. Renal cell carcinoma (RCC) is by far the most common type of kidney cancer, accounting for 90% of renal malignancies. Cancers of the renal pelvis, ureter, and bladder are predominantly urothelial carcinoma (UC; formerly known as transitional cell carcinoma) and also represent a major source of morbidity and mortality.

RCC and UC differ in their presentation and management. In the current era, RCC is most often detected incidentally during the imaging work-up for unrelated symptoms.

Disclosure Statement: None.
[a] Glickman Urological and Kidney Institute, Cleveland Clinic, 9500 Euclid Avenue, Q10-1, Cleveland, OH 44195, USA; [b] Center for Urologic Oncology, Glickman Urological and Kidney Institute, Cleveland Clinic, 9500 Euclid Avenue, Q10-1, Cleveland, OH 44195, USA
* Corresponding author.
E-mail address: campbes3@ccf.org

Med Clin N Am 102 (2018) 231–249
https://doi.org/10.1016/j.mcna.2017.10.002
0025-7125/18/© 2017 Elsevier Inc. All rights reserved.

In contrast, patients with UC often present with gross or microscopic hematuria. Even though UC of the upper urinary tract and bladder are histologically similar, they differ in their management and prognosis. A high index of suspicion with prompt referral to an experienced urologist is critical for early detection and treatment, and to prevent local or systemic progression of these malignancies. The objective of this article is to provide an overview of the evaluation and management of malignancies of the urinary tract.

KIDNEY CANCER: RENAL CELL CARCINOMA

The term renal mass encompasses a biologically diverse group of tumors ranging from benign lesions to aggressive cancers.[1–3] The incidence of RCC in the United States has been increasing in recent decades with nearly 64,000 new cases and more than 14,000 deaths expected in 2017.[4] Increased use of imaging studies resulting in increased early-stage detection is a suggested contributor to the increased incidence of renal masses.[5] The major environmental risk factors for RCC include smoking, hypertension, and obesity.[6–9] Acquired renal cystic disease, often presenting in end-stage renal disease patients, also confers an increased risk for RCC, specifically papillary RCC.[3] RCC can be hereditary in 3% to 5% of cases and, in this setting, typically presents in a younger age group and may be part of a clinical syndrome complex.

Patient History

Historically, renal masses were diagnosed with the classic triad of symptoms: flank pain, hematuria, and a palpable abdominal or flank mass. Currently, more than 50% of renal masses are diagnosed incidentally during imaging studies, with only 10% or less presenting with the classic triad, which often indicates locally advanced or metastatic disease.[3] Despite increased detection of renal masses at earlier stages, the incidence of metastatic disease on initial presentation has remained 20% to 30% across population-based studies.[1,10] RCC can present with several paraneoplastic conditions, including anemia, polycythemia, hypercalcemia, constitutional symptoms (fever, weight loss, cachexia), and elevated erythrocyte sedimentation rate or C-reactive protein.[3] A reversible hepatitis (Stauffer syndrome) may also be observed in RCC even in the absence of liver metastases, and elevated liver enzyme levels may improve after tumor resection. RCC has been termed the internist's tumor owing to the diversity of potential presentations related to these paraneoplastic syndromes.

Pathophysiology

The major subtypes of RCC are clear cell, papillary, chromophobe, and collecting duct. These subtypes differ in their genetic origin, histologic appearance, and metastatic potential (**Table 1**).[3,11,12] Familial hereditary syndromes can present with either renal-related symptoms or extrarenal manifestations, such as skin lesions or spontaneous pneumothoraces, and are typically associated with specific subtypes of RCC (**Table 2**).

RCC is often associated with increased tumor neovascularity, particularly for clear cell variants. Inactivation of the *VHL* tumor suppressor gene results in the accumulation of hypoxia-inducible factor (HIF)-related proteins, which leads to overexpression of vascular endothelial growth factor (VEGF) and increased angiogenesis.[3] Another important pathway is that of mammalian target of rapamycin (mTOR) kinase, an upstream activator of HIF-1 protein expression that leads to cell growth and angiogenesis.[3,13] Many of these pathways can now be targeted with tyrosine kinase or mTOR inhibitors, improving outcomes for patients with advanced RCC.

Table 1
Major histologic classification of renal cell carcinoma

Pathologic Assessment	Facts and Features
Clear Cell	• Most common variant of RCC • Arises from proximal convoluted tubule • Associated with mutation or loss of *VHL* gene • Also seen in von Hippel-Lindau (VHL) syndrome • Highly vascular • Most likely to respond to tyrosine kinase inhibitors • Relatively aggressive
Papillary	• Arises from proximal convoluted tubule • Commonly seen in patients with acquired cystic kidney disease from chronic renal failure • Type 1: associated with polysomy 7 & 17, loss of Y, and MET mutations, typically less aggressive, but often multifocal • Type 2: tend to be high-grade, aggressive, worse prognosis
Chromophobe	• Arises from the collecting duct • Associated with multiple chromosomal deletions and genetic changes • Generally good prognosis; tend to grow to large size while remaining organ confined • Small proportion have sarcomatoid differentiation and worse prognosis
Collecting Duct	• Rare, aggressive, and poor prognosis • Arises from the collecting duct • May respond to conventional chemotherapy
Renal Medullary	• Rare form of collecting duct carcinoma • Occurs primarily in young adults, African descent, and with sickle cell trait • Rarely responds to chemotherapy or radiation, poor prognosis
Unclassified	• Histology not belonging entirely to one of the previous subtypes • Difficult to predict clinical outcome, but generally more aggressive

Physical Examination

Physical examination of a patient with known or suspected RCC involves assessment of blood pressure, skin, and lymph nodes, in addition to the abdomen and flanks. Certain skin lesions may be present in association with RCC, most notably in hereditary syndromes. Neurologic examination is also important and positive findings may indicate metastatic disease. Lower extremity edema can suggest the presence of an inferior vena caval (IVC) tumor thrombus causing central venous obstruction, which is occasionally seen with locally advanced RCC.

Diagnostic Testing and Imaging Studies

Patients with suspicion for renal malignancy should be evaluated initially with a comprehensive metabolic panel, complete blood count, urinalysis, and high-quality multiphase, cross-sectional abdominal imaging. These data are essential not only for staging disease but for facilitating patient-driven decision-making and provider counseling because they often elucidate extrarenal manifestations of RCC, identify patients with poor health, and stratify patients at risk for worsening kidney function (**Fig. 1**). It is imperative to evaluate renal function in this population because it influences the selection of treatment modalities.[10,14–17] At times, the initial evaluation may identify those with underlying chronic kidney disease (CKD); it is often beneficial to involve a nephrologist early in the evaluation and care of these patients. Imaging,

Table 2
More common familial renal cell carcinoma syndromes

Syndrome	Key Features
VHL Syndrome	• Mechanism: VHL tumor suppressor gene mutation (chromosome 3p), resulting in intracellular accumulation of hypoxia-inducible factor, which leads to increased angiogenesis and increased vascularity. • Clear cell RCC, typically bilateral and multifocal • Other clinical manifestations: retinal angiomas, central nervous system hemangioblastomas, pancreatic cysts, pheochromocytomas
Birt-Hogg-Dubé Syndrome	• Mechanism: folliculin tumor suppressor mutation (chromosome 17p) • Chromophobe RCC, often bilateral and multifocal • Also oncocytomas, and hybrid tumors with features of oncocytoma and chromophobe • May also develop clear cell RCC and other variants of RCC • Other clinical manifestations: fibrofolliculomas of head and neck, pulmonary cysts, and spontaneous pneumothoraces
Hereditary Leiomyoma RCC	• Mechanism: fumarate hydratase tumor suppressor mutation (chromosome 1q) • Characterized by type 2 papillary RCC, very aggressive, and managed more proactively • Other clinical manifestations: painful cutaneous and uterine leiomyomas
Hereditary Papillary RCC	• Mechanism: cMET protooncogene mutation (chromosome 7q) • Type 1 papillary RCC, often bilateral and multifocal • Often no extrarenal manifestations
Tuberous Sclerosis	• Mechanism: mutations of TSC1 (chromosome 9) or TSC2 (chromosome 16) genes • Associated with development of angiomyolipomas (multiple, bilateral), RCC, or renal cysts • Classic triad of developmental delay, seizures, skin findings (adenoma sebaceum, ash-leaf spots, shagreen patches), but many patients do not have complete penetrance for all 3 manifestations

either by computed tomography (CT) or MRI, assesses important characteristics of renal masses, such as tumor complexity, extension into the renal vein or IVC, and involvement of contiguous organs.[18–21] The presence of adipose tissue in the renal mass suggests that the lesion is a benign angiomyolipoma rather than RCC, both of which are often detected incidentally on imaging studies. Characteristic cross-sectional imaging findings of RCC are shown in **Fig. 2**A,B. Metastatic evaluation should include chest imaging to determine the presence of pulmonary metastases because the lungs are the most common sites of metastatic disease. Tumor-node-metastasis (TNM) staging should be assigned according to the American Joint Committee on Cancer (AJCC) (**Table 3**).

The role of renal mass biopsy (RMB) continues to evolve as a tool in the urologist's armamentarium when evaluating a renal mass. The decision to pursue RMB is complex and, in general, RMB should be done when the practitioner is concerned that the mass may be hematologic, metastatic, infectious, or inflammatory in origin, and only if the information obtained may direct clinical management. Early referral to a urologist for counseling about RMB and further evaluation should be considered given some of the nuances about the utility and performance characteristics of this procedure. The recently updated 2017 American Urological Association Guidelines for Renal Mass and Localized Renal Cancer provide an in-depth overview for the primary care

Renal Mass and Localized Renal Cancer

Evaluation/Diagnosis

1. Obtain high quality, multiphase, cross-sectional abdominal imaging to optimally characterize/stage the renal mass.
2. Obtain CMP, CBC, and UA. If malignancy suspected, metastatic evaluation should include chest imaging and careful review of abdominal imaging.
3. Assign CKD stage based on GFR and degree of proteinuria.

Counseling

1. A urologist should lead the counseling process and should consider all management strategies. A multidisciplinary team should be included when necessary.
2. Counseling should include current perspectives about tumor biology and a patient-specific oncologic risk assessment. For cT1a tumors, the low oncologic risk of many small renal masses should be reviewed.
3. Counseling should review the most common and serious urologic and non-urologic morbidities of each treatment pathway and the importance of patient age, comorbidities/frailty, and life expectancy.
4. Physicians should review the importance of renal functional recovery related to renal mass management, including risk of progressive CKD, potential short/long-term need for dialysis, and long-term overall survival considerations.
5. Consider referral to nephrology in patients with a high risk of CKD progression, including those with GFR < 45 mL/min/1.73m², confirmed proteinuria, diabetics with preexisting CKD, or whenever GFR is expected to be <30 mL/min/1.73m² after intervention.
6. Recommend genetic counseling for all patients ≤ 46 y of age and consider genetic counseling for patients with multifocal or bilateral renal masses, or if personal/family history suggests a familial renal neoplastic syndrome.

Renal Mass Biopsy (RMB)

1. RMB should be considered when a mass is suspected to be hematologic, metastatic, inflammatory, or infectious.
2. RMB is not required for young/healthy patients who are not willing to accept the uncertainties associated with RMB or for older/frail patients who will be managed conservatively independent of RMB.
3. Counsel regarding rationale, positive/negative predictive values, potential risks and non-diagnostic rates of RMB.
4. Multiple core biopsies are preferred over FNA.

Active Surveillance (AS)

1. For patients with renal masses suspicious for cancer, especially those <2 cm, AS is an option for initial management.
2. Prioritize AS/Expectant Management when the anticipated risk of intervention or competing risks of death outweigh the potential oncologic benefits of active treatment.
3. When the risk/benefit analysis for treatment is equivocal and the patient prefers AS, physicians should repeat imaging in 3–6 mo to assess for interval growth and may consider RMB for additional risk stratification.
4. When the oncologic benefits of intervention outweigh the risks of treatment and competing risks of death, physicians should recommend active treatment. In this setting, AS may be pursued only if the patient understands and is willing to accept the associated oncologic risk

Factors Favoring AS/Expectant Management	
Patient-related	**Tumor-related**
Elderly	Tumor size <3 cm
Life expectancy <5 y	Tumor growth <5 mm/year
High comorbidities	Non-infiltrative
Excessive perioperative risk	Low complexity
Frailty (poor functional status)	Favorable histology
Patient preference for AS	
Marginal renal function	

Management

Thermal Ablation (TA)

1. Consider TA an alternate approach for management of cT1a renal masses <3 cm in size. A percutaneous approach is preferred to TA.
2. Both radiofrequency ablation and cryoablation are options.
3. A RMB should be performed prior to TA to include information regarding increased likelihood of tumor persistence/recurrence after primary TA, which may be addressed with repeat TA if further intervention is elected.
4. Counseling about TA should include information regarding increased likelihood of tumor persistence/recurrence after primary TA, which may be addressed with repeat TA if further intervention is elected.

Radical Nephrectomy (RN)

1. Physicians should consider RN for patients where increased oncologic potential is suggested by tumor size, RMB, and/or imaging characteristics. In this setting, RN is preferred if all of the following criteria are met: 1) high tumor complexity and PN would be challenging even in experienced hands; 2) no preexisting CKD/proteinuria; and 3) normal contralateral kidney and new baseline eGFR will likely be >45 mL/min/1.73m²

Surgical Principles

1. In the presence of clinically concerning regional lymphadenopathy, lymph node dissection should be performed for staging purposes.
2. Adrenalectomy should be performed if imaging and/or intraoperative findings suggest metastasis or direct invasion.
3. A minimally invasive approach should be considered when it would not compromise oncologic, functional and perioperative outcomes.
4. Pathologic evaluation of the adjacent renal parenchyma should be performed after PN or RN to assess for possible nephropathic disease, particularly for patients with CKD or risk factors for developing CKD.

Partial Nephrectomy (PN) and Nephron-Sparing Approaches

1. Prioritize PN for the management of the cT1a renal mass when intervention is indicated.
2. Prioritize nephron-sparing approaches for patients with an anatomic or functionally solitary kidney, bilateral tumors, known familial RCC, preexisting CKD, or proteinuria.
3. Consider nephron-sparing approaches for patients who are young, have multifocal masses, or comorbidities that are likely to impact renal function in the future

Principles Related to PN

1. Prioritize preservation of renal function through efforts to optimize nephron mass preservation and avoidance of prolonged warm ischemia.
2. Negative surgical margins should be a priority. The extent of normal parenchyma removed should be determined by surgeon discretion taking into account the clinical situation; tumor characteristics including growth pattern, and interface with normal tissue. Enucleation should be considered in patients with familial RCC, multifocal disease, or severe CKD to optimize parenchymal mass preservation.

Fig. 1. Guidelines for evaluation and management of renal mass and localized renal cancer, from the American Urologic Association. Focus is on clinically localized renal masses suspicious for RCC in adults, including solid enhanced tumors and Bosniak 3 and 4 complex cystic lesions. CBC, complete blood count; CKD, chronic kidney disease; CMP, comprehensive metabolic panel; eGFR, endothelial growth factor receptor; FNA, Fine Needle Aspiration; GFR, growth factor receptor; UA, Urinalysis. (*From* Campbell S, Uzzo RG, Allaf ME, et al. Renal mass and localized renal cancer: AUA guideline. J Urol 2017;198(3):522; with permission.)

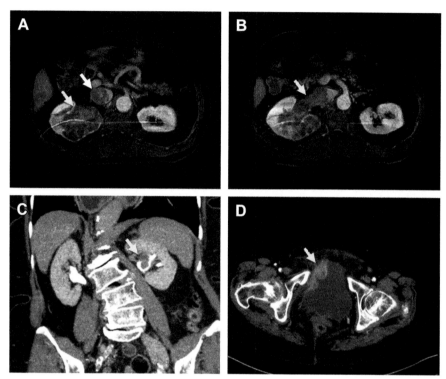

Fig. 2. Characteristic cross-sectional imaging findings for RCC and UC. (*A*) MRI demonstrating large, infiltrative renal mass in the posterior portion of the right kidney, consistent with renal cell carcinoma (*yellow arrow*) with IVC thrombus (*white arrow*). (*B*) Caudal cross-sections show contiguous RCC tumor involvement from primary tumor with extension into renal vein (*yellow arrow*) and IVC. (*C*) Coronal cross-section of CT urogram excretory phase demonstrating filling defect derived from the urothelial lining (*yellow arrow*) in the left renal pelvis consistent with upper tract urothelial carcinoma. (*D*) CT urogram with soft tissue mass (*yellow arrow*) in the right anterior aspect of the urinary bladder. Characteristically, conventional imaging demonstrates that most tumor growth occur intraluminally owing to its origin within the urothelial lining of the bladder.

physician and urologist alike to better understand the multifaceted decision-making process involved in the diagnosis, counseling, and management for localized renal masses (see **Fig. 1**).[22]

Differential Diagnosis

The differential diagnosis for renal masses includes several benign and malignant renal tumors in addition to RCC (**Table 4**).[3,23]

Treatment

In this era when an increased number of renal masses are being discovered incidentally, many are small and benign or indolent, and may not require immediate surgical intervention. Active surveillance (AS) has emerged as a management strategy for small renal masses, particularly those less than 2 cm. AS can also be considered for larger tumors and is especially pertinent for individuals with significant comorbidities, and for whom ablation or surgery poses an increased risk of complications.[24,25]

Table 3
American Joint Committee on Cancer tumor-node-metastasis staging for renal cell carcinoma with associated 5-year survival

Tumor Characteristics	T	N	M	5-y Survival (%)
Confined to kidney	T1–2	N0	M0	70–90
≤4.0 cm	T1a	N0	M0	90–100
>4.0 cm but ≤7.0 cm	T1b	N0	M0	80–90
>7.0 cm but ≤10.0 cm	T2a	N0	M0	65–80
>10.0 cm	T2b	N0	M0	50–70
Extends beyond kidney into major veins or perinephric tissues but confined to Gerota's fascia	T3	N0	M0	—
Extends into renal vein or segmental branches or invades perirenal or renal sinus	T3a	N0	M0	40–70
Extends into IVC below diaphragm	T3b	N0	M0	30–50
Extends into IVC above diaphragm or invades IVC wall	T3c	N0	M0	20–40
Extends beyond Gerota's fascia, including ipsilateral adrenal gland	T4	N0	M0	0–20
Lymph node involvement	T1–4	N1	M0–1	0–20
Distant Metastasis	T1–4	N0–1	M1	0–10

Adapted from Campbell SC, Lane BR. Malignant renal tumors. In: Wein AJ, Kavoussi LR, Partin AW, et al, editors. Campbell-Walsh urology. 11th edition. Philadelphia: Elsevier; 2016. p. 1339; with permission.

Other factors to consider when deciding whether to offer AS are outlined in **Fig. 1**.[26–28]

The surgical treatment options for renal masses include partial nephrectomy (PN) and radical nephrectomy (RN). PN entails excision of the tumor with organ reconstruction, with the goals of negative surgical margins and optimal preservation of renal function. PN is the standard of care for small renal masses.[29] PN is particularly indicated in

Table 4
Differential diagnosis for renal masses

Malignant	Renal cell carcinoma (solid and cystic)
	Urothelial carcinoma
	Sarcoma
	Lymphoma or leukemia
	Metastasis; eg, lung, breast
	Wilms tumor (more common in pediatric population)
	Other
Benign	Epithelial: oncocytoma, papillary adenoma
	Mesenchymal: angiomyolipoma, reninoma, schwannoma
	Mixed epithelial or mesenchymal: mixed epithelial and stromal tumor, cystic nephroma
	Metanephric: metanephric adenoma, adenofibroma
	Benign cysts

Adapted from Campbell SC, Lane BR. Malignant renal tumors. In: Wein AJ, Kavoussi LR, Partin AW, et al, editors. Campbell-Walsh urology. 11th edition. Philadelphia: Elsevier; 2016. p. 1315; with permission.

the setting of a solitary kidney, bilateral renal tumors, and advanced CKD but is also useful in patients with hereditary cancer syndromes or multifocal disease, both of which may require frequent reoperation.[30–33] It is this preservation in renal function that has led several investigators to suggest improved overall survival with PN compared with RN, though this remains contested.[34–36] In general, RN is reserved for larger tumors or tumors thought to have increased oncological potential based on tumor size, RMB, or imaging characteristics such as infiltrative appearance. RN is the preferred operative approach in cases in which the following conditions are met: the patient does not have preexisting CKD or proteinuria, the renal mass is highly complex (PN may be challenging even for experienced urologic surgeons), and the contralateral kidney is otherwise normal with an expected postoperative estimated glomerular filtration rate of greater than 45 mL/min/1.73 m^2.[22] Both PN and RN can be performed using either an open or minimally invasive approach (ie, laparoscopic or robotic) with comparable oncological outcomes in appropriately selected patients.[32,37] Regardless of treatment modality, serial follow-up evaluations, including physical examinations, repeat blood work, and serial imaging to assess for recurrence and metastases, are required.

Thermal ablation (TA) has emerged as an alternative approach to renal surgery for managing small renal masses less than 3 cm. Cancer-specific survival rates for PN and TA are comparable with a favorable morbidity profile for TA compared with PN and RN.[15] Counseling about TA should include a discussion about the increased risk of persistent disease or disease recurrence after treatment, with need for possible repeat TA. Current recommendations suggest obtaining an RMB before TA to confirm histologic diagnosis because TA induces tissue necrosis, significantly hampering the chance of identifying residual or recurrent disease posttreatment. Renal function outcomes after ablation are similar to PN.[15,38] The need for extended surveillance after TA continues to remain an area of investigation.[39]

After nephrectomy, 20% of patients with localized disease will eventually develop metastasis and about 20% of patients will present with metastatic disease at time of diagnosis.[40] Based on the molecular mechanisms involved in the pathogenesis of RCC, VEGF and mTOR-targeted therapies are the mainstay for treatment of advanced RCC. These drugs include sunitinib, pazopanib, and axitinib (tyrosine kinase inhibitors that reduce angiogenesis via the VEGF pathway); interferon along with bevacizumab (a recombinant antibody that sequesters VEGF); and temsirolimus and everolimus (mTOR inhibitors). Despite these advances in medical therapy, RCC continues to be predominantly a surgical disease, and patients with a solitary metastatic lesion are still often considered for surgical resection. Unlike most other types of cancers, certain patients with metastatic RCC may also benefit from cytoreductive surgery.[41,42] Patient selection is critical to success with cytoreductive nephrectomy because better outcomes are observed in patients with good performance status, absence of brain or liver metastasis, and in whom the main tumor bulk is within the retroperitoneum, thus leading to substantial reduction of the disease burden. Recently, immunotherapy agents such as checkpoint inhibitors have begun to change the landscape of metastatic RCC.[43,44] However, survival remains poor for locally advanced and metastatic disease, and current systemic treatments are rarely curative (see **Table 3**).

UPPER URINARY TRACT AND BLADDER CANCER: UROTHELIAL CARCINOMA

Cancer of the renal pelvis, ureter, and bladder most commonly originates from the urothelium (luminal lining) of the genitourinary tract. Upper tract UC (UTUC) refers to urothelial neoplasms that arise anywhere from the intrarenal collecting system to the distal insertion of the ureter into the bladder. UC of the renal pelvis accounts for 7% of all kidney tumors and is the most common site for UTUC, followed by the distal ureter. Noninvasive UTUC may be curable in up to 90% of cases, whereas those that are invasive may only be curable 40% to 50% of the time. Bladder cancer is the fourth most common cancer in men, and the eighth most common cause of cancer death for men in the United States.[4,45] UC of the bladder accounts for 99% of bladder cancers and is 3 to 4 times more common in men than women. However, women tend to have a poorer prognosis and less favorable tumor characteristics at the time cancer is discovered because bladder symptoms in women are often attributed to urinary tract infections, resulting in a delay in diagnosis.[46]

Treatment outcomes and prognosis of UC depend on the depth of invasion of the tumor. Seventy-five percent of patients with bladder cancer have disease confined to the mucosa or submucosa at presentation.[47] In contrast, UTUC generally presents at more advanced stages due to the thin submucosal and muscular layers of the ureters.

Prompt work-up of concerning symptoms with referral to a urologist is a key component for improving the survival of UC. Unfortunately, there is no good screening test for UC, so it is critical to recognize potential clinical symptoms to make the proper diagnosis at an early stage.

Patient History

The most common presenting symptom of UC is painless gross or microscopic hematuria.[48–50] Approximately 10% to 20% of patients with gross hematuria may be found to have bladder cancer compared with 2% to 5% of patients with microscopic hematuria.[51,52] However, the extent of hematuria does not correlate with disease severity, and hematuria can be intermittent.[53] Voiding symptoms, including dysuria, frequency, and urgency may also occur with bladder cancer; however, patients with UTUC without bladder involvement rarely present with such symptoms. Flank pain due to hydronephrosis is less common with bladder cancer but when present is typically associated with locally advanced disease. Flank pain is a more common presenting symptom in UTUC (second to hematuria) due to progressive obstruction leading to hydronephrosis and may be present in approximately 30% of cases. Not all patients with UTUC present with symptoms; approximately 15% of UTUC patients may be completely asymptomatic. A pertinent review of symptoms is an important component of the clinical evaluation of patients with suspected genitourinary malignancy because constitutional symptoms, including weight loss, fatigue, anemia, or bone pain, may indicate advanced disease.[54]

Pathophysiology

UC is the prototype of an environmentally related cancer and is only due to identified genetic causes in a small minority of cases. Tobacco use is the most common risk factor for the development of UC, which is believed to be due to urinary secretion of aromatic amines and their metabolites. In the bladder, smoking increases the risk of cancer development 2-fold to 4-fold in a dose-dependent manner. Chronic exposure to certain medicinal, chemical, and industrial compounds also represents an important risk factor for the development of UC, including cyclophosphamide, arsenic, phenacetin, aniline dyes, and other carcinogens. These environmental exposures are generally found in the textile, asphalt, petroleum, metallurgy, rubber, dye, leather, dry cleaning, and painting industries.[47,55–57] Albeit uncommon, a history of therapeutic radiation exposure also increases the risk for development of bladder cancer. Chronic inflammation due to chronic bacterial infection, calculi, indwelling catheters, or Schistosoma haematobium (bilharzial) infection may also increase risk for development of the squamous cell carcinoma subtype of bladder cancer.[58] The etiologic factors of UTUC are hereditary in a small proportion of patients. Subjects with hereditary nonpolyposis colorectal carcinoma, also known as Lynch Syndrome, are predisposed to develop UTUC. These patients are typically younger at diagnosis, more likely to be female patients, and have a predilection for development of bilateral disease.[59]

In any patient with UC, there is an increased rate of malignant transformation of adjacent noncancerous mucosal tissue, resulting in synchronous or metachronous primary tumors that may be present anywhere along the urothelium from the renal pelvis to the proximal urethra.[60] This is due to the field cancerization effect of UC, similar to certain biliary and respiratory epithelial cancers. It necessitates evaluation of the entire genitourinary tract when hematuria is present or UC is suspected, or in any patient with a history of UC.[61–64]

Physical Examination

A general physical examination should be performed with special emphasis on abdominal, pelvic, genital, and rectal examinations. A bimanual examination should be performed to provide information for the clinical staging of bladder cancer. Digital rectal examination in men is also recommended to evaluate for presence of concomitant prostate cancer. Evaluation of lymph nodes in the supraclavicular, axillary, and groin regions should be performed to assess for possible metastatic disease. A negative physical examination should not preclude further work-up because many patients with UC will not have abnormal physical findings.

Diagnostic Testing and Imaging

In the presence of hematuria, urinalysis with microscopic examination should be obtained.[65] The presence of greater than 3 red blood cells per high-powered field raises the suspicion for malignancy. Urinalysis by dipstick alone cannot quantify the number of red blood cells and also cannot differentiate between true hematuria and false-positive results, emphasizing the importance of incorporating microscopic examination. Urine culture should be performed whenever urinalysis is suspicious for urinary tract infection.[65] Voided urine cytology should also be obtained for patients who have had gross hematuria because it is highly specific for high-grade disease and can be positive even when occult UC is present.[47,53] Cytology has a lower sensitivity in UTUC (50%–60%) and is generally not able to localize the site of disease.[66] Another urine-based test is fluorescence in situ hybridization (FISH), which is used to detect aneuploidy of chromosomes. FISH has a higher sensitivity than cytology but its role in first-line settings remains controversial.[67] The development of urine-based biomarkers with high sensitivity and specificity is an area of active investigation.[68,69]

If hematuria (gross or microscopic) is documented, or if UC is suspected for any other reason, prompt referral to a urologist is strongly recommended. Initial evaluation includes blood tests (complete blood count, blood urea nitrogen, creatinine, liver function tests), cystoscopy, and cross-sectional abdominal radiological evaluation. CT urogram has supplanted intravenous urogram as a more sensitive and specific modality for detecting UC. Characteristic images of UC in the upper urinary tract and bladder are shown in **Fig. 2**C,D, respectively. MR urogram is also an acceptable alternative, specifically in patients in whom use of iodinated intravenous contrast dye is contraindicated. Additionally, CT imaging is used to assess for lymphadenopathy or distant metastatic disease. If CT imaging or MRI is unavailable, cystoscopy and retrograde pyelogram with renal ultrasound may also be used for selected patients. Potential imaging findings include a renal pelvis, ureteral, or bladder intraluminal mass; prominent pelvic or retroperitoneal lymph nodes; intraluminal filling defects; or hydronephrosis.[70,71]

Cystoscopy, or endoscopic evaluation of the bladder, is a crucial part of the urologic evaluation in hematuria and/or suspected UC. Even if upper tract disease is suspected or already discovered on radiological studies, cystoscopy is still important to rule out concomitant bladder tumor, which may occur in up to 17% of cases of UTUC.[72–75] This is typically undertaken in the office using a flexible cystoscope and local anesthetic. Only limited biopsies may be obtained in this setting; findings of intravesical tumor usually warrant further management in the operating room. If upper tract disease is suspected with positive findings on radiological studies, endoscopic visualization of the ureters and renal pelvis (known as ureteroscopy or ureteropyeloscopy) allows the urologist to identify sessile lesions and perform biopsies of suspicious areas to provide a pathologic diagnosis.[76,77] The histologic appearance determines whether a tumor is classified as low-grade or high-grade, which correlates strongly with stage. Examination by an experienced pathologist is an essential step because treatment plans and prognosis vary between low-grade and high-grade disease, and up to 30% of tumors may be inaccurately staged and graded based on gross appearance alone.[78] High-grade UC has increased rates of progression and metastatic potential compared with low-grade disease. Although a biopsy often provides vital pathologic information, it may not provide accurate staging information due to limitations of tumor sampling and inaccuracy of evaluating depth of invasion.[79]

Differential Diagnosis

Differential diagnosis of a mass in the upper urinary tract or bladder in the setting of hematuria includes calculus and a variety of uncommon benign entities such as papilloma, leiomyoma, nephrogenic adenoma, or other inflammatory lesions. The diagnosis of papilloma can only be confirmed on biopsy.[80] Leiomyomas are the most common benign bladder tumor and are similar to leiomyomas of the uterus. These most commonly present in women of childbearing age.[81] Nephrogenic adenomas are rare, metaplastic lesions that form as a result of trauma or inflammation, including prior surgery, and recur frequently. These patients may have urinary symptoms and are at increased risk for urinary tract infections.[82,83]

The AJCC TNM system is used for staging of UC and is similar for both upper tract and bladder disease (**Table 5**).[84] Pathologic staging of bladder specimens obtained by endoscopic resection is an important step in patient evaluation. Clinical staging, which is determined by cystoscopy, bimanual examination, and radiographic analysis, is often inaccurate for predicting disease severity and prognosis.[85] Generally, bladder UC is divided into 2 groups, depending on whether it invades into the muscularis propria. Stages Ta and T1, and carcinoma in situ (CIS), are considered non-muscle invasive bladder cancer (NMIBC).[47,53] Muscle-invasive bladder cancer consists of stage T2 and higher. At presentation, approximately 75% of patients are diagnosed with NMIBC and 25% with either muscle-invasive or metastatic disease.[47,86] CIS lesions are flat, high-grade tumors confined to the mucosa, and their presence in the urothelial tract carries great significance. The term in situ in this setting can be misleading because molecular studies have demonstrated that these lesions have highly malignant potential.[47] CIS is typically multifocal and can be missed on cystoscopy. It may occur in the bladder, upper urinary tract, prostatic ducts, and prostatic urethra.

Table 5
American Joint Committee on cancer tumor-node-metastasis staging for urothelial carcinoma

	UTUC	Bladder UC
Primary Tumor (T)		
Tx	Primary tumor cannot be assessed	
T0	No evidence of primary tumor	
Ta	Papillary noninvasive carcinoma	
Tis	Carcinoma in situ; flat tumor	
T1	Tumor invades subepithelial connective tissue	
T2	Tumor invades muscularis propria	
T2A	—	Tumor invades superficial muscle (inner half)
T2B	—	Tumor invades deep muscle (outer half)
T3	For renal pelvis: tumor invades beyond muscularis propria into peripelvic fat or renal parenchyma. For ureter: tumor invades beyond muscularis propria into periureteric fat	Tumor invades into perivesical tissue
T3A	—	Microscopic invasion
T3B	—	Microscopic invasion
T4	Tumor invades adjacent organs, or through the kidney into the perinephric fat	Tumor invades any of the following: prostate, uterus, vagina, pelvic wall, abdominal wall
T4A	—	Tumor invades prostate, uterus or vagina
T4B	—	Tumor invades pelvic wall or abdominal wall
Regional Lymph Nodes (N)		
Nx	Regional lymph nodes cannot be assessed	
N0	No regional lymph node metastasis	
N1	Metastasis in a single lymph node, ≤2 cm in greatest dimension	Metastasis in a single lymph node in the true pelvis (hypogastric, obturator, external iliac or presacral)
N2	Metastasis in a single lymph node, >2 cm; or multiple lymph nodes	Metastasis in multiple lymph nodes in the true pelvis (hypogastric, obturator, external iliac, or presacral)
N3	Metastasis in a lymph node, more than 5 cm in greatest dimension	Metastasis in common iliac lymph nodes
Distant Metastasis (M)		
M0	No distant metastasis	
M1	Distant metastasis	

Data from McKiernan J, Hansel D, Bochner B. Renal Pelvis and Ureter. In: Amin MB, Edge SB, Greene F, et al, editors. AJCC Cancer Staging Manual, 8th edition. New York: Springer; 2017. p. 754, 763–64.

UC can progress locally through direct extension into adjacent structures or systemically through lymphatic or hematogenous routes. The most common sites of metastasis are the lungs, liver, bones, and regional lymph nodes. If invasive or metastatic disease is suspected, further evaluation includes liver function tests and chest imaging, with additional studies based on specific symptoms.

Treatment of Bladder Urothelial Carcinoma

Initial operative management for concerning lesions in the upper tract or bladder involves complete endoscopic resection with diagnostic as well as therapeutic intent. Primary transurethral resection of bladder tumor (TURBT) is done in the operating room for a visible tumor seen on office cystoscopy. A restaging TURBT should be performed within 2 to 6 weeks of the first resection in cases of incomplete initial resection, when tumor invades the submucosal layer, or the muscularis propria layer is not available in the specimen to accurately determine the depth of invasion.[47] After TURBT, intravesical chemotherapy administered in the recovery room is generally recommended to reduce local recurrence of tumors. Intravesical instillation of Bacille Calmette-Guerin (BCG) is used when tumor recurrences are frequent or in cases of high-grade NMIBC to delay or prevent disease progression.[87–89] BCG is a live attenuated strain of *Mycobacterium bovis* that stimulates the immune system to develop a vigorous inflammatory response in the bladder to reduce the risk of tumor recurrence and progression. It represents one of the earliest examples of the potential beneficial effects of immunotherapy for the treatment of human cancers. In cases of low-grade and noninvasive high-grade lesions, life-long close surveillance is required. The first surveillance cystoscopy after TURBT is usually done at 3 months postoperatively because it provides important prognostic information.[90] Surveillance for bladder cancer is more intensive than for almost any other malignancy.

For patients with muscle-invasive UC of the bladder (stage T2 and higher) or BCG-refractory tumors, the recommended treatment is radical cystectomy with pelvic lymphadenectomy and urinary diversion.[47] Chemotherapy with platinum-based agents has shown survival benefits when administered before radical cystectomy.[91] In men, radical cystectomy includes removal of the prostate and seminal vesicles. In women, the anterior vagina, uterus, Fallopian tubes, and ovaries are removed. For patients who are poor surgical candidates for radical cystectomy, bladder-preserving approaches with chemotherapy plus radiation may be offered.[81] Partial cystectomy can also be considered, but only in very select situations. After radical cystectomy, a urinary diversion using a segment of the gastrointestinal tract is performed with the following diversion options:

- Ileal conduit: drains continuously through cutaneous stoma (requires an external drainage bag)
- Continent catheterizable reservoir (Indiana pouch): internal pouch that is catheterized via cutaneous stoma every 4 to 6 hours (does not require an external drainage bag)
- Orthotopic neobladder: patient voids through native urethra with no external stoma.

Treatment of Upper Tract Urothelial Carcinoma

Standard treatment of localized UTUC is en bloc excision of the kidney and ipsilateral ureter with a small margin or cuff of bladder from around the adjacent ureteral orifice. This procedure is known as a nephroureterectomy. It should include excision of adjacent lymph nodes, particularly in high-grade, high-stage cancer.[92] Surgical approaches include open, laparoscopic, and robotic-assisted modalities. A renal scan may be obtained preoperatively to assess the function of the contralateral kidney. In selected patients with disease localized to the distal segment of the ureter, segmental excision via distal ureterectomy with concomitant ureteral implant into the bladder may be offered to preserve renal function. Endoscopic ablation of UTUC is reserved for subjects with low-grade cancer, poor renal function, or bilateral tumors; or those who would otherwise be poor surgical candidates. Because accurate grading and staging information cannot be obtained by endoscopic biopsies, there is an increased risk of recurrence and progression with endoscopic treatment. If the tumor seems to be invasive or locally advanced, neoadjuvant chemotherapy should be administered before nephroureterectomy. The treatment regimens used are most often derived from the bladder UC literature, and are cisplatin-based.[93] Adjuvant radiation therapy may reduce local recurrence but has no proven survival benefit.[94,95]

Life-long follow-up is needed after the treatment of UC, the details of which depend on risk category, tumor stage, and prior treatment.[81] This includes history, physical examination, blood tests, urinalysis, and urine cytology, as well as cross-sectional imaging of the abdomen and pelvis at periodic intervals, more frequently in the first year and less often thereafter. Cystoscopy should be included in any follow-up protocol in the setting of bladder-sparing therapy. The most important prognostic factor in UC pathogenesis is tumor stage, although tumor grade is also highly relevant for clinical decision-making.[96] In the case of locally advanced nonmetastatic T2 to T4 tumors, the prognosis is remarkably grim with a high rate of distant recurrence and poor survival.[97] In advanced, recurrent, or metastatic disease, systemic chemotherapy with cisplatin-based treatment regimens should be offered. Immunotherapy based on T-cell programmed death receptors (PD-1) have recently been approved by the FDA for patients who cannot receive chemotherapy due to side effects, poor renal function, or who progress while on chemotherapy.[98]

SUMMARY

Kidney cancers are increasingly being detected incidentally and can be cured with early surgical interventions. Preservation of renal function is important whenever feasible. There is substantial heterogeneity in the tumor biology of renal masses, ranging from benign to highly aggressive, highlighting the need for risk stratification and appropriate management. Newer targeted drug therapies have become available and can prolong survival in cases of advanced and metastatic disease, although generally these patients are incurable with occasional exceptions. UC typically presents with symptoms that include hematuria. There is a high risk of local recurrence and progression. Early intervention with a combination of surgery and selective utilization of chemotherapy provides the best chance of cure, though life-long surveillance is needed. There are also emerging immunotherapy regimens being developed to treat advanced UC; however, survival is poor for advanced and metastatic disease. Newer checkpoint inhibitors are starting to move the needle toward improved management of patients with advanced disease for both of these malignancies. Physicians should have a high index of suspicion for RCC and UC, and prompt referral to a urologist should be prioritized to facilitate early intervention and optimize treatment outcomes.

REFERENCES

1. Thompson RH, Hill JR, Babayev Y, et al. Metastatic renal cell carcinoma risk according to tumor size. J Urol 2009;182(1):41–5.
2. Kutikov A, Fossett LK, Ramchandani P, et al. Incidence of benign pathologic findings at partial nephrectomy for solitary renal mass presumed to be renal cell carcinoma on preoperative imaging. Urology 2006;68(4):737–40.
3. Campbell S, Lane B. Malignant renal tumors. In: Wein AJ, Kavoussi LR, Partin AW, et al, editors. Campbell-walsh urology. 11th edition. Philadelphia: Elsevier; 2016. p. 1314–64.
4. Siegel RL, Miller KD, Jemal A. Cancer statistics, 2017. CA Cancer J Clin 2017; 67(1):7–30.
5. Znaor A, Lortet-Tieulent J, Laversanne M, et al. International variations and trends in renal cell carcinoma incidence and mortality. Eur Urol 2015;67(3):519–30.

6. Tsivian M, Moreira DM, Caso JR, et al. Cigarette smoking is associated with advanced renal cell carcinoma. J Clin Oncol 2011;29(15):2027–31.
7. Adams KF, Leitzmann MF, Albanes D, et al. Body Size and renal cell cancer incidence in a large US cohort study. Am J Epidemiol 2008;168(3):268–77.
8. Mandel JS, McLaughlin JK, Schlehofer B, et al. International renal-cell cancer study. IV. Occupation. Int J Cancer 1995;61(5):601–5.
9. Leibovich BC, Lohse CM, Crispen PL, et al. Histological subtype is an independent predictor of outcome for patients with renal cell carcinoma. J Urol 2010; 183(4):1309–16.
10. Frank I, Blute ML, Cheville JC, et al. Solid renal tumors: an analysis of pathological features related to tumor size. J Urol 2003;170(6 Pt 1):2217–20.
11. Srigley JR, Delahunt B, Eble JN, et al. The International Society of Urological Pathology (ISUP) vancouver classification of renal neoplasia. Am J Surg Pathol 2013;37(10):1469–89.
12. Linehan WM. Genetic basis of kidney cancer: role of genomics for the development of disease-based therapeutics. Genome Res 2012;22(11):2089–100.
13. Gnarra JR, Zhou S, Merrill MJ, et al. Post-transcriptional regulation of vascular endothelial growth factor mRNA by the product of the VHL tumor suppressor gene. Proc Natl Acad Sci U S A 1996;93(20):10589–94.
14. Hallan SI, Ritz E, Lydersen S, et al. Combining GFR and albuminuria to classify CKD improves prediction of ESRD. J Am Soc Nephrol 2009;20(5):1069–77.
15. Pierorazio PM, Johnson MH, Patel HD, et al. Management of renal masses and localized renal cancer: systematic review and meta-analysis. J Urol 2016; 196(4):989–99.
16. Kutikov A, Egleston BL, Canter D, et al. Competing risks of death in patients with localized renal cell carcinoma: a comorbidity based model. J Urol 2012;188(6): 2077–83.
17. Mir MC, Ercole C, Takagi T, et al. Decline in renal function after partial nephrectomy: etiology and prevention. J Urol 2015;193(6):1889–98.
18. Kopp RP, Aganovic L, Palazzi KL, et al. Differentiation of clear from non-clear cell renal cell carcinoma using CT washout formula. Can J Urol 2013;20(3):6790–7.
19. Young JR, Margolis D, Sauk S, et al. Clear cell renal cell carcinoma: discrimination from other renal cell carcinoma subtypes and oncocytoma at multiphasic multidetector CT. Radiology 2013;267(2):444–53.
20. Kutikov A, Smaldone MC, Egleston BL, et al. Anatomic features of enhancing renal masses predict malignant and high-grade pathology: a preoperative nomogram using the RENAL Nephrometry score. Eur Urol 2011;60(2):241–8.
21. Mehrazin R, Palazzi KL, Kopp RP, et al. Impact of tumour morphology on renal function decline after partial nephrectomy. BJU Int 2013;111(8):E374–82.
22. Campbell S, Uzzo RG, Allaf ME, et al. Renal mass and localized renal cancer: AUA guideline. J Urol 2017;198(3):520–9.
23. Margulis V, Karam J, Matin S, et al. Benign renal tumors. In: Wein AJ, Kavoussi LR, Partin AW, et al, editors. Campbell-Walsh urology. 11th edition. Philadelphia: Elsevier; 2016. p. 1300–13.
24. Smaldone MC, Corcoran AT, Uzzo RG. Active surveillance of small renal masses. Nat Rev Urol 2013;10(5):266–74.
25. Crispen PL, Viterbo R, Boorjian SA, et al. Natural history, growth kinetics, and outcomes of untreated clinically localized renal tumors under active surveillance. Cancer 2009;115(13):2844–52.
26. Kunkle DA, Egleston BL, Uzzo RG. Excise, ablate or observe: the small renal mass dilemma—A meta-analysis and review. J Urol 2008;179(4):1227–34.

27. Jewett MAS, Mattar K, Basiuk J, et al. Active surveillance of small renal masses: progression patterns of early stage kidney cancer. Eur Urol 2011;60(1):39–44.

28. Mason RJ, Abdolell M, Trottier G, et al. Growth kinetics of renal masses: analysis of a prospective cohort of patients undergoing active surveillance. Eur Urol 2011; 59(5):863–7.

29. Campbell SC, Novick AC, Belldegrun A, et al. Guideline for management of the clinical T1 renal mass. J Urol 2009;182(4):1271–9.

30. Minervini A, Tuccio A, Masieri L, et al. Endoscopic robot-assisted simple enucleation (ERASE) for clinical T1 renal masses: description of the technique and early postoperative results. Surg Endosc 2015;29(5):1241–9.

31. Leibovich BC, Blute ML, Cheville JC, et al. Nephron sparing surgery for appropriately selected renal cell carcinoma between 4 and 7 cm results in outcome similar to radical nephrectomy. J Urol 2004;171(3):1066–70.

32. Gill IS, Eisenberg MS, Aron M, et al. "Zero ischemia" partial nephrectomy: novel laparoscopic and robotic technique. Eur Urol 2011;59(1):128–34.

33. Huang WC, Levey AS, Serio AM, et al. Chronic kidney disease after nephrectomy in patients with renal cortical tumours: a retrospective cohort study. Lancet Oncol 2006;7(9):735–40.

34. Kim SP, Murad MH, Thompson RH, et al. Comparative effectiveness for survival and renal function of partial and radical nephrectomy for localized renal tumors: a systematic review and meta-analysis. J Urol 2012;188(1):51–7.

35. Huang WC, Elkin EB, Levey AS, et al. Partial nephrectomy versus radical nephrectomy in patients with small renal tumors—Is there a difference in mortality and cardiovascular outcomes? J Urol 2009;181(1):55–62.

36. Van Poppel H, Da Pozzo L, Albrecht W, et al. A prospective, randomised EORTC intergroup phase 3 study comparing the oncologic outcome of elective nephron-sparing surgery and radical nephrectomy for low-stage renal cell carcinoma. Eur Urol 2011;59(4):543–52.

37. Gill IS, Kavoussi LR, Lane BR, et al. Comparison of 1,800 laparoscopic and open partial nephrectomies for single renal tumors. J Urol 2007;178(1):41–6.

38. Atwell TD, Callstrom MR, Farrell MA, et al. Percutaneous renal cryoablation: local control at mean 26 months of followup. J Urol 2010;184(4):1291–5.

39. Stewart SB, Thompson RH, Psutka SP, et al. Evaluation of the National Comprehensive Cancer Network and American Urological Association renal cell carcinoma surveillance guidelines. J Clin Oncol 2014;32(36):4059–65.

40. Janzen NK, Kim HL, Figlin RA, et al. Surveillance after radical or partial nephrectomy for localized renal cell carcinoma and management of recurrent disease. Urol Clin North Am 2003;30(4):843–52.

41. Flanigan RC, Salmon SE, Blumenstein BA, et al. Nephrectomy followed by interferon alfa-2b compared with interferon alfa-2b alone for metastatic renal-cell cancer. N Engl J Med 2001;345(23):1655–9.

42. Mickisch GH, Garin A, van Poppel H, et al, European Organisation for Research and Treatment of Cancer (EORTC) Genitourinary Group. Radical nephrectomy plus interferon-alfa-based immunotherapy compared with interferon alfa alone in metastatic renal-cell carcinoma: a randomised trial. Lancet 2001;358(9286): 966–70.

43. Goebell PJ, Doehn C, Grüllich C, et al. The PAZOREAL noninterventional study to assess effectiveness and safety of pazopanib and everolimus in the changing metastatic renal cell carcinoma treatment landscape. Future Oncol 2017; 13(17):1463–71.

44. Unverzagt S, Moldenhauer I, Nothacker M, et al. Immunotherapy for metastatic renal cell carcinoma. Cochrane Database Syst Rev 2017;(5):CD011673.
45. Pawinski A, Sylvester R, Kurth KH, et al. A combined analysis of European Organization for Research and Treatment of Cancer, and Medical Research Council randomized clinical trials for the prophylactic treatment of stage TaT1 bladder cancer. J Urol 1996;156(6):1934–41.
46. Fajkovic H, Halpern JA, Cha EK, et al. Impact of gender on bladder cancer incidence, staging, and prognosis. World J Urol 2011;29(4):457–63.
47. Babjuk M, Böhle A, Burger M, et al. EAU guidelines on non–muscle-invasive urothelial carcinoma of the bladder: update 2016. Eur Urol 2017;71(3):447–61.
48. Murphy DM, Zincke H, Furlow WL. Management of high grade transitional cell cancer of the upper urinary tract. J Urol 1981;125(1):25–9.
49. Guinan P, Volgelzang NJ, Randazzo R, et al. Renal pelvic transitional cell carcinoma. The role of the kidney in tumor-node-metastasis staging. Cancer 1992; 69(7):1773–5.
50. Raabe NK, Fosså SD, Bjerkehagen B. Carcinoma of the renal pelvis. Experience of 80 cases. Scand J Urol Nephrol 1992;26(4):357–61.
51. Mariani AJ, Mariani MC, Macchioni C, et al. The significance of adult hematuria: 1,000 hematuria evaluations including a risk-benefit and cost-effectiveness analysis. J Urol 1989;141(2):350–5.
52. Khadra MH, Pickard RS, Charlton M, et al. A prospective analysis of 1,930 patients with hematuria to evaluate current diagnostic practice. J Urol 2000; 163(2):524–7.
53. Oosterlinck W, Lobel B, Jakse G, et al, European Association of Urology (EAU) Working Group on Oncological Urology. Guidelines on bladder cancer. Eur Urol 2002;41(2):105–12.
54. Resseguie LJ, Nobrega FT, Farrow GM, et al. Epidemiology of renal and ureteral cancer in Rochester, Minnesota, 1950-1974, with special reference to clinical and pathologic features. Mayo Clin Proc 1978;53(8):503–10.
55. Jensen OM, Knudsen JB, McLaughlin JK, et al. The Copenhagen case-control study of renal pelvis and ureter cancer: role of smoking and occupational exposures. Int J Cancer 1988;41(4):557–61.
56. Colin P, Koenig P, Ouzzane A, et al. Environmental factors involved in carcinogenesis of urothelial cell carcinomas of the upper urinary tract. BJU Int 2009;104(10): 1436–40.
57. Burger M, Catto JWF, Dalbagni G, et al. Epidemiology and risk factors of urothelial bladder cancer. Eur Urol 2013;63(2):234–41.
58. Sagalowsky AI, Jarrett TW, Flanigan RC. Urothelial tumors of the upper urinary tract and ureter. In: Wein AJ, Kavoussi LR, Partin AW, et al, editors. Campbell-Walsh urology. 11th edition. Philadelphia: Elsevier; 2012. p. 1516–53.e7.
59. Lynch HT, Ens JA, Lynch JF. The Lynch syndrome II and urological malignancies. J Urol 1990;143(1):24–8.
60. Jones TD, Wang M, Eble JN, et al. Molecular evidence supporting field effect in urothelial carcinogenesis. Clin Cancer Res 2005;11(18):6512–9.
61. Wright JL, Hotaling J, Porter MP. Predictors of upper tract urothelial cell carcinoma after primary bladder cancer: a population based analysis. J Urol 2009; 181:1035–9.
62. Picozzi S, Ricci C, Gaeta M, et al. Upper urinary tract recurrence following radical cystectomy for bladder cancer: a meta-analysis on 13,185 patients. J Urol 2012; 188(6):2046–54.

63. Slaughter DP, Southwick HW, Smejkal W. Field cancerization in oral stratified squamous epithelium; clinical implications of multicentric origin. Cancer 1953; 6(5):963–8.

64. Lochhead P, Chan AT, Nishihara R, et al. Etiologic field effect: reappraisal of the field effect concept in cancer predisposition and progression. Mod Pathol 2015; 28(1):14–29.

65. Davis R, Jones JS, Barocas DA, et al. Diagnosis, evaluation and follow-up of asymptomatic microhematuria (AMH) in adults: AUA guideline. J Urol 2012; 188(6):2473–81.

66. Konety BR, Getzenberg RH. Urine based markers of urological malignancy. J Urol 2001;165(2):600–11.

67. Luo B, Li W, Deng C-H, et al. Utility of fluorescence in situ hybridization in the diagnosis of upper urinary tract urothelial carcinoma. Cancer Genet Cytogenet 2009;189(2):93–7.

68. Marín-Aguilera M, Mengual L, Ribal MJ, et al. Utility of fluorescence in situ hybridization as a non-invasive technique in the diagnosis of upper urinary tract urothelial carcinoma. Eur Urol 2007;51(2):409–15.

69. Lotan Y, O'Sullivan P, Raman JD, et al. Clinical comparison of noninvasive urine tests for ruling out recurrent urothelial carcinoma. Urol Oncol 2017;35(8): 531.e15-22.

70. Stein JP, Lieskovsky G, Cote R, et al. Radical cystectomy in the treatment of invasive bladder cancer: long-term results in 1,054 patients. J Clin Oncol 2001;19(3): 666–75.

71. Shariat SF, Karakiewicz PI, Palapattu GS, et al. Outcomes of radical cystectomy for transitional cell carcinoma of the bladder: a contemporary series from the Bladder Cancer Research Consortium. J Urol 2006;176(6):2414–22.

72. McTavish JD, Jinzaki M, Zou KH, et al. Multi-detector row CT urography: comparison of strategies for depicting the normal urinary collecting system. Radiology 2002;225(3):783–90.

73. Raman SP, Fishman EK. Upper and lower tract urothelial imaging using computed tomography urography. Radiol Clin North Am 2017;55(2):225–41.

74. Anderson EM, Murphy R, Rennie ATM, et al. Multidetector computed tomography urography (MDCTU) for diagnosing urothelial malignancy. Clin Radiol 2007;62(4): 324–32.

75. Jinzaki M, Kikuchi E, Akita H, et al. Role of computed tomography urography in the clinical evaluation of upper tract urothelial carcinoma. Int J Urol 2016;23(4): 284–98.

76. Soderdahl DW, Fabrizio MD, Rahman NU, et al. Endoscopic treatment of upper tract transitional cell carcinoma. Urol Oncol 2005;23(2):114–22.

77. Keeley FX, Kulp DA, Bibbo M, et al. Diagnostic accuracy of ureteroscopic biopsy in upper tract transitional cell carcinoma. J Urol 1997;157(1):33–7.

78. El-Hakim A, Weiss GH, Lee BR, et al. Correlation of ureteroscopic appearance with histologic grade of upper tract transitional cell carcinoma. Urology 2004; 63(4):647–50.

79. Smith AK, Stephenson AJ, Lane BR, et al. Inadequacy of biopsy for diagnosis of upper tract urothelial carcinoma: implications for conservative management. Urology 2011;78(1):82–6.

80. Batata M, Grabstald H. Upper urinary tract urothelial tumors. Urol Clin North Am 1976;3(1):79–86.

81. Goel R, Thupili CR. Bladder leiomyoma. J Urol 2013;189(4):1536–7.

82. Montironi R, Lopez-Beltran A. The 2004 WHO classification of bladder tumors: a summary and commentary. Int J Surg Pathol 2005;13(2):143–53.
83. Pavlidakey PG, MacLennan GT, Goldman HB. Nephrogenic adenoma of the bladder. J Urol 2010;184(6):2535–6.
84. McKiernan J, Hansel D, Bochner B. Renal pelvis and ureter. In: Amin MB, Edge SB, Greene F, et al, editors. AJCC cancer staging manual. 8th edition. New York: Elsevier; 2017. p. 749.
85. Reuter VE, Grossman HB, Blute ML, et al. The pathology of bladder cancer. Urology 2006;67(3 SUPPL. 1):11–8.
86. Kamat AM, Hahn NM, Efstathiou JA, et al. Bladder cancer. Lancet 2016; 388(10061):2796–810.
87. Sylvester RJ, van der Meijden APM, Witjes JA, et al. *Bacillus calmette-guerin* versus chemotherapy for the intravesical treatment of patients with carcinoma in situ of the bladder: a meta-analysis of the published results of randomized clinical trials. J Urol 2005;174(1):86–91.
88. Malmstrom PU, Sylvester RJ, Crawford DE, et al. An individual patient data meta-analysis of the long-term outcome of randomised studies comparing intravesical mitomycin C versus bacillus Calmette-Guerin for non-muscle-invasive bladder cancer. Eur Urol 2009;56(2):247–56.
89. Shelley MD, Kynaston H, Court J, et al. A systematic review of intravesical bacillus Calmette-Guérin plus transurethral resection vs transurethral resection alone in Ta and T1 bladder cancer. BJU Int 2001;88(3):209–16.
90. Palou J, Rodríguez-Rubio F, Millán F, et al. Recurrence at three months and high-grade recurrence as prognostic factor of progression in multivariate analysis of T1G2 bladder tumors. Urology 2009;73(6):1313–7.
91. Green DA, Rink M, Xylinas E, et al. Urothelial carcinoma of the bladder and the upper tract: disparate twins. J Urol 2013;189(4):1214–21.
92. Messing EM, Catalona WJ. Urothelial tumors of the urinary tract. In: Walsh P, Retik A, Vaughan E, editors. Campbell's urology. 7th edition. Philadelphia: Saunders; 1998. p. 2327–410.
93. Hellenthal NJ, Shariat SF, Margulis V, et al. Adjuvant chemotherapy for high risk upper tract urothelial carcinoma: results from the Upper Tract Urothelial Carcinoma Collaboration. J Urol 2009;182(3):900–6.
94. Czito B, Zietman A, Kaufman D, et al. Adjuvant radiotherapy with and without concurrent chemotherapy for locally advanced transitional cell carcinoma of the renal pelvis and ureter. J Urol 2004;172(4 Pt 1):1271–5.
95. Cozad SC, Smalley SR, Austenfeld M, et al. Adjuvant radiotherapy in high stage transitional cell carcinoma of the renal pelvis and ureter. Int J Radiat Oncol Biol Phys 1992;24(4):743–5.
96. Edge, S, Byrd, DR, Compton, CC, et al. AJCC cancer staging manual | Stephen Edge | Springer. Springer.
97. Skinner DG, Lieskovsky G. Contemporary cystectomy with pelvic node dissection compared to preoperative radiation therapy plus cystectomy in management of invasive bladder cancer. J Urol 1984;131(6):1069–72.
98. Bellmunt J, Powles T, Vogelzang NJ. A review on the evolution of PD-1/PD-L1 immunotherapy for bladder cancer: the future is now. Cancer Treat Rev 2017; 54:58–67.

Testicular Cancer
Epidemiology, Diagnosis, and Management

Zachary L. Smith, MD*, Ryan P. Werntz, MD, Scott E. Eggener, MD

KEYWORDS

- Testicular cancer • Germ cell tumors • Seminoma • Nonseminoma • Chemotherapy
- Radiation therapy • Orchiectomy • Retroperitoneal lymph node dissection

KEY POINTS

- Testicular cancer (TC) is a rare malignancy, generally occurring in younger men.
- Substantial treatment advances have been made in recent decades that have made TC the most curable solid malignancy.
- Survivorship is an important consideration because TC management can impact fertility, quality of life, and long-term health for many decades.
- An individualized approach must be taken with patients based on their clinical and pathologic findings, with counseling on the risks and benefits of each method.

INTRODUCTION AND EPIDEMIOLOGY

In 2016, there were an estimated 8700 new cases of testicular cancer (TC) in the United States and 380 deaths.[1] Although TC is a rare disease, accounting for only approximately 1% of all male tumors,[1] the incidence has been steadily increasing from 5.7 per 100,000 in 1992 to 6.8 per 100,000 in 2009.[2] Fortunately, substantial advances in the management of TC have occurred over the last few decades. The 5-year relative survival rates have improved from 83% in 1975 to 1977 to 97% in 2005 to 2011.[1]

CAUSE AND RISK FACTORS

There are several environmental risk factors independently associated with TC. The most common include cryptorchidism (odds ratio [OR] 4.3, 95% confidence interval

Disclosure Statement: The authors have nothing to disclose.
Section of Urology, Department of Surgery, The University of Chicago Medicine, 5841 South Maryland Avenue, MC 6038, Chicago, IL 60637, USA
* Corresponding author.
E-mail address: zachary.smith@uchospitals.edu

Med Clin N Am 102 (2018) 251–264
https://doi.org/10.1016/j.mcna.2017.10.003
0025-7125/18/© 2017 Elsevier Inc. All rights reserved.

[CI] 3.6–5.1), low birth weight (OR 1.3, 95% CI 1.1–1.7), short gestational age (OR 1.3, 95% CI 1.1–1.6), and twinning (OR 1.2, 95% CI 1.0–1.4).[3]

Cryptorchidism increases the risk of both ipsilateral and contralateral TC. Historically, it was thought that the primary benefit of surgical correction (orchiopexy) was to allow for the examination of the testis for TC screening, and that it does not necessarily decrease the risk of TC development.[4]

Testicular microlithiasis (calcifications in the seminiferous tubules) is an incidental finding on ultrasound (US) characterized by multiple small echogenic foci within the testicular parenchyma. It is present in approximately 5% of men aged 18 to 35 years.[5] There is no definitive evidence microlithiasis is a premalignant condition, although it often coexists in the setting of malignancy.[6] Prospective studies have suggested incidentally detected microlithiasis is not a risk factor for developing TC.[7] However, there are some data to suggest an association between testicular microlithiasis and carcinoma in situ (CIS) in patients with a history of TC.[8] Based on the available data, routine testicular self-examination is a reasonable surveillance strategy for individuals with microlithiasis[8] and surveillance US are probably unnecessary.

There are also genetic factors that play a role in the development of TC, though less than 5% of all men diagnosed with TC are thought to have a hereditary cause. Having a brother or a father with TC increases one's risk by 8 to 10 or 4 to 6 fold, respectively.[9] Additionally, genetic disorders, such as Down syndrome and testicular dysgenesis syndrome, are also associated with increased risks of TC.[10]

SYMPTOMS AND PRESENTATION

Most patients with TC present with a painless testicular mass. Cryptorchidism is more commonly right sided, thus, so is TC. Occasionally, patients with a testicular tumor may develop a reactive hydrocele. However, if this is associated with painful testicular swelling, it is more likely to represent an infectious cause. Testicular masses are often noticed following local trauma. Regardless of the described mechanism of injury, any palpable nodule in the testicle should be treated as TC until proven otherwise.

If patients have metastatic disease at the time of diagnosis, they may present with symptoms pursuant to the location of disease. Although most metastatic locations will not be palpable, if patients have metastasis to the supraclavicular lymph nodes, they may feel a mass in the left neck. Pulmonary metastases may present with symptoms of shortness of breath or, rarely, hemoptysis. If patients have extensive retroperitoneal disease, they may experience symptoms of compression of surrounding organs (ie, flank pain from obstructive uropathy) or back pain. Lastly, although rare, brain metastasis may present with a variety of neurologic symptoms.

DIAGNOSTIC TESTS

With suspicion of a testicular mass, the first test ordered is generally a scrotal US. This test should be ordered expeditiously, as TCs often exhibit a rapid growth rate. When the US confirms a concerning intratesticular lesion, patients should have a prompt referral to a urologist for evaluation and management. For detection of a testicular malignancy, US carries a sensitivity and specificity of 92% to 98% and 95% to 99%, respectively.[11] A biopsy of a testicular lesion should *never* be performed. Serum tumor markers (STMs), beta-human chorionic gonadotropin (hCG), alpha-fetoprotein (AFP), and lactate dehydrogenase (LDH) should be ordered before orchiectomy. Although hCG and AFP may provide information on the histology of the tumor, LDH is a nonspecific marker that may be representative of a global tumor burden.

Practice patterns vary in regard to staging evaluation. In clinically stable patients, imaging may be performed before or after orchiectomy and should never delay the time to orchiectomy. Imaging at a minimum should include a computed tomography (CT) scan of the abdomen/pelvis with intravenous contrast and a chest radiograph (CXR). If STMs are elevated or metastatic disease is seen on the CT abdomen/pelvis or CXR, a noncontrast chest CT should be performed.[12] Brain imaging should be obtained if the primary tumor has a significant component of choriocarcinoma or there are signs or symptoms suggestive of brain metastases.

Given the proclivity for TC to metastasize to the retroperitoneum, any patient between 15 and 44 years of age with a retroperitoneal mass should undergo evaluation with STMs, a testicular examination, and a scrotal US. If the clinical diagnosis of TC is made, patients do not require a biopsy or surgical exploration of the retroperitoneal lesion.

DIFFERENTIAL DIAGNOSIS

The differential diagnosis of a scrotal mass can be wide and varied. Extratesticular and paratesticular masses are generally benign. Similarly, painful testicular enlargement is generally infectious or inflammatory. However, a mass in the testicular body is TC until proven otherwise. Greater than 95% of intra testicular masses are malignant, and this should be made clear to the patient who may ardently rationalize avoidance of an orchiectomy.

Germ cell tumors (GCTs) account for 95% of TCs. These tumors are classified as either seminoma or nonseminoma (nonseminomatous GCT [NSGCT]). The remaining 5% of tumors are generally gonadal stromal tumors (Leydig cell, Sertoli cell, granulosa cell), which tend to be benign but occasionally have malignant potential. Malignant lymphoma is occasionally seen in older men and should be suspected if bilateral tumors are seen. Rare situations exist whereby an intratesticular lesion proves to be benign. Fortunately, these lesions have characteristic findings on US that lend to the diagnosis. These characteristics include epidermoid cysts (onion-ring appearance on US) or infarcts (avascular wedge-shaped defect on US).

STAGING

TC staging is done according to the American Joint Committee on Cancer classification.[13] Clinical stage (CS) is assigned based on the TNM system (**Box 1**). CS I is disease confined to the testis; CS II is disease in the retroperitoneal lymph nodes, and CS III is distant metastatic disease (**Table 1**). The International Germ Cell Cancer Collaborative Group (IGCCCG) classification is also used to stratify patients by risk[14]: good (95% cure), intermediate (80%–90% cure), and poor risk (50% cure) (**Table 2**).

PATHOLOGY
Germ Cell Tumors

As mentioned previously, GCTs account for 95% of TCs; in clinical practice, TC and GCT are typically used synonymously. **Table 3** summarizes the diagnostic cues of the different types of GCT.

Intratubular germ cell neoplasia
Intratubular germ cell neoplasia (IGCN) is a noninvasive, premalignant precursor to GCTs, alternatively referred to as CIS of the testis. When untreated, up to 50% of testes with IGCN will develop GCT. However, biopsy of the contralateral testis (during orchiectomy for TC) looking for IGCN is controversial and reserved for rare

---

Box 1
The American Joint Committee on Cancer TNM staging system

Primary tumor (T)

pTX	Primary tumor cannot be assessed
pT0	No evidence of primary tumor
pTis	Intratubular germ cell neoplasia
pT1	Tumor limited to the testis and epididymis or tumor invasion into the tunica albuginea only
pT2	Tumor extending through the tunica albuginea with involvement of the tunica vaginalis
pT3	Tumor invades the spermatic cord
pT4	Tumor invades the scrotum

Regional lymph nodes: clinical staging (N)

NX	Regional lymph nodes cannot be assessed
N0	No regional lymph node metastasis
N1	Metastases to single or multiple lymph nodes, each less than 2 cm in size
N2	Metastases to single or multiple lymph nodes, greater than 2 cm but less than 5 cm in size
N3	Metastases to lymph node, greater than 5 cm in greatest dimension

Regional lymph nodes: pathologic staging (pN)

pNX	Regional lymph nodes cannot be assessed
pN0	No regional lymph node metastasis
pN1	Metastases to single or multiple lymph nodes, each less than 2 cm in size and 5 or less nodes positive
pN2	Metastases to single or multiple lymph nodes, greater than 2 cm but less than 5 cm in size; or greater than 5 nodes positive; or extranodal extension of tumor
pN3	Metastases to lymph node, greater than 5 cm in size

Distant metastasis (M)

MX	Distant metastasis cannot be assessed
M0	No distant metastasis
M1	Distant metastasis
M1a	Nonregional nodal or pulmonary metastasis
M1b	Distant metastasis other than to nonregional lymph nodes and lungs

Serum tumor markers (S): based off nadir value after orchiectomy

SX	Markers not available				
	LDH		hCG (IU/mL)		AFP (ng/mL)
S0	Normal	&	Normal	&	Normal
S1	<1.5 × ULN	&	<5000	&	<1000
S2	1.5–10 × ULN	or	5000–50,000	or	1000–10,000
S3	>10 × ULN	or	>50,000	or	>10,000

Abbreviation: ULN, upper limit of normal.

Data from Amin MB, Edge S, Greene F, et al. editors. AJCC cancer staging manual. 8th edition. New York: Springer; 2017.

---

circumstances. It is also controversial whether IGCN needs to be treated, as it is unclear whether treating IGCN improves survival over treating a GCT if it arises.

Seminoma

Seminoma is the most common TC in adults, and the most common in patients with cryptorchidism. *Classic seminoma* accounts for 95% of cases and *spermatocytic seminoma* for 5%. Classic seminoma can present at any age, most commonly at 30 to 40 years of age. Spermatocytic seminoma generally presents at greater than 50 years of age and is of very low metastatic potential. Seminoma produces hCG approximately 10% of the time but *never* produces AFP. If patients have pure

Table 1
The American Joint Committee on Cancer clinical stage grouping

Stage Group	T	N	M	S
CS 0	pTis	N0	M0	S0
CS I	pT1-4	N0	M0	SX
IA	pT1	N0	M0	S0
IB	pT2	N0	M0	S0
	pT3	N0	M0	S0
	pT4	N0	M0	S0
IS	Any pT/TX	N0	M0	S1-3
CS II	Any pT/TX	N1-3	M0	SX
IIA	Any pT/TX	N1	M0	S0
	Any pT/TX	N1	M0	S1
IIB	Any pT/TX	N2	M0	S0
	Any pT/TX	N2	M0	S1
IIC	Any pT/TX	N3	M0	S0
	Any pT/TX	N3	M0	S1
CS III	Any pT/TX	Any N	M1	SX
IIIA	Any pT/TX	Any N	M1a	S0
	Any pT/TX	Any N	M1a	S1
IIIB	Any pT/TX	N1-3	M0	S2
	Any pT/TX	Any N	M1a	S2
IIIC	Any pT/TX	N1-3	M0	S3
	Any pT/TX	Any N	M1a	S3
	Any pT/TX	Any N	M1b	Any S

Data from Amin MB, Edge S, Greene F, et al. editors. AJCC cancer staging manual. 8th edition. New York: Springer; 2017.

Table 2
International Germ Cell Cancer Collaborative Group classification for clinical stage IIC and III germ cell tumors

Group	Nonseminoma	Seminoma
Good risk	All of the following criteria • Testis/retroperitoneal primary • M0 or M1a • S0 or S1	All of the following criteria • M0 or M1a • Normal AFP
Intermediate risk	All of the following criteria • Testis/retroperitoneal primary • M0 or M1a • S2	All of the following criteria • M1b • Normal AFP
Poor risk	Any of the following criteria • Mediastinal primary • M1b • S3	No seminoma patients classified as poor risk

Data from International Germ Cell Consensus Classification: a prognostic factor-based staging system for metastatic germ cell cancers. International Germ Cell Cancer Collaborative Group. J Clin Oncol 1997;15(2):594–603.

Table 3 Presentation characteristics of germ cell tumors		
Tumor Type	**AFP**	**hCG**
Classic seminoma	Never	Sometimes
Yolk sac tumor	Sometimes	Sometimes
Choriocarcinoma	Never	Always
Embryonal carcinoma	Sometimes	Sometimes
Teratoma	Never	Never

seminoma on orchiectomy and an elevated serum AFP level (>25 IU/mL), they should be treated as patients with NSGCT, as these elements were either missed on pathologic analysis or are present in metastatic lesions.

Nonseminoma

NSGCT may be present as pure (only one histologic subtype) or mixed (multiple histologic subtypes, which may include elements of seminoma). Mixed lesions are treated as NSGCT. There are multiple histologic subtypes of NSGCT, which may each carry unique presentation, behavior, and risk profiles.

Yolk sac tumor (YST), also referred to as endodermal sinus tumor, is often a component of mixed GCTs. When a tumor is pure YST, it typically presents in children younger than 10 years. It may secrete AFP and/or hCG. It often exhibits hematogenous metastasis.

Choriocarcinoma never secretes AFP and *always* secretes hCG. Choriocarcinoma carries the worst prognosis of all GCT, often exhibiting early hematogenous metastases to multiple locations, most commonly the lungs. When present, even as a component of mixed GCT, brain imaging should be considered.

Embryonal carcinoma (EC) may secrete AFP and/or hCG. A predominance of EC in the orchiectomy specimen is a risk factor for microscopic metastases.

Teratoma is often cystic and composed of tissue from multiple germ cell layers (endoderm, mesoderm, and ectoderm). It has a predilection for invasive local growth into surrounding organs and requires surgical resection for cure, as it is both chemoresistant and radioresistant.

Gonadal Stromal Tumors

Leydig cell and Sertoli cell

Leydig cell and Sertoli cell tumors may each secrete either androgen or estrogen byproducts and, therefore, have varied presentations. In prepubertal boys, they may show virilizing or feminizing symptoms based on tumor activity. In adults, androgen-secreting tumors are generally asymptomatic, whereas estrogen-secreting tumors may present with loss of libido, impotence, or feminization. Only 10% of Leydig cell or Sertoli cell tumors are malignant. Both are generally cured with orchiectomy; however, patients may have persistent virilizing or feminizing features given the irreversibility of some of these changes.

Granulosa cell

Granulosa cell tumors are almost always diagnosed in the neonatal period and are always benign. They are typically asymptomatic, although it is possible for them to secrete estrogen and have pursuant physiologic effects. Extremely rarely, granulosa cell tumors have been reported in adults and can carry malignant potential.

Other Tumors

Lymphoma

Lymphoma typically presents in men greater than 50 years. It is the most common metastatic tumor found in the testis and also the most common bilateral tumor of the testis. Primary testicular lymphoma occurs very rarely and is more common in men greater than 60 years of age. Histology is generally diffuse large B-cell lymphoma in primary cases; but in secondary (metastatic) involvement, it may be any of the other histologies but particularly Burkitt lymphoma.[15]

Gonadoblastoma

Gonadoblastoma is a rare tumor that occurs almost exclusively in patients with gonadal dysgenesis secondary to disorders of sexual differentiation (previously referred to as intersex). Although gonadoblastoma is a benign entity, it carries a high risk of malignant transformation (>50%); therefore, prophylactic bilateral gonadectomy is recommended.

INITIAL MANAGEMENT OF A TESTICULAR MASS
General Considerations

After a solid intratesticular mass is identified on physical examination and confirmed on scrotal US, patients should be promptly referred to a urologist. The reason for avoidance of a biopsy is twofold. First, the diagnosis of TC can virtually always be made by US. Second, trans-scrotal biopsies may alter the lymphatic drainage pattern of the testis (to the inguinal lymph nodes), making surveillance and treatment more complicated.

Fertility Considerations

Because most patients with TC are of reproductive age, fertility considerations are paramount. Patients with TC often require chemotherapy, radiation therapy (RT), and/or retroperitoneal lymph node dissection (RPLND) that may have substantial impacts on fertility. The germinal epithelium is exquisitely sensitive to both platinum-based chemotherapy and RT. Nearly all patients will become azoospermic after chemotherapy, with 50% and 80% of patients returning to preoperative sperm counts within 2 and 5 years, respectively.[16,17] Similarly, patients who receive RT may require 2 to 3 years to recover spermatogenesis.[18] RPLND may result in ejaculatory dysfunction secondary to injury of the sympathetic nerves along their course (sympathetic chain → postganglionic sympathetic nerves → hypogastric plexus). Given these potential impacts on fertility, all men should be counseled and strongly recommended to undergo semen cryopreservation (SCP) before treatment is initiated. However, SCP may be carried out before or after radical orchiectomy.

Radical Orchiectomy

The first step in the treatment of nearly every patient with TC is to perform a radical orchiectomy through an inguinal incision. The spermatic cord is ligated high (at the peritoneal reflection) with a permanent suture. If patients later require RPNLD, the distal extent of the spermatic cord remnant can be identified by this suture and removed. A testicular prosthesis may be offered to patients and safely performed at the time of orchiectomy or at a later date if desired. Partial orchiectomy (removal of the tumor from the testis) is only performed in extenuating circumstances and generally reserved for patients with a solitary testis. If the orchiectomy specimen reveals TC, patients are then staged using the surgical pathological diagnosis, imaging, and STM results.

SEMINOMA: CLINICAL STAGE IA OR IB

Patients with CS I seminomas are typically offered 3 management options: surveillance, RT, or adjuvant chemotherapy. Importantly, cancer-specific survival (CSS) for each option approaches 99% (**Table 4**).[19] The rationale for surveillance is avoidance of unnecessary treatment. The retroperitoneal nodes will harbor micrometastatic disease in approximately 20% of patients; therefore, if all patients with CS I seminoma receive upfront treatment, 80% will be overtreated. However, this means that patients who elect surveillance carry a relapse rate of up to 20%, most commonly in the retroperitoneum. Patients who relapse typically require full induction chemotherapy with bleomycin, etoposide, and cisplatin (BEP) or RT in some situations.[20]

Seminomas are exquisitely radiosensitive. Patients who elect to undergo RT to the retroperitoneum require less intensive follow-up with CT scans. The relapse rate following adjuvant RT is around 3% to 5% and recurrences usually occur outside of the retroperitoneum (most commonly the lungs).[21,22] The disadvantages of this approach include overtreatment, an increased risk of death from cardiac disease, and the risk of secondary malignancy in the treatment field.[20]

The third option is adjuvant chemotherapy with 1 cycle of carboplatin. This approach carries the lowest relapse rate (approximately 4%–5%).[23] If patients relapse, it typically occurs in the retroperitoneum. Therefore, patients require close surveillance with abdominal imaging (but less frequent than patients who elected for surveillance). Short-term toxicity of chemotherapy includes myelosuppression, infertility, and fatigue. Long-term toxicity is poorly defined.

Because CS IA and IB seminoma carry such a good prognosis, surveillance is the preferred option for most patients. The National Comprehensive Cancer Network (NCCN) recommends surveillance for all compliant patients with CS IA or IB pure seminoma. Surveillance regimens vary but include frequent physical examination, STMs, abdominal imaging, and chest imaging for at least 5 years.

SEMINOMA: CLINICAL STAGE IIA, IIB, OR IS

Patients with CS IIA, IIB, or IS seminoma, clinical evidence of metastatic disease either with persistently elevated postorchiectomy STMs (IS) or disease in the retroperitoneum (IIA: N1; IIB: N2), are offered either RT to the retroperitoneum (plus/minus ipsilateral iliac lymph nodes) or chemotherapy. Full induction chemotherapy (EP × 4 cycles or BEP × 3 cycles) is the preferred option for patients with IIB or IS. With this approach, cure rates are greater than 95%.[20]

Table 4
Seminoma clinical stage I treatment outcomes

	Surveillance	Radiation	Chemotherapy
CSS (%)	99	99	99
5-y risk of relapse (%)	15	3–5	2–5
Relapse site	Retroperitoneum	Outside retroperitoneum	Retroperitoneum
Treatment if relapse	Chemotherapy or radiation	Chemotherapy	Chemotherapy or radiation

SEMINOMA: CLINICAL STAGE IIC OR III

Patients with more extensive metastatic disease are treated with induction chemotherapy. Patients with IGCCCG good-risk disease receive BEP × 3 cycles or EP × 4 cycles. Patients with IGCCCG intermediate -risk disease receive BEP × 4 cycles. Even with advanced disease, no patients with seminoma are considered a poor risk. After chemotherapy, these patients should be followed closely with frequent physical examination, STMs, abdominal imaging, and chest imaging for at least 5 years.

Five-year survival is approximately 90% and 80% for good-risk and intermediate-risk patients, respectively.[24,25] Patients who relapse with seminoma after induction chemotherapy typically relapse in the retroperitoneum. Relapse in patients with seminoma is treated much differently than a relapse with NSGCT because of the potential histologies of the postchemotherapy residual mass (**Table 5**). Postchemotherapy masses in patients with seminoma are necrosis/fibrosis 80% to 90% of the time, with only 10% to 20% viable GCT.[26–28] Teratoma is exceedingly rare in this setting. Given the high likelihood of benign findings, the management of postchemotherapy masses can be challenging, particularly because postchemotherapy residual masses in patients with seminoma are notoriously difficult to surgically remove because of an intense desmoplastic reaction that surrounds the tissues. For these reasons, the current guidelines recommend observing masses less than 3 cm and obtaining a PET scan for masses that are 3 cm or greater at least 6 weeks after chemotherapy.[29] If the PET scan is positive or the mass is growing, resection is considered.[26]

NONSEMINOMATOUS GERM CELL TUMOR: CLINICAL STAGE IA/IB

Patients with CS I NSGCT have 3 management options: surveillance, adjuvant chemotherapy, and RPLND. All 3 management strategies carry similar 5-year CSS of approximately 99% (**Table 6**). The counseling process is very important for these patients because each option carries specific risks and benefits.

Patients with CS I NSGCT harbor micrometastatic disease in the retroperitoneum 25% to 30% of the time. Concordantly, the relapse rate with surveillance is 25% to 30%. If lymphovascular invasion (LVI) is present in the primary tumor, the likelihood of relapse approaches 50%.[30] In the absence of LVI, the relapse rate is 15% to 20%. A predominance of EC in the primary tumor is generally thought to increase the risk of relapse. Around one-third of surveillance patients who relapse and receive chemotherapy will subsequently also require postchemotherapy RPLND.[26] Therefore, patients with LVI may not represent the best candidates for surveillance, as this may subject them to more treatment than upfront chemotherapy or RPLND. Thus, the ideal candidates for surveillance with CS I NSGCT are medically compliant patients who will adhere to the strict surveillance protocol and who have no presence of LVI in the primary tumor. Surveillance is the preferred treatment strategy by the NCCN for CS IA.

Table 5
Histology of postchemotherapy retroperitoneal masses

	Seminoma	Nonseminoma
Teratoma (%)	0	40–50
Viable GCT (%)	10–20	10–20
Fibrosis/necrosis (%)	80–90	30–40

Table 6
Nonseminoma clinical stage I treatment outcomes

	Surveillance	RPLND	Chemotherapy
CSS (%)	99	99	99
5-y risk of relapse (%)	25–30	10	3
Relapse site	Retroperitoneum	Outside retroperitoneum	Retroperitoneum
Treatment if relapse	Chemotherapy	Chemotherapy	RPLND

Although surveillance is an option for compliant CS IB patients, adjuvant treatments (chemotherapy or surgery) are often considered given the significant risk of relapse.

The rationale for primary RPLND in CS I NSGCT is accurate staging, cure of micrometastatic disease, less intensive follow-up needed, and a significant reduction in the lifetime risk of requiring chemotherapy. A primary RPLND is less morbid than in the postchemotherapy setting, and the frequency of CT scans can be reduced significantly. The disadvantages are 50% to 80% undergoing an unnecessary operation, a risk of ejaculatory dysfunction (1%–2%), and a low risk of surgical complications. Sensible candidates for primary RPLND are patients with LVI (CS IB), primarily teratoma in the orchiectomy specimen, or patients who are either anxious about the risk of relapse or are noncompliant.[31] Patients with teratoma in the primary tumor are more likely (but not guaranteed) to harbor teratoma in the retroperitoneum, which is both chemoresistant and radioresistant, and may, therefore, benefit from upfront RPLND.[32] The overall relapse rate for primary RPLND is around 10%, and relapses are outside the retroperitoneum. Virtually all relapses are salvaged with chemotherapy.

Lastly, chemotherapy (1 or 2 cycles of BEP) is another option for CS IA or IB. Chemotherapy carries the lowest risk of relapse of the 3 treatment strategies at around 3%, with relapses typically occurring in the retroperitoneum and salvaged with RPLND.[20] The rationale for upfront chemotherapy is that it is less invasive than RPLND, micrometastases are treated even outside the retroperitoneum, and it decreases the intensity of follow-up. However, it does not treat teratoma, there is a significant risk of infertility and long-term risks of secondary malignancy or cardiovascular toxicity. Additionally, there are potential long-term side effects specific to each agent.

NONSEMINOMATOUS GERM CELL TUMOR: CLINICAL STAGE IS

CS IS NSGCT is defined as no identifiable disease on imaging, but patients have persistently elevated STMs following orchiectomy. Patients with CS IS are thought to have micrometastatic disease and are treated with chemotherapy.

NONSEMINOMATOUS GERM CELL TUMOR: CLINICAL STAGE IIA OR IIB

Patients with limited retroperitoneal disease but no metastasis outside of the retroperitoneum are categorized at CS IIA or IIB. The treatment options include RPLND or chemotherapy (BEP × 3 cycles or EP × 4 cycles) for those with negative STMs (if S1, patients should receive chemotherapy). Survival remains excellent in this patient population (>95%) with either choice.[19] If an RPLND is performed, the cure rate is approximately 70% to 90% when pathology returns as pN1; therefore, no adjuvant chemotherapy is recommended.[33] Only 50% of patients are cured when pN2-3 is discovered; therefore, adjuvant chemotherapy (BEP × 2 cycles) may be offered to further reduce the relapse rate. Although induction chemotherapy or RPLND are both appropriate options for CS IIA and CS IIB patients with negative STMs, the NCCN recommends chemotherapy as the preferred choice for CS IIB because these patients have a higher likelihood of microscopic metastases elsewhere.

NONSEMINOMATOUS GERM CELL TUMOR: CS IIC OR III

Patients with NSGCT with CS IIC or III signify the most advanced presentation, with high-volume retroperitoneal disease, distant metastatic disease, and/or profoundly elevated STMs. The treatment of this stage is induction chemotherapy. IGCCCG good-risk patients receive BEP × 3 cycles or EP × 4 cycles, whereas intermediate- or poor-risk patients receive BEP × 4 cycles. The 5-year overall survival is approximately 95%, 80%, and 50% for good, intermediate, and poor risk, respectively.[19,24]

NONSEMINOMATOUS GERM CELL TUMOR: MANAGEMENT OF POSTCHEMOTHERAPY RECURRENCE

All patients with NSGCT with a persistent or recurrent retroperitoneal mass greater than 1 cm following chemotherapy for any CS should undergo a postchemotherapy RPLND.[26] This treatment is done when STMs are negative. If STMs remain elevated, they typically receive salvage chemotherapy. The composition of a postchemotherapy mass in patients with NSGCT is much different than patients with seminoma (see **Table 5**). At the time of RPLND, 40% to 50% of masses will have teratoma, 15% to 20% viable GCT, and 40% to 50% fibrosis/necrosis.[22,27,34] PET scans are not indicated in the management of NSGCT. Around one-third of patients who receive induction chemotherapy for a CS IIC or III disease will require a postchemotherapy RPLND.[26] The rationale for surgery in this setting is because 50% to 70% of patients will have either teratoma or viable GCT in the retroperitoneum. Resecting teratoma is particularly important because these tumors have the potential for malignant degeneration into different types of more aggressive tumors, such as sarcomas or neuroendocrine tumors, that are often resistant to salvage treatments.[35] Fortunately, most patients will be cured with postchemotherapy RPLND; however, if viable GCT is found in the specimen, then additional salvage chemotherapy may be required.

NONSEMINOMATOUS GERM CELL TUMOR: SALVAGE SETTINGS
Salvage Chemotherapy

Patients who progress on primary chemotherapy or who relapse after primary chemotherapy with viable GCT will require salvage chemotherapy. This therapy typically consists of 4 cycles of etoposide, ifosfamide, and cisplatin; vinblastine, ifosfamide, and cisplatin; paclitaxel, ifosfamide, and cisplatin; or paclitaxel, ifosfamide, carboplatin, and etoposide. Around 50% achieve a complete radiographic or STM response; however, half of these patients will relapse again.[36]

Desperation Retroperitoneal Lymph Node Dissection

A desperation RPLND is indicated in patients who have persistently elevated STMs and a growing retroperitoneal mass after exhausting all chemotherapeutic regimens. These findings represent a poor prognostic sign; these patients typically have very aggressive tumors, often with distant micrometastatic disease. However, 47% to 60% will have normalization of STMs; long-term survival has been reported in 33% to 57% of patients.[31]

LATE RELAPSES

Because most TC recurrences occur within 2 years, a late relapse is defined as any that occurs beyond 2 years after completion of primary therapy. This late relapse happens in 3% of patients. Late relapses are best managed with surgical resection rather than salvage chemotherapy, particularly if they have already received chemotherapy.[26] Another option that has shown promise in the clinical trial setting is gemcitabine with paclitaxel. Unfortunately, many of these late relapses do not respond to salvage treatment, and survival is poor. Therefore, patients in this setting are often encouraged to consider a clinical trial.

TREATMENT-RELATED SEQUELAE

Many long-term sequelae have been reported in TC survivors, including peripheral neuropathy, hearing loss, hypogonadism, infertility, secondary malignancies, and cardiovascular disease. Hearing loss from cisplatin-based chemotherapy regimens has been reported in up to 20% to 40% of men.[37,38] Sexual dysfunction and infertility affect 20% to 25% of men treated with first-line chemotherapy.[17] Of particular concern is the impact of treatments on secondary malignancies and cardiovascular disease. Large population-based studies of GCT survivors have reported an increased risk of death from gastrointestinal and cardiovascular disease after RT and an increased risk of death from cardiovascular and pulmonary disease after chemotherapy.[39] The causes of the cardiovascular injury are not well understood, but it is thought the treatment causes vascular injury as well as a metabolic syndrome.[40,41]

Patients who undergo treatment with RT or chemotherapy are both at an increased risk for secondary malignancies. The incidence of non–germ cell malignancies is thought to be 60% to 100% higher in TC survivors treated with cisplatin-based chemotherapy or RT compared with the general population and roughly 200% higher if patients receive both RT and chemotherapy.[42] Given the young age of most patients with TC, these issues are extremely important to consider when counseling men on their treatment options.

SUMMARY

Metastatic TC was once uniformly fatal. Today, TC is one of the most curable malignancies because of the multimodal approach and introduction of cisplatin-based chemotherapy with consolidative surgery. Despite the significant survival improvements over the last 40 years, much work remains on maximizing the treatment efficacy while minimizing the morbidity associated with treatment in these young men.

REFERENCES

1. Siegel RL, Miller KD, Jemal A. Cancer statistics, 2016. CA Cancer J Clin 2016; 66(1):7–30.
2. Nigam M, Aschebrook-Kilfoy B, Shikanov S, et al. Increasing incidence of testicular cancer in the United States and Europe between 1992 and 2009. World J Urol 2015;33(5):623–31.
3. Cook MB, Akre O, Forman D, et al. A systematic review and meta-analysis of perinatal variables in relation to the risk of testicular cancer–experiences of the son. Int J Epidemiol 2010;39(6):1605–18.
4. Pettersson A, Richiardi L, Nordenskjold A, et al. Age at surgery for undescended testis and risk of testicular cancer. N Engl J Med 2007;356(18):1835–41.

5. Peterson AC, Bauman JM, Light DE, et al. The prevalence of testicular microlithiasis in an asymptomatic population of men 18 to 35 years old. J Urol 2001;166(6): 2061–4.

6. Dogra VS, Gottlieb RH, Oka M, et al. Sonography of the scrotum. Radiology 2003; 227(1):18–36.

7. DeCastro BJ, Peterson AC, Costabile RA. A 5-year follow-up study of asymptomatic men with testicular microlithiasis. J Urol 2008;179(4):1420–3 [discussion: 1423].

8. Costabile RA. How worrisome is testicular microlithiasis? Curr Opin Urol 2007; 17(6):419–23.

9. Hemminki K, Li X. Familial risk in testicular cancer as a clue to a heritable and environmental aetiology. Br J Cancer 2004;90(9):1765–70.

10. Dalgaard MD, Weinhold N, Edsgärd D, et al. A genome-wide association study of men with symptoms of testicular dysgenesis syndrome and its network biology interpretation. J Med Genet 2012;49(1):58–65.

11. Coursey Moreno C, Small WC, Camacho JC, et al. Testicular tumors: what radiologists need to know–differential diagnosis, staging, and management. Radiographics 2015;35(2):400–15.

12. See WA, Hoxie L. Chest staging in testis cancer patients: imaging modality selection based upon risk assessment as determined by abdominal computerized tomography scan results. J Urol 1993;150(3):874–8.

13. Amin MB, Edge S, Greene F, et al. editors. AJCC cancer staging manual. 8th edition. New York: Springer; 2017.

14. International germ cell consensus classification: a prognostic factor-based staging system for metastatic germ cell cancers. International Germ Cell Cancer Collaborative Group. J Clin Oncol 1997;15(2):594–603.

15. Vitolo U, Ferreri AJM, Zucca E. Primary testicular lymphoma. Crit Rev Oncol Hematol 2008;65(2):183–9.

16. Bujan L, Walschaerts M, Moinard N, et al. Impact of chemotherapy and radiotherapy for testicular germ cell tumors on spermatogenesis and sperm DNA: a multicenter prospective study from the CECOS network. Fertil Sterility 2013; 100(3):673–80.

17. Hartmann JT, Albrecht C, Schmoll HJ, et al. Long-term effects on sexual function and fertility after treatment of testicular cancer. Br J Cancer 1999;80(5–6):801–7.

18. Fosså SD, Dahl AA, Haaland CF. Health-related quality of life in patients treated for testicular cancer. Curr Opin Urol 1999;9(5):425–9.

19. van Dijk MR, Steyerberg EW, Habbema JDF. Survival of non-seminomatous germ cell cancer patients according to the IGCC classification: an update based on meta-analysis. Eur J Cancer 2006;42(7):820–6.

20. Chovanec M, Hanna N, Cary KC, et al. Management of stage I testicular germ cell tumours. Nat Rev Urol 2016;13(11):663–73.

21. Jones WG, Fosså SD, Mead GM, et al. Randomized trial of 30 versus 20 Gy in the adjuvant treatment of stage I testicular seminoma: a report on medical research council trial TE18, European Organisation for the Research and Treatment of Cancer Trial 30942 (ISRCTN18525328). J Clin Oncol 2005;23(6):1200–8.

22. Kollmannsberger C, Tandstad T, Bedard PL, et al. Patterns of relapse in patients with clinical stage I testicular cancer managed with active surveillance. J Clin Oncol 2015;33(1):51–7.

23. Oliver RTD, Mead GM, Rustin GJS, et al. Randomized trial of carboplatin versus radiotherapy for stage I seminoma: mature results on relapse and contralateral

testis cancer rates in MRC TE19/EORTC 30982 study (ISRCTN27163214). J Clin Oncol 2011;29(8):957–62.

24. Albers P, Albrecht W, Algaba F, et al. Guidelines on testicular cancer: 2015 update. Eur Urol 2015;68(6):1054–68.

25. Rajpert-De Meyts E, McGlynn KA, Okamoto K, et al. Testicular germ cell tumours. Lancet 2016;387(10029):1762–74.

26. Daneshmand S, Albers P, Fosså SD, et al. Contemporary management of post-chemotherapy testis cancer. Eur Urol 2012;62(5):867–76.

27. Sheinfeld J, Bajorin D. Management of the postchemotherapy residual mass. Urol Clin North Am 1993;20(1):133–43.

28. Schultz SM, Einhorn LH, Conces DJ, et al. Management of postchemotherapy residual mass in patients with advanced seminoma: Indiana University experience. J Clin Oncol 1989;7(10):1497–503.

29. Bantis A, Sountoulides P, Metaxa L, et al. The diagnostic yield of fluorine-18 fluorodeoxyglucose positron emission tomography-computed tomography in recurrent testicular seminoma. Urol Ann 2016;8(4):496–9.

30. Albers P, Siener R, Kliesch S, et al. Risk factors for relapse in clinical stage I nonseminomatous testicular germ cell tumors: results of the German testicular cancer study group trial. J Clin Oncol 2003;21(8):1505–12.

31. Beck SDW, Foster RS, Bihrle R, et al. Pathologic findings and therapeutic outcome of desperation post-chemotherapy retroperitoneal lymph node dissection in advanced germ cell cancer. Uro 2005;23(6):423–30.

32. Heidenreich A, Moul JW, McLeod DG, et al. The role of retroperitoneal lymphadenectomy in mature teratoma of the testis. J Urol 1997;157(1):160–3.

33. Sheinfeld J, Motzer RJ, Rabbani F, et al. Incidence and clinical outcome of patients with teratoma in the retroperitoneum following primary retroperitoneal lymph node dissection for clinical stages I and IIA nonseminomatous germ cell tumors. J Urol 2003;170(4 Pt 1):1159–62.

34. Donohue JP, Foster RS. Management of retroperitoneal recurrences. Seminoma and nonseminoma. Urol Clin NA 1994;21(4):761–72.

35. Beck SDW, Foster RS, Bihrle R, et al. Teratoma in the orchiectomy specimen and volume of metastasis are predictors of retroperitoneal teratoma in post-chemotherapy nonseminomatous testis cancer. J Urol 2002;168(4 Pt 1):1402–4.

36. Feldman DR, Bosl GJ, Sheinfeld J, et al. Medical treatment of advanced testicular cancer. Jama 2008;299(6):672–84.

37. Brydøy M, Oldenburg J, Klepp O, et al. Observational study of prevalence of long-term Raynaud-like phenomena and neurological side effects in testicular cancer survivors. J Natl Cancer Inst 2009;101(24):1682–95.

38. Rossen PB, Pedersen AF, Zachariae R, et al. Health-related quality of life in long-term survivors of testicular cancer. J Clin Oncol 2009;27(35):5993–9.

39. Fosså SD, Gilbert E, Dores GM, et al. Noncancer causes of death in survivors of testicular cancer. J Natl Cancer Inst 2007;99(7):533–44.

40. Altena R, de Haas EC, Nuver J, et al. Evaluation of sub-acute changes in cardiac function after cisplatin-based combination chemotherapy for testicular cancer. Br J Cancer 2009;100(12):1861–6.

41. Nuver J, Smit AJ, Wolffenbuttel BH, et al. The metabolic syndrome and disturbances in hormone levels in long-term survivors of disseminated testicular cancer. J Clin Oncol 2005;23(16):3718–25.

42. Travis LB, Fosså SD, Schonfeld SJ, et al. Second cancers among 40,576 testicular cancer patients: focus on long-term survivors. J Natl Cancer Inst 2005; 97(18):1354–65.

Urinary Stone Disease
Diagnosis, Medical Therapy, and Surgical Management

Wesley W. Ludwig, MD*, Brian R. Matlaga, MD, MPH

KEYWORDS

- Urolithiasis • Dietary therapy • Medical therapy
- Extracorporeal shockwave lithotripsy • Ureteroscopy
- Percutaneous nephrolithotomy

KEY POINTS

- Low-dose computed tomography (CT) scan is the first-line imaging modality for diagnosis of urolithiasis in nonpregnant, adult patients.
- Patients with calcium stones should reduce dietary sodium and maintain normal dietary calcium. If dietary modification fails, thiazide and citrate therapy may be beneficial.
- Uric acid and cystine stones benefit from urinary alkalinization.
- Ureteroscopy (URS) and extracorporeal shockwave lithotripsy (SWL) can be used for ureteral stones. URS is associated with a better stone-free rate.
- Lower-pole renal stones less than 10 mm can be treated with URS or SWL, whereas those greater than 10 mm should be treated with URS or percutaneous nephrolithotomy (PCNL). Non–lower-pole stones less than 2 cm are best treated with URS or SWL, whereas those greater than 2 cm are best treated with PCNL.

INTRODUCTION

Urolithiasis is highly prevalent in the United States and is commonly encountered by both primary care physicians and specialists. Based on the latest National Health and Nutrition Examination Survey, the prevalence of kidney stones in the United States is 8.8%, or nearly 1 in 11 Americans.[1] The increasing prevalence of urolithiasis is thought to be driven in part by the skyrocketing rates of obesity and diabetes, which continues to be a difficult public health crisis to manage.[2] In addition, the frequent use of cross-sectional imaging has led to the common incidental diagnosis of urolithiasis.[3]

Disclosure Statement: The authors have no conflicts of interest to disclose.
Department of Urology, The James Buchanan Brady Urological Institute, Johns Hopkins Hospital, The Johns Hopkins University School of Medicine, 600 North Wolfe Street, Marburg 134, Baltimore, MD 21287, USA
* Corresponding author.
E-mail address: wludwig1@jhmi.edu

Med Clin N Am 102 (2018) 265–277
https://doi.org/10.1016/j.mcna.2017.10.004
0025-7125/18/© 2017 Elsevier Inc. All rights reserved.

There have been several recent advancements in the imaging, medical, and surgical management of urolithiasis, which are reviewed in this article.

DIAGNOSIS
Presentation

Patients with stone disease typically seek medical attention due to pain. Colicky flank pain is typically due to ureteral obstruction and can be associated with a variety of symptoms, including abdominal, flank, or pelvic pain, dysuria, hematuria, fever, nausea, or vomiting.[4] This array of symptoms has a broad differential diagnosis, including urinary tract infection, interstitial cystitis, vaginitis, prostatitis, benign prostatic hyperplasia/lower urinary tract symptoms, glomerular disease, urothelial cancer, gastrointestinal disease, and musculoskeletal pain, among many others.[5]

Clinical Evaluation

A patient suspected of urolithiasis should have a complete medical history performed; this may reveal predisposing conditions, such as diabetes, primary hyperparathyroidism, gout, renal tubular acidosis type I, obesity, and diagnoses related to gastrointestinal malabsorption.[6] A thorough dietary history should be obtained, including intake of calcium, sodium, fluid, fruits, vegetables, animal protein, oxalate-rich foods, over-the-counter dietary supplements, vitamin C, and vitamin D.[6] A careful medication review should be performed because a variety of medications can predispose to urolithiasis. Some medications induce metabolic changes that predispose to stone development, such as loop diuretics, carbonic anhydrase inhibitors, and laxatives. Other medications lead to stone formation due to urinary supersaturation of the drug or metabolite, including ciprofloxacin, magnesium trisilicate, sulfa medications, triamterene, indinavir, guaifenesin, and ephedrine.[7]

Imaging

Computed tomography

When there is clinical suspicion for urinary stone disease, low-dose noncontrast computed tomography (CT) is the preferred diagnostic method for most nonobese individuals.[8] Obese individuals typically require standard-dose noncontrast CT. CT is frequently used because it has an estimated sensitivity and specificity for stone detection of nearly 100%.[9] The only stone type that cannot be visualized using CT is one formed from protease-inhibitor medications.[10] In addition, CT provides an attenuation measurement in the form of Hounsfield units, which aid in determination of stone composition.[11] Uric acid calculi are typically less than 400 HU, whereas calcium oxalate calculi are 600 to 1200 HU.[12] Because of the diagnostic accuracy and ability to aid in management planning, both the American College of Radiology and the American Urological Association recommend CT as the first-line imaging modality for patients presenting with renal colic.[13,14] The drawbacks of CT imaging are radiation exposure and higher cost compared with ultrasound (US) and MRI. There are some clinical scenarios in which CT is not an appropriate first-line imaging choice.

Ultrasound

To avoid unnecessary radiation exposure, US is the preferred first-line diagnostic test for pediatric and pregnant patients with suspected stone disease.[15,16] An additional benefit is US's significantly lower cost compared with CT, which has become an important factor as high-value care is increasingly stressed.[17] A wide range of sensitivities and specificities has been reported for the ability of US to detect urinary stones, likely because of variations in technique. A meta-analysis of studies examining stone detection using US found a median sensitivity and specificity of 61% and 97%, respectively.[14] An additional downside of US is that it does not reliably measure stone size. Typically, US overestimates stone size by approximately 2 mm, and overestimation increases by about 20% with each 2-cm increase in depth.[18] Methods have been developed to improve stone size measurements on US, such as measuring stone shadow width, yet inaccuracies remain.[19] Of note, CT may be equivalent to US in the initial diagnosis of nephrolithiasis in an emergency department setting. A trial randomized patients in an emergency department with suspected nephrolithiasis to CT or ultrasonography and found no significant differences in diagnostic accuracy, adverse events, pain scores, or hospitalizations.[20]

MRI

MRI is used in a very limited fashion in the diagnosis of urolithiasis. MRI has a median sensitivity and specificity for detecting kidney stones of 82% and 98%, respectively.[14] MRI is typically recommended for pregnant individuals in their first trimester after an equivocal US.[21] However, its role outside of this setting is limited due to high cost and long acquisition time.

Laboratory Evaluation

At the initial visit following a diagnosis of urolithiasis, a serum chemistry and urinalysis should be obtained. If a patient has signs or symptoms consistent with primary hyperparathyroidism, a serum-intact parathyroid level is required.[6] Twenty-four-hour urine studies may help guide therapy decisions for patients that are recurrent stone formers, high risk for a metabolic abnormality, or particularly interested.[22] Twenty-four-hour urine studies should be collected while the patient remains on a regular diet. At a minimum, volume, pH, calcium, uric acid, oxalate, citrate, sodium, potassium, and creatinine should be measured, because these metrics can reveal contributors to stone formation.[6] Similarly, passed stones should be sent for analysis because stone type may change preventive strategies, which is particularly true for uric acid, cystine, struvite or calcium phosphate stones.[23] In the past, calcium loading tests were common to distinguish between different types of hypercalciuria. This practice is no longer recommended because it does not change clinical management.[24]

DIETARY AND MEDICAL THERAPY

Dietary modifications are likely beneficial for all patients with urolithiasis, whereas medical therapy is indicated in the setting of recurrent stone disease without appropriate response to dietary modifications. The type of medical therapy largely depends on urinary electrolyte abnormalities and stone composition. In the following section, medical expulsive therapies for ureteral stones and medical therapies for specific stone types with indications and evidence for their use are presented.

Medical Expulsive Therapy for Ureteral Stones

Multiple randomized trials have been performed evaluating the effect of medical expulsive therapy (MET) on stone passage rate, often resulting in conflicting conclusions. A *Cochrane Review* of 32 randomized trials evaluating alpha-blockers found an improvement in stone-free rate in the alpha-blocker group compared with standard therapy.[25] Patients receiving alpha-blockers experienced stone expulsion nearly 3 days earlier and reduced the number of painful episodes, analgesic use, and hospitalization rate. There is consistent evidence that MET helps in the passage of distal ureteral stones. A recent trial randomized patients with a unilateral ureteral stone to silodosin (a selective alpha-blocker) or placebo. Although there were no significant differences in the passage rate for all stones, there was a significantly greater rate of passage for distal ureteral stones.[26] However, other well-designed studies have found no benefit for MET even within subgroups. A multicenter, randomized trial of patients with a single ureteral stone was randomized to tamsulosin, nifedipine, or placebo and found that neither drug was effective in decreasing need for further treatment, regardless of stone location or size.[27]

Urine Volume

Regardless of stone type, patients should strive for a fluid intake that results in a urine volume greater than 2.5 L daily.[6] All stones form because of elevated urinary concentration of particular metabolites, and decreasing urine concentration benefits all stone types. A trial randomizing stone-forming patients to fluid intake resulting in urine volume greater than 2 L daily or no intervention resulted in decreased recurrences and prolonged interval between stone episodes in the increased urine volume cohort.[28]

Calcium Stones

Dietary intervention

Current evidence suggests that patients with calcium stones and hypercalciuria should maintain a dietary calcium intake of 1000 to 1200 mg per day (recommended daily allowance) and limit sodium intake.[6] Dietary sodium increases urinary calcium excretion, and a randomized trial has found a low-salt diet reduces both urinary calcium and oxalate.[29] Perhaps counterintuitively, a low-calcium diet does not prevent calcium stone formation. A randomized trial found a normal calcium diet in men with calcium oxalate nephrolithiasis reduced the risk of stone recurrence compared with a low calcium diet.[30] For patients with calcium oxalate stones, dietary oxalate should be limited, because elevated urinary oxalate levels are associated with an increased risk of stone disease.[31] In addition, patients with calcium stones and hypocitraturia should increase intake of fruits and vegetables and limit protein from nondairy animal sources. Fruits and vegetables provide an alkali load that increases urinary citrate, whereas animal protein creates an acid load leading to a decrease in urinary citrate.[32]

Thiazides

Thiazide diuretics decrease urinary calcium and are appropriate for individuals with hypercalciuria that have experienced stone recurrence despite dietary modifications. There have been 6 fair-quality trials randomizing patients with recurrent calcium stone disease to a thiazide diuretic or placebo. A meta-analysis of these studies found thiazide administration significantly reduced the risk of stone recurrence over placebo.[33] Thiazides may also be appropriate for recurrent calcium stone formers that do not have a specific metabolic abnormality.[34]

Citrate

For individuals with recurrent calcium stones, there have been 6 randomized trials evaluating the role of citrate for individuals with recurrent calcium stones. Most of these studies included recommendations for increased fluid intake, but no other dietary or medical manipulations. Most trials found a decreased risk of stone recurrence for individuals administered citrate.[33] Importantly, different types of citrate appear to have equivalent effectiveness, including potassium citrate, potassium-sodium citrate, and potassium-magnesium citrate. Perhaps the best study was done by Barcelo and colleagues[35] and randomized patients with recurrent urolithiasis and hypocitraturia to daily potassium citrate or placebo. Patients receiving potassium citrate had a significantly lower rate of stone formation and elevated levels of urine citrate, pH, and potassium. Potassium citrate is also appropriate for recurrent calcium stone formers that do not have identified metabolic abnormalities.[36]

Allopurinol

Allopurinol is indicated for patients with calcium oxalate stones, hyperuricosuria, and normocalciuria. A trial randomized patients that met the above criteria to allopurinol or placebo and found fewer stone recurrences and longer time to recurrence in the allopurinol cohort.[37]

Uric Acid Stones

Dietary intervention

Patients with uric acid stone disease commonly have low urine pH, which greatly decreases the solubility of uric acid.[38] Thus, reducing dietary animal protein and increasing consumption of foods with a high alkali load are beneficial.[39] Unfortunately, there is little evidence that dietary modification improves clinical outcomes for patients with uric acid stones.

Medical therapy

If dietary modification fails to prevent stone recurrence, potassium citrate should be prescribed.[6] Potassium citrate raises urinary pH, increasing the solubility of urine uric acid.[40] The goal of alkali therapy is to increase urine pH to 6.0, which results in a more than 10-fold increase in uric acid solubility compared with a urine pH of 5.0.[41] In addition, urinary alkalinization can dissolve existing uric acid stones and may successfully do so in up to 70% of patients.[42] Allopurinol should not be prescribed in a first-line fashion because the major metabolic abnormality is low urinary pH and not hyperuricosuria.[6] If urinary alkalinization is unsuccessful in preventing stone recurrence or a patient has significant hyperuricosuria, allopurinol is an appropriate choice.[43]

Cystine Stones

Dietary intervention

Cystinuria is due to an autosomal-recessive disease that results in impaired reabsorption of cystine, ornithine, lysine, and arginine.[44] Cystinuria leads to an elevated urinary concentration of cystine with subsequent stone formation often presenting in adolescence.[45] Patients with cystine stones benefit from reducing dietary sodium and protein. Animal protein is rich in cystine and methionine, which is metabolized to cystine and increases urinary excretion of sodium.[46] In addition, sodium promotes urinary cystine excretion.[47] Elevated cystine concentration leads to the formation of cystine stones, making increasing urine volume of great importance. To achieve this, it is recommended that patients consume more than 4 L of fluid daily.[6]

Medical therapy

The solubility of cystine increases with higher urinary pH, in a fashion similar to uric acid. Thus, potassium citrate should be prescribed for individuals with cystine stones in an attempt to maintain a urine pH of 7.0.[48] Increasing urine pH with citrate can potentially lead to stone dissolution, but is unlikely.[49] Cystine-binding thiol drugs should be administered to patients that fail urinary alkalinization or have particularly large recurrent stone burdens.[6] Cystine-binding drugs include tiopronin, D-penicillamine, and captopril. These drugs are reducing agents that undergo disulfide exchange to convert water-insoluble cystine to water-soluble cysteine. Tiopronin is the preferred agent, because it has been shown to be more efficacious than D-penicillamine and has a better side-effect profile.[50] However, toxicity associated with both tiopronin and D-penicillamine is common and has led to a high discontinuation rate for both drugs.[51] Captopril is a thiol drug commonly used to treat hypertension and has far fewer side effects compared with tiopronin and D-penicillamine.[52] Currently, there is insufficient evidence that captopril provides clinical benefit for patients with recurrent cystine stones, which may be due to insufficient urinary excretion to significantly bind cystine.[53]

Struvite Stones

Struvite (magnesium ammonium phosphate) stones form because of infection of the urinary tract with urease-producing bacteria. The mainstay of treatment is complete surgical stone removal to eliminate a nidus for future stone formation.[54] If a patient cannot tolerate a complete stone removal procedure, medical therapy in the form of acetohydroxamic acid (AHA) may be indicated. AHA irreversibly inhibits bacterial urease and is used to prevent struvite stone recurrence and progression. A randomized trial of AHA for struvite stones found stone growth occurred in 17% in the AHA group compared with 46% in the placebo cohort.[55] However, adverse events associated with AHA are common and can be severe, including hypercoagulability and neurologic symptoms.[56] Approximately a quarter of patients on AHA will experience intolerable side effects; thus, every effort should be made to achieve a fist-line surgical cure before initiating medical therapy.[55]

SHOCKWAVE LITHOTRIPSY AND SURGICAL MANAGEMENT

Surgical stone management largely depends on stone size and location. For a given stone, there are often multiple appropriate treatment modalities, and selection typically depends on surgeon preference and comfort. There are few high-quality studies comparing surgical modalities for particular stone locations, making evidence-based decision making challenging. The 3 main treatment modalities are extracorporeal shockwave lithotripsy (SWL), ureteroscopy (URS), and percutaneous nephrolithotomy (PCNL), which are discussed in the following sections.

Stone Management Techniques

Ureteroscopy

URS is an endoscopic approach to urolithiasis, typically involving laser stone fragmentation and basket extraction. URS offers excellent stone-free rates and low complication rates for most stone types, which has led to an increase in the use of URS by more than 250% in the previous 8 years.[57] URS is now the most common modality of definitive stone treatment in many locations, and more recently, trained urologists use URS for more than 70% of stone-related cases.[58,59] URS is the treatment modality of choice for individuals with bleeding diatheses or those unable to stop anticoagulant/antiplatelet therapy, because the risk of bleeding or hematoma formation is acceptably low.[60]

Percutaneous nephrolithotomy

PCNL is a minimally invasive, endoscopic procedure in which a needle is used to percutaneously access the collecting system. The needle tract is dilated, and a sheath is placed to allow a nephroscope to easily access the collecting system for stone fragmentation and removal. PCNL is frequently used for stone burdens greater than 2 cm, with excellent stone-free rates and a low rate of serious complications.[61] Currently, the minimally invasive profile of PCNL is improving even further as "mini" PCNL is becoming more widely used and permits usage of a smaller tract size.[62] PCNL cannot be safely used in some patients because of use of anticoagulants, bleeding disorders, or severe contractions or flexion deformities. In these patients, staged and repeated URS may be attempted to clear all stones.[63,64]

Shockwave lithotripsy
SWL is a noninvasive technology that uses shock waves to achieve stone fragmentation. SWL was popularized in the 1980s, but its use has been declining recently because URS is increasingly disseminated.[57] Following SWL, alpha-blockers are frequently prescribed to facilitate stone fragment passage. A meta-analysis of randomized trials found that alpha-blockers improved both stone-free rate and decreased time to achieve stone-free status.[65] SWL cannot be used in patients with an anatomic or functional obstruction distal to the stone, because fragments will not be effectively cleared.[66] If a particular stone has failed initial treatment with SWL, endoscopic therapy should be used as opposed to repeated SWL. URS and PCNL after failed SWL have stone-free rates up to 100%, whereas repeat SWL stone-free rates are substantially lower.[67,68]

Nonendoscopic surgery
Open, laparoscopic, and robotic surgery are options for patients with anatomic abnormalities that preclude the use of less invasive options.[69] Nonendoscopic surgery is not used as first-line treatment for the vast majority of stones because of increased invasiveness, higher complication rates, and worse recuperative profile. However, for patients that require concomitant reconstructive procedures, such as pyeloplasty or ureteral stricture treatment, a nonendoscopic procedure is indicated.[70]

Treatment by Stone Location

Ureteral stones
Patients with asymptomatic ureteral stones less than 10 mm may safely undergo observation with MET, particularly in the setting of a distal ureteral stone.[71] Based on experimental data, patients that fail to pass a ureteral stone within 6 weeks should undergo definitive treatment to avoid irreversible renal damage.[72] A patient with an obstructing ureteral stone and suspicion of a urinary tract infection should undergo drainage of the collecting system with a nephrostomy tube or a ureteral stent and should undergo stone extraction only after documented clearance of the infection.[73] URS and SWL are most commonly used for the treatment of ureteral stones. Complication rates between URS and SWL are similar; however, URS has a higher rate of ureteral perforation compared with SWL.[74] Furthermore, although both have excellent stone-free rates, URS has a better stone-free rate when data across multiple studies are analyzed.[65] URS is favored for mid to distal ureteral stones and stones composed of cystine or uric acid, which are denser and less likely to be effectively treated by SWL.[65,75] Following URS, a ureteral stent is typically left in place for a short period of time, and alpha-blockers or antimuscarinic therapy may be prescribed because these agents have been shown to reduce stent-related discomfort in randomized trials.[76,77] Very large or complex ureteral stones may require PCNL, laparoscopic, robotic, or open stone extraction in rare situations.[78,79] However, these approaches are uncommon and should not be used as first-line therapy.

Renal stones
The treatment of renal stones largely depends on polar location and stone size. Small, nonobstructing caliceal stones can be safely observed. However, numerous retrospective studies have found that 10% of asymptomatic stones necessitate intervention per year, and 30% to 46% experience stone growth.[80–82] Stones located in the lower pole and greater than 4 mm in size are more likely to become symptomatic

and should be observed with increased caution.[81] Observed stones should be actively followed with imaging to ensure significant growth or new stone formation is not occurring.

Symptomatic lower-pole stones less than 10 mm can be treated with SWL or URS. A randomized trial comparing these modalities found that stone-free rates are equivalent. URS is associated with slightly higher complication rates, and SWL is associated with better patient satisfaction.[83] However, for symptomatic lower-pole stones greater than 10 mm, SWL is not the optimal treatment because stone clearance is difficult due to the dependent nature of the lower pole. A randomized trial of PCNL versus SWL for lower-pole stones greater than 10 mm found the difference in success rates to be 91% versus 21%, respectively.[84] Not surprisingly, the complication rate for PCNL is higher than SWL.

Stones located outside of the lower pole and less than 2 cm should be treated with SWL or URS. PCNL is an option, but SWL and URS achieve similar stone-free rates with less associated morbidity.[85] PCNL is the preferred therapy for stones larger than 2 cm, and SWL should be avoided because of poor stone clearance.[86] Two randomized trials have compared PCNL to URS for stones larger than 2 cm and found PCNL was associated with better stone-free rate, need for fewer subsequent procedures, and need shorter treatment time.[87,88] Nephrectomy is an option for a large stone in a poorly functioning kidney, because there is no benefit to preserving the kidney.[89]

Staghorn calculi are large stones that conform to the shape of multiple calyces, and PCNL is typically indicated even if the stone is asymptomatic. Multiple studies have shown that untreated staghorn stones are associated with declining renal function, infections, and even death.[90,91]

SUMMARY

Obstructive urolithiasis typically presents with colicky flank pain but can involve a wide variety of symptoms. Initial evaluation should include a thorough history and physical, including a careful review of medical conditions, medications, and dietary history. Low-dose CT is the first-line imaging modality for most individuals when there is clinical suspicion of urolithiasis. US is indicated for pregnant or pediatric patients, in order to avoid radiation exposure. When a stone is detected, MET may be beneficial for facilitating passage of distal ureteral stones, but its utility is questionable in other settings. Regardless of stone type, patients should strive for a fluid intake that results in urine volume of greater than 2.5 L daily. For individuals with calcium stones, patients should maintain a low-sodium, normal calcium diet. If stones continue to recur, patients can be treated with thiazide diuretics if hypercalciuria is present or citrate therapy. Individuals with uric acid stones benefit from reducing dietary animal protein and increasing foods with high alkali content. If dietary modification fails, potassium citrate should be prescribed to increase urinary pH. Patients with cystine stones benefit from reducing dietary sodium and protein, and administration of a cystine-binding thiol drug if dietary therapy is unsuccessful. Struvite stones are primarily managed with surgical therapy, but AHA can be prescribed if a patient is not a surgical candidate. In terms of treatment, ureteral stones less than 10 mm can be observed in an attempt to achieve spontaneous passage, and URS or SWL may be indicated if observation is unsuccessful. Lower-pole renal stones less than 10 mm can be treated with URS or SWL, whereas those greater than 10 mm should be treated with URS or PCNL. Non–lower-pole stones less than 2 cm are best treated with URS or SWL, whereas those greater than 2 cm are best treated with PCNL.

REFERENCES

1. Scales CD, Smith AC, Hanley JM, et al. Prevalence of kidney stones in the United States. Eur Urol 2012;62:160–5.
2. Shoag J, Tasian GE, Goldfarb DS, et al. The new epidemiology of nephrolithiasis. Adv Chronic Kidney Dis 2015;22:273–8.
3. Boyce CJ, Pickhardt PJ, Lawrence EM, et al. Prevalence of urolithiasis in asymptomatic adults: objective determination using low dose noncontrast computerized tomography. J Urol 2010;183:1017–21.
4. Pietrow PK, Karellas ME. Medical management of common urinary calculi. Am Fam Physician 2006;74:86–94.
5. Frassetto L, Kohlstadt I. Treatment and prevention of kidney stones: an update. Am Fam Physician 2011;84:1234–42.
6. Pearle MS, Goldfarb DS, Assimos DG, et al. Medical management of kidney stones: AUA guideline. J Urol 2014;192:316–24.
7. Matlaga B, Shah O, Assimos DG. Drug-induced urinary calculi. Rev Urol 2003;5:227–31.
8. Türk C, Petřík A, Sarica K, et al. EAU guidelines on diagnosis and conservative management of urolithiasis. Eur Urol 2016;69(3):468–74.
9. Rob S, Bryant T, Wilson I, et al. Ultra-low-dose, low-dose, and standard-dose CT of the kidney, ureters, and bladder: is there a difference? Results from a systematic review of the literature. Clin Radiol 2017;72(1):11–5.
10. Wu DS, Stoller ML. Indinavir urolithiasis. Curr Opin Urol 2000;10:557–61.
11. Kawahara T, Miyamoto H, Ito H, et al. Predicting the mineral composition of ureteral stone using non-contrast computed tomography. Urolithiasis 2016;44:231–9.
12. Nakada SY, Hoff DG, Attai S, et al. Determination of stone composition by non-contrast spiral computed tomography in the clinical setting. Urology 2000;55:816–9.
13. Coursey C, Casalino DD, Remer EM, et al. ACR Appropriateness Criteria® acute onset flank pain–suspicion of stone disease. Ultrasound Q 2012;28:227–33.
14. Fulgham PF, Assimos DG, Pearle MS, et al. Clinical effectiveness protocols for imaging in the management of ureteral calculous disease: AUA technology assessment. J Urol 2013;189:1203–13.
15. Masselli G, Weston M, Spencer J. The role of imaging in the diagnosis and management of renal stone disease in pregnancy. Clin Radiol 2015;70:1462–71.
16. Colleran GC, Callahan MJ, Paltiel HJ, et al. Imaging in the diagnosis of pediatric urolithiasis. Pediatr Radiol 2017;47:5–16.
17. Melnikow J, Xing G, Cox G, et al. Cost analysis of the STONE randomized trial can health care costs be reduced one test at a time? Med Care 2016;54:337–42.
18. Dunmire B, Lee FC, Hsi RS, et al. Tools to improve the accuracy of kidney stone sizing with ultrasound. J Endourol 2015;29:147–52.
19. Dunmire B, Harper JD, Cunitz BW, et al. Use of the acoustic shadow width to determine kidney stone size with ultrasound. J Urol 2016;195:171–6.
20. Smith-Bindman R, Aubin C, Bailitz J, et al. Ultrasonography versus computed tomography for suspected nephrolithiasis. N Engl J Med 2014;371:1100–10.
21. Brisbane W, Bailey M, Sorenson M. An overview of kidney stone imaging techniques. Nat Rev Urol 2016;13:654–62.
22. Kocvara R, Plasgura P, Petřík A, et al. A prospective study of nonmedical prophylaxis after a first kidney stone. Br J Urol 1999;84:393–8.

23. Pak CY, Poindexter JR, Adams-Huet B, et al. Predictive value of kidney stone composition in the detection of metabolic abnormalities. Am J Med 2003;115: 26–32.

24. Lein JW, Keane PM. Limitations of the oral calcium loading test in the management of the recurrent calcareous renal stone former. Am J Kidney Dis 1983;3: 76–9.

25. Campschroer T, Zhu Y, Duijvesz D, et al. Alpha-blockers as medical expulsive therapy for ureteral stones. Cochrane Database Syst Rev 2014;(4):CD008509.

26. Sur RL, Shore N, L'Esperance J, et al. Silodosin to facilitate passage of ureteral stones: a multi-institutional, randomized, double-blinded, placebo-controlled trial. Eur Urol 2015;67:959–64.

27. Pickard R, Starr K, MacLennan G, et al. Medical expulsive therapy in adults with ureteric colic: a multicentre, randomised, placebo-controlled trial. Lancet 2015; 386:341–9.

28. Borghi L, Meschi T, Amato F, et al. Urinary volume, water and recurrences in idiopathic calcium nephrolithiasis: a 5-year randomized prospective study. J Urol 1996;155:839–43.

29. Nouvenne A, Meschi T, Prati B, et al. Effects of a low-salt diet on idiopathic hypercalciuria in calcium-oxalate stone formers: a 3-mo randomized controlled trial. Am J Clin Nutr 2010;91:565–70.

30. Borghi L, Schianchi T, Meschi T, et al. Comparison of two diets for the prevention of recurrent stones in idiopathic hypercalciuria. N Engl J Med 2002;346:77–84.

31. Taylor EN, Curhan GC. Oxalate intake and the risk for nephrolithiasis. J Am Soc Nephrol 2007;18:2198–204.

32. Trinchieri A, Lizzano R, Marchesotti F, et al. Effect of potential renal acid load of foods on urinary citrate excretion in calcium renal stone formers. Urol Res 2006;34:1–7.

33. Fink HA, Wilt TJ, Eidman KE, et al. Medical management to prevent recurrent nephrolithiasis in adults: a systematic review for an American College of Physicians Clinical Guideline. Ann Intern Med 2013;158:535–43.

34. Ettinger B, Citron JT, Livermore B, et al. Chlorthalidone reduces calcium oxalate calculous recurrence but magnesium hydroxide does not. J Urol 1988;139: 679–84.

35. Barcelo P, Wuhl O, Servitge E, et al. Randomized double-blind study of potassium citrate in idiopathic hypocitraturic calcium nephrolithiasis. J Urol 1993;150: 1761–4.

36. Ettinger B, Pak CY, Citron JT, et al. Potassium-magnesium citrate is an effective prophylaxis against recurrent calcium oxalate nephrolithiasis. J Urol 1997;158: 2069–73.

37. Ettinger B, Tang A, Citron JT, et al. Randomized trial of allopurinol in the prevention of calcium oxalate calculi. N Engl J Med 1986;315:1386–9.

38. Trinchieri A, Montanari E. Biochemical and dietary factors of uric acid stone formation. Urolithiasis 2017;1–6. [Epub ahead of print].

39. Bobulescu IA, Moe OW. Renal transport of uric acid: evolving concepts and uncertainties. Adv Chronic Kidney Dis 2012;19:358–71.

40. Pak CY, Sakhaee K, Fuller C. Successful management of uric acid nephrolithiasis with potassium citrate. Kidney Int 1986;30:422–8.

41. Rodman JS. Intermittent versus continuous alkaline therapy for uric acid stones and ureteral stones of uncertain composition. Urology 2002;60:378–82.

42. Moran ME, Abrahams HM, Burday DE, et al. Utility of oral dissolution therapy in the management of referred patients with secondarily treated uric acid stones. Urology 2002;59:206–10.

43. Heilberg I. Treatment of patients with uric acid stones. Urolithiasis 2016;44:57–63.

44. Andreassen KH, Pedersen KV, Osther SS, et al. How should patients with cystine stone disease be evaluated and treated in the twenty-first century? Urolithiasis 2016;44:65–76.

45. Rogers A, Kalakish S, Desai R, et al. Management of cystinuria. Urol Clin North Am 2007;34:347–62.

46. Rodman JS, Blackburn P, Williams JJ, et al. The effect of dietary protein on cystine excretion in patients with cystinuria. Clin Nephrol 1984;22:273–8.

47. Jaeger P, Portmann L, Saunders A, et al. Anticystinuric effects of glutamine and of dietary sodium restriction. N Engl J Med 1986;315:1120–3.

48. Tekin A, Tekgul S, Atsu N, et al. Cystine calculi in children: the results of a metabolic evaluation and response to medical therapy. J Urol 2001;165:2328–30.

49. Smith AD, Lange PH, Miller RP, et al. Dissolution of cystine calculi by irrigation with acetylcysteine through percutaneous nephrostomy. Urology 1979;13:422–3.

50. Pak CY, Fuller C, Sakhaee K, et al. Management of cystine nephrolithiasis with alpha-mercaptopropionylglycine. J Urol 1986;136:1003–8.

51. Fattah H, Hambaroush Y, Goldfarb DS. Cystine nephrolithiasis. Transl Androl Urol 2014;3:228–33.

52. Chow GK, Streem SB. Medical treatment of cystinuria: results of contemporary clinical practice. J Urol 1996;156:1576–8.

53. Michelakakis H, Delis D, Anastasiadou V, et al. Ineffectiveness of captopril in reducing cystine excretion in cystinuric children. J Inherit Metab Disord 1993; 16:1042–3.

54. Marien T, Miller NL. Treatment of the infected stone. Urol Clin North America 2015; 42:459–72.

55. Griffith DP, Gleeson MJ, Lee H, et al. Randomized, double-blind trial of Lithostat (acetohydroxamic acid) in the palliative treatment of infection-induced urinary calculi. Eur Urol 1991;20:243–7.

56. Rodman JS, Williams JJ, Jones RL. Hypercoagulability produced by treatment with acetohydroxamic acid. Clin Pharmacol Ther 1987;42:346–50.

57. Geraghty R, Jones P, Somani B. Worldwide trends of urinary stone disease treatment over the last two decades: a systematic review. J Endourol 2017;31(6): 547–56.

58. Oberlin DT, Flum AS, Bachrach L, et al. Contemporary surgical trends in the management of upper tract calculi. J Urol 2015;193:880–4.

59. Marchini GS, Mello MF, Levy R, et al. Contemporary trends of inpatient surgical management of stone disease: national analysis in an economic growth scenario. J Endourol 2015;29:956–62.

60. Turna B, Stein RJ, Smaldone MC, et al. Safety and efficacy of flexible ureterorenoscopy and holmium:yag lithotripsy for intrarenal stones in anticoagulated cases. J Urol 2008;179:1415–9.

61. De S, Autorino R, Kim FJ, et al. Percutaneous nephrolithotomy versus retrograde intrarenal surgery: a systematic review and meta-analysis. Eur Urol 2015;67: 125–37.

62. Druskin SC, Ziemba JB. Minimally invasive ('Mini') percutaneous nephrolithotomy: classification, indications, and outcomes. Curr Urol Rep 2016;17:30.

63. Grasso M, Conlin M, Bagley D. Retrograde ureteropyeloscopic treatment of 2 cm. or greater upper urinary tract and minor staghorn calculi. J Urol 1998;160: 346–51.

64. Cohen J, Cohen S, Grasso M. Ureteropyeloscopic treatment of large, complex intrarenal and proximal ureteral calculi. BJU Int 2013;111(3 Pt B):E127–31.

65. Assimos D, Krambeck A, Miller NL, et al. Surgical management of stones: AUA/Endourology Society Guideline. J Urol 2016;196:1153–60.

66. Gallucci M, Vincenzoni A, Schettini M, et al. Extracorporeal shock wave lithotripsy in ureteral and kidney. Urol Int 2001;66:61–5.

67. Pace KT, Weir MJ, Tariq N, et al. Low success rate of repeat shock wave lithotripsy for ureteral stones after failed initial treatment. J Urol 2000;164:1905–7.

68. Tugcu V, Gürbüz G, Aras B, et al. Primary ureteroscopy for distal-ureteral stones compared with ureteroscopy after failed extracorporeal lithotripsy. J Endourol 2006;20:1025–9.

69. Li S, Liu TZ, Wang XH, et al. Randomized controlled trial comparing retroperitoneal laparoscopic pyelolithotomy versus percutaneous nephrolithotomy for the treatment of large renal pelvic calculi: a pilot study. J Endourol 2014;28:946–50.

70. Zheng J, Yan J, Zhou Z, et al. Concomitant treatment of ureteropelvic junction obstruction and renal calculi with robotic laparoscopic surgery and rigid nephroscopy. Urology 2014;83:237–42.

71. Hubner WA, Irby P, Stoller ML. Natural history and current concepts for the treatment of small ureteral calculi. Eur Urol 1993;24:172–6.

72. Vaughan E, Gillenwater J. Recovery following complete chronic unilateral ureteral occlusion: functional, radiographic and pathologic alterations. J Urol 1973;100: 27.

73. Borofsky MS, Walter D, Shah O, et al. Surgical decompression is associated with decreased mortality in patients with sepsis and ureteral calculi. J Urol 2013;189: 946–51.

74. Aboumarzouk O, Kata S, Keeley FX, et al. Extracorporeal shock wave lithotripsy (ESWL) versus ureteroscopic management for ureteric calculi. Cochrane Database Syst Rev 2012;(16):CD006029.

75. Zhong P, Preminger GM. Mechanisms of differing stone fragility in extracorporeal shockwave lithotripsy. J Endourol 1994;8:263–8.

76. Zhou L, Cai X, Li H, et al. Effects of α-blockers, antimuscarinics, or combination therapy in relieving ureteral stent-related symptoms: a meta-analysis. J Endourol 2015;29:650–6.

77. Yakoubi R, Lemdani M, Monga M, et al. Is there a role for alpha-blockers in ureteral stent related symptoms? A systematic review and meta-analysis. J Urol 2011;186:928–34.

78. Basiri A, Simforoosh N, Ziaee A, et al. Retrograde, antegrade, and laparoscopic approaches for the management of large, proximal ureteral stones: a randomized clinical trial. J Endourol 2008;22:2677–80.

79. Falahatkar S, Khosropanah I, Allahkhah A, et al. Open surgery, laparoscopic surgery, or transureteral lithotripsy–which method? Comparison of ureteral stone management outcomes. J Endourol 2011;25:31–4.

80. Glowacki LS, Beecroft ML, Cook RJ, et al. The natural history of asymptomatic urolithiasis. J Urol 1992;147:319–21.

81. Burgher A, Beman M, Holtzman JL, et al. Progression of nephrolithiasis: long-term outcomes with observation of asymptomatic calculi. J Endourol 2004; 18:534–9.

82. Koh LT, Ng FC, Ng KK. Outcomes of long-term follow-up of patients with conservative management of asymptomatic renal calculi. BJU Int 2012;109:622–5.
83. Pearle MS, Lingeman JE, Leveillee R, et al. Prospective randomized trial comparing shock wave lithotripsy and ureteroscopy for lower pole caliceal calculi 1 cm or less. J Urol 2008;179:69–73.
84. Albala DM, Assimos DG, Clayman RV, et al. Lower pole I: a prospective randomized trial of extracorporeal shock wave lithotripsy and percutaneous nephrostolithotomy for lower pole nephrolithiasis-initial results. J Urol 2001;166:2072–80.
85. Srisubat A, Potisat S, Lojanapiwat B, et al. Extracorporeal shock wave lithotripsy (ESWL) versus percutaneous nephrolithotomy (PCNL) or retrograde intrarenal surgery (RIRS) for kidney stones. Cochrane Database Syst Rev 2014;(11):CD007044.
86. Lam HS, Lingeman JE, Barron M, et al. Staghorn calculi: analysis of treatment results between initial percutaneous nephrostolithotomy and extracorporeal shock wave lithotripsy monotherapy with reference to surface area. J Urol 1992;147:1219–25.
87. Karakoyunlu N, Goktug G, Şener NC, et al. A comparison of standard PCNL and staged retrograde FURS in pelvis stones over 2 cm in diameter: a prospective randomized study. Urolithiasis 2015;43:283–7.
88. Bryniarski P, Paradysz A, Zyczkowski M, et al. A randomized controlled study to analyze the safety and efficacy of percutaneous nephrolithotripsy and retrograde intrarenal surgery in the management of renal stones more than 2 cm in diameter. J Endourol 2012;26:52–7.
89. Zelhof B, McIntyre IG, Fowler SM, et al. Nephrectomy for benign disease in the UK: results from the British Association of Urological Surgeons nephrectomy database. BJU Int 2016;117:138–44.
90. Rous SN, Turner WR. Retrospective study of 95 patients with staghorn calculus disease. J Urol 1977;118:902–4.
91. Teichman JM, Long RD, Hulbert JC. Long-term renal fate and prognosis after staghorn calculus management. J Urol 1995;153:1403–7.

Cutaneous Lesions of the External Genitalia

Emily Yura, MD, Sarah Flury, MD*

KEYWORDS

- Cutaneous lesion • Dermatosis • Genitalia • Sexually transmitted infection
- Malignancy • Urology • Dermatology

KEY POINTS

- Widespread dermatoses may also affect the skin of the genitals, and these lesions may have distinct or atypical morphology compared with extragenital lesions.
- Malignant transformation may occur in background of benign conditions.
- Uncircumcised men are at increased risk for developing malignancy of the genitalia.
- Lesions that do not respond as expected to indicated treatment should be referred to a specialist because of concern for premalignant or malignant changes.

INITIAL EVALUATION

Individuals with cutaneous diseases of the external genitalia often initially present to their primary care provider. When present, these conditions may be associated with considerable physical symptoms and psychological distress. Initial evaluation of these patients requires obtaining a complete history with attention to associated symptoms, including sexual or urinary dysfunction, circumcision status, sexual history including contraceptive use, personal and family history, medications, and drug use. A thorough genital examination and a complete skin survey are necessary.

GENITAL INVOLVEMENT OF SYSTEMIC SKIN DISEASES

Many systemic dermatoses have genital manifestations that resemble their extragenital counterparts and thus are excluded from this review. However, some skin conditions have distinct or atypical genital lesions that differ from those located on extragenital sites. Occasionally, the genital lesion is the first or only manifestation of the systemic condition.

Disclosure Statement: The authors have no disclosures.
Department of Urology, Northwestern University, Tarry Building Room 16-703, 300 East Superior Street, Chicago, IL 60611, USA
* Corresponding author.
E-mail address: Sflury@nm.org

Med Clin N Am 102 (2018) 279–300
https://doi.org/10.1016/j.mcna.2017.10.012
0025-7125/18/© 2017 Elsevier Inc. All rights reserved.

Psoriasis

The characteristic lesion of psoriasis is a sharply demarcated, erythematous plaque with silvery-white scales, often affecting the extensor surfaces of the skin. Genital involvement in this condition is common affecting 30% to 40% of patients[1] and is typically in the context of extragenital lesions. Lesions on the genitals have variable appearance depending on their site. When located in intertrigonal regions (inguinal folds, intergluteal cleft, under preputial skin, on the labia), lesions tend to weep instead of scale.[2,3] When found on the glans or corona of circumcised men, plaques typically scale (**Fig. 1**); lesions may involve the entire penis and scrotum.[3]

Diagnosis of genital psoriasis can usually be made clinically; if associated with intertrigonal lesions, fungal infection should be ruled out. Mainstay of treatment is low-potency topical steroid for a short course (maximum of 2 weeks). Other approaches include topical vitamin D_3 analogues, topical calcineurin inhibitors, and low-potency retinoids.[4]

Lichen Planus

Lichen planus (LP) is an idiopathic inflammatory disease affecting the skin and mucous membranes with genital involvement in 25% of cases.[5,6] Lesions typical of LP are small, polygonal, violaceous flat-topped papules that commonly involve the flexor surfaces of the extremities, trunk, and lumbrosacral area. Oral mucosa may also be involved. When involving the genitalia, the appearance is variable and may include isolated or grouped papules, a white reticular pattern (known as Wickham striae; **Fig. 2**), or an annular arrangement of papules with or without ulceration.[7] Genital lesions may be associated with pruritus, pain, or burning, or may be asymptomatic. In men, the glans of the penis is most often involved and may have an erosive component; in women, lesions mainly involve the labia minora and the vaginal introitus and may erode, leading to pain, burning with urination, and dyspareunia. In long-standing LP, white plaques may develop around erosive lesions. Lesions often resolve spontaneously after a year; however, isolated cases of squamous cell carcinoma (SCC) arising in chronic genital lesions has been reported.[8]

Diagnosis of LP involving the genitals is clinical, but biopsy may be performed to establish the diagnosis, particularly if the lesions are noncharacteristic or isolated to the genitalia.[3] The mainstay of treatment of symptomatic genital LP is short course of high-potency topical corticosteroid (ie, clobetasol, 0.05% or halobetasol, 0.05%). Topical calcineurin inhibitors may also be used.[9] Systemic corticosteroid therapy

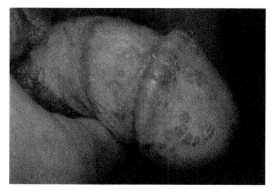

Fig. 1. Psoriasis on a circumcised phallus. (*From* English JC, Laws RA, Keough GC, et al. Dermatoses of the glans penis and prepuce. J Am Acad Dermatol 1997;37(1):14; with permission.)

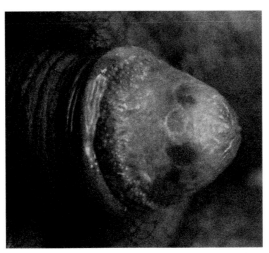

Fig. 2. Lichen planus, with Wickham striae. (*From* Andreassi L, Bilenchi R. Non-infectious inflammatory genital lesions. Clin Dermatol 2014;32(2):309; with permission.)

may shorten the time course to clearance of lesions in those with widespread involvement.

Lichen Sclerosus/Balanitis Xerotica Obliterans

Lichen sclerosus (LS) is a chronic inflammatory skin disease with a predilection for the external genitalia; the condition has a relapsing and remitting course, ultimately leading to scarring of the affected tissue. LS is more common in women than in men and has a bimodal age distribution, occurring most commonly in prepubertal years and around the time of menopause (in women) or after the age of 60 (in men).[10] Appearance of genital lesions is variable, with atrophic white patches or plaques on the glans or prepuce, or fine scaly lilac-colored patches.[11] Associated symptoms include dyspareunia, pruritus, burning, bleeding, dysuria, and in men may be associated with changes in urinary stream. Late manifestations include scarring leading to phimosis and urethral strictures in men (**Fig. 3**), or vulvar adhesions with labial fusion, clitoral

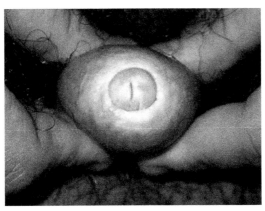

Fig. 3. Lichen sclerosus with phimosis and meatal stenosis. (*From* Micali G, Nasca MR, Innocenzi D, et al. Penile cancer. J Am Acad Dermatol 2006;54(3):373; with permission.)

phimosis, and vaginal obstruction in women. Extragenital disease occurs in 15% to 20% of patients.[10] There exists an association with SCC of the penis and vulva and thus LS may represent a premalignant condition.[9]

Although diagnosis may be made clinically, biopsy may be worthwhile to confirm the diagnosis and exclude malignant change. Treatment of LS involves high-potency topical corticosteroids for prolonged course (2–3 months). Patients with symptoms refractory to topical therapy, or those with phimosis, meatal stenosis, or urethral stricture should be referred to a surgical specialist, and urgent referral should be made in those with erosive, hyperkeratotic, or verrucous changes because of concern for neoplastic condition.[12]

Erythema Multiforme

Erythema multiforme (EM) is a self-limited skin condition characterized by acute development of symmetric fixed red papules that may evolve into "target" lesions. These lesions are often grouped and may arise anywhere on the body, including the genitalia. Lesions often arise on the palms and soles and the oral mucosa. In most extreme manifestations, EM is called Stevens-Johnson syndrome, which has a high mortality rate and requires inpatient admission to a burn unit. Stevens-Johnson syndrome genital manifestations include erythema and erosions of the labia, penis, and perianal region. Long-term complications include labial adhesions, stenosis of the vagina and urethral meatus, and anal strictures; these complications may ultimately require surgical management.[13]

In recurrent cases of EM minor, there is an association with herpes simplex virus (HSV), and thus suppressive acyclovir may thwart the appearance of EM lesions.[14] Treatment otherwise is supportive as the lesions regress spontaneously over several weeks. Inciting drugs should be avoided; nonsteroidal anti-inflammatory drugs, various antibiotics, and anticonvulsants are the typical culprits and should be discontinued immediately in patients with Stevens-Johnson syndrome.[9]

Reactive Arthritis (Formerly Reiter Syndrome)

Reactive arthritis is characterized by the triad of nongonococcal urethritis, arthritis, and conjunctivitis. Dermatologic involvement is also common. Involvement of the male genitalia, known as balanitis circinata, is reported in 12% to 70% of men with this condition.[5] These lesions are dry and hyperkeratotic plaques with similar appearance to psoriasis on circumcised patients; on the uncircumcised, lesions begin as small vesicles or pustules on the glans that rupture and form painless superficial erosions with a scalloped or serpiginous pattern (**Fig. 4**).[15] The condition is less common in females but has similar morphology to balanitis circinata, and may be associated with vaginal discharge. This condition typically self-resolves over the course of a few weeks to months. Low-potency topical steroids may be used.[9]

Fixed Drug Eruption

A fixed drug eruption occurs 1 to 2 weeks following initial exposure to an oral medication; with subsequent exposures, the lesion recurs in the exact same location within 24 hours. Typical sites of involvement include the lips, face, hands, feet, and genitalia.[9] The lesions are usually solitary, violaceous inflammatory plaques on the penile shaft or glans with clear borders (**Fig. 5**) and may blister and erode and be associated with pain and pruritus.[16] Lesions heal with time but may leave hyperpigmented patches. Barbiturates, sulfonamides, salicylates, nonsteroidal anti-inflammatory drugs, and tetracyclines are commonly implicated in causing these reactions and should be avoided.[3]

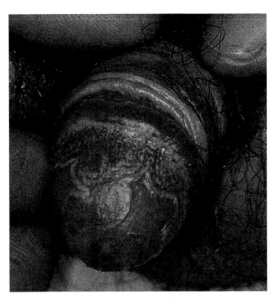

Fig. 4. Balanitis circinata of reactive arthritis. (*From* Wu IB, Schwartz RA. Reiter's syndrome: the classic triad and more. J Am Acad Dermatol 2008;59(1):117; with permission.)

NONINFECTIOUS ULCERS
Behçet Disease

Behçet disease (BD) is a chronic relapsing systemic vasculitis of small vessels that may have a genetic predisposition; the classic triad includes oral aphthous ulcers, genital ulcers, and uveitis but widespread manifestations include involvement of the joints and neurologic, gastrointestinal, pulmonary, vascular, genitourinary, and cardiac systems.[17] Genital lesions are generally painful and may be the initial presenting sign in 18% of patients.[17] Such lesions are oval or round with a gray-yellow necrotic base, with an erythematous halo or rim (**Fig. 6**).[17] In men, lesions most commonly occur on the scrotum and less often on the glans and shaft; in women lesions are often located on the labia and vaginal mucosa and sometimes on the cervix. Genital ulcers

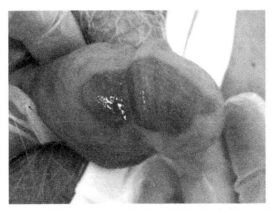

Fig. 5. Fixed drug eruption. (*From* Andreassi L, Bilenchi R. Non-infectious inflammatory genital lesions. Clin Dermatol 2014;32(2):311; with permission.)

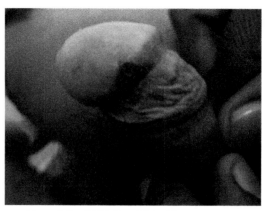

Fig. 6. Behçet disease. (*From* Sehgal VN, Pandhi D, Khurana A. Nonspecific genital ulcers. Clin Dermatol 2014;32(2):262; with permission.)

typically persist for 10 to 30 days and often scar, so in the absence of active lesions, clinicians should look for evidence of scar when suspecting BD.[17]

There is no specific diagnostic test for BD; diagnosis is made on the aggregate of findings and relies heavily on the presence of mucocutaneous signs, but other causes of genital ulceration (chancre, chancroid, HSV) should be considered before a diagnosis of BD is made. Rheumatologic evaluation is advised when BD is suspected. Treatment of genital ulcers includes topical corticosteroids, dapsone, colchicine, 5-aminosalicylic acid derivatives, cyclosporine A, and tumor necrosis factor-α inhibitors.[9]

Pyoderma Gangrenosum

Pyoderma gangrenosum is an ulcerative skin condition associated with systemic illness including inflammatory bowel disease, collagen vascular disease, arthritis, human immunodeficiency virus (HIV), hepatitis, and myeloproliferative disease. The condition can involve the penis, scrotum, vulva, and peristomal sites; genital lesions are commonly ulcerative with a raised, dusky-red border and a boggy, necrotic base, but may have a bright red halo that extends 2 cm into neighboring, apparently normal skin.[9] No specific diagnostic study or clinical feature is pathognomonic for this condition, and diagnosis of pyoderma gangrenosum requires satisfaction of various criteria. Biopsy is not necessary but further testing (eg, endoscopic evaluation, serum protein electropheresis [SPEP]) to evaluate for associated conditions should be undertaken. Topical steroids, tacrolimus, and imiquimod may be prescribed for local disease, but severe disease may warrant systemic therapy with oral corticosteroid or cyclosporine.[9]

INFECTIOUS DISORDERS
Genital Herpes

Genital herpes is a chronic recurring condition arising from HSV 1 or 2 infection. Most transmissions of anogenital herpes occur from individuals who do not know they are infected.[18] Classic initial presentation occurs 4 to 7 days following exposure and is characterized by clusters of erythematous papules and vesicles on the external genitalia (**Fig. 7**); atypical lesions may resemble furuncles or fissures.[19] These lesions may progress and coalesce into ulcers before crusting and healing. Recurrent episodes tend to be milder than the initial infection and may not involve the genitals.

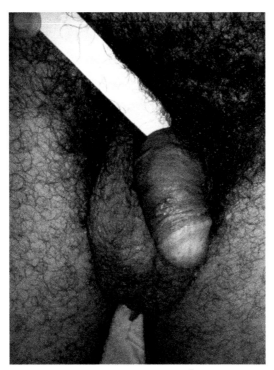

Fig. 7. Genital herpes infection. (*From* Basta-Juzbašić A, Čeović R. Chancroid, lymphogranuloma venereum, granuloma inguinale, genital herpes simplex infection, and molluscum contagiosum. Clin Dermatol 2014;32(2):294; with permission.)

Diagnosis of HSV may be performed by viral culture or polymerase chain reaction assay of fluid from the base of a lesion; this method is more accurate in initial episodes and declines as lesions heal or in recurrent episodes. Tzanck preparation should not be relied on.[20] Type-specific HSV serologic antibodies should be pursued in the following scenarios: (1) recurrent genital symptoms or atypical symptoms with negative HSV polymerase chain reaction or culture, (2) clinical diagnosis of genital herpes without laboratory confirmation, and (3) patients whose partner has genital herpes. It should also be considered in individuals presenting for a sexually transmitted disease evaluation (especially if have multiple sex partners), persons with HIV infection, and men who have sex with men at increased risk for HIV acquisition.[18] It should not be used for screening the general population. Treatment of HSV does not eradicate the infection nor does it affect the risk, frequency, or severity of recurrence after the drug is discontinued. It may provide symptomatic relief and reduce the recurrence of new lesions.[19] Topical therapy offers minimal clinical benefit and is discouraged. **Table 1** outlines the treatments of choice as described by the Centers for Disease Control and Prevention.

Genital Warts/Human Papilloma Virus

Most human papilloma virus (HPV) infections are self-limited and asymptomatic. More than 50% of sexually active persons become infected in their lifetime.[19] Transmission can occur from symptomatic, asymptomatic, or subclinical patients. The HPV vaccine can prevent genital warts but does not treat existing conditions.[18] Most (90%) of these

Table 1
Treatment of genital herpes

	First Episode	Suppressive Therapy	Episodic Treatment
Acyclovir	400 mg po bid × 7–10 d 200 mg po 5 ×/d × 7–10 d	400 mg po bid	400 mg po tid × 5 d 800 mg po bid × 5 d 800 mg po tid × 2 d
Valacyclovir	1 g po bid × 7–10 d	500 mg po qd[a] 1 g po qd	500 mg po bid × 3 d 1 g po qd × 5 d
Famciclovir	250 mg po tid × 7–10 d	250 mg po bid	125 mg bid × 5 d 1 g po qd × 1 d 500 mg po once, then 250 mg po bid × 2 d

[a] Valacyclovir, 500 mg po daily, may be less effective than 1 g po daily if patient has frequent recurrences.
Adapted from Workowski KA, Bolan GA, Centers for Disease Control and Prevention. Sexually transmitted diseases treatment guidelines, 2015. MMWR Recomm Rep 2015;64(RR-03):1–137.

infections resolve spontaneously in 2 years. The appearance of anogenital warts is variable, with flat, papular, or pedunculated growths (**Fig. 8**). Lesions are typically asymptomatic but may be painful or pruritic depending on the size and location. Common sites include around the vaginal introitus, under the foreskin of the uncircumcised penis, and on the shaft of the circumcised penis.[21] They may also occur within the urethra, vagina, or anus.[18]

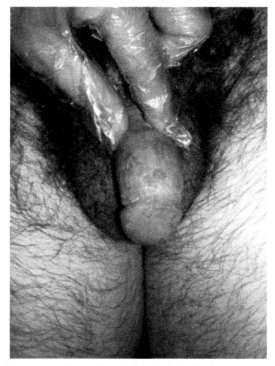

Fig. 8. Penile condyloma acuminata. (*From* Ljubojevic S, Skerlev M. HPV-associated diseases. Clin Dermatol 2014;32(2):228; with permission.)

Diagnosis of anogenital warts is made clinically but may be confirmed by biopsy, which is indicated in the following scenarios[18]:

1. The diagnosis is uncertain
2. The patient is immunocompromised
3. The lesions are pigmented, indurated, or fixed
4. The lesion does not respond or worsens with standard treatment
5. There is persistent ulceration or bleeding

Use of acetic acid to detect nonvisible skin lesions is not recommended because of low specificity.[19] If left untreated, most lesions resolve spontaneously, but they may remain unchanged or increase in size or number. Treatment options are outlined in **Table 2**.

Syphilis

Syphilis is a systemic disease caused by infection by *Treponema pallidum*, and anogenital cutaneous lesions are typical of primary and secondary syphilis. Primary syphilis is marked by a single chancre at the site of infection that appears 9 to 90 days after the infection.[19] The chancre is a solitary painless, indurated, firm, and round lesion with a clean base (**Fig. 9**); it may also be associated with nontender lymphadenopathy. In men, lesions are typically located on the glans or in the coronal or perineal area; in women, lesions are often on the labia or perianal skin. The chancre lasts 3 to 6 weeks and heals regardless of whether a person is treated or not.[19] Secondary syphilis appears 3 to 5 months following initial infection and is characterized by a maculopapular rash that may be widespread and involve the scalp, palms and soles. The rash may ulcerate and lead to wart-like lesions (condyloma lata), which are raised, large gray

Table 2
Treatment of external anogenital warts

Patient Applied	Provider Administered
Imiquimod	Cryotherapy
5% cream: apply qh 3 ×/wk	May repeat application q 1–2 wk
3.75% cream: qh every night	Surgical removal
Wash with soap and water 6–10 h after	Direct excision, shave excision, curettage,
application	laser
Use for up to 16 wk	Trichloroacetic acid or bichloroacetic acid
Podofilox	80%–90% solution
0.5% solution or gel	Apply small amount to warts and allow
Apply to lesions bid for 3 d, followed by	to dry until develops white frost
4 d of no therapy, and repeat up to	before the patient stands
four cycles	If too much acid applied, neutralize with
Limit total volume applied to 0.5 mL/d,	baking soda or liquid soap
and total wart area not to exceed	preparations
10 cm²	May repeat weekly if necessary
Sinecatechins	Podophyllin resin
15% ointment	10%–25% in tincture of benzoin
Apply 0.5-cm strand of ointment to each	Limit to area <10 cm² or <0.5 mL used, to
wart tid with a finger until complete	areas without open lesions or wounds
clearance is achieved, but should not	
exceed 16 wk	
Do not wash after application	

Adapted from Workowski KA, Bolan GA, Centers for Disease Control and Prevention. Sexually transmitted diseases treatment guidelines, 2015. MMWR Recomm Rep 2015;64(RR-03):1–137.

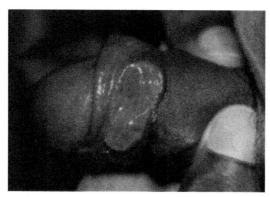

Fig. 9. Penile chancre. (*From* English JC, Laws RA, Keough GC, et al. Dermatoses of the glans penis and prepuce. J Am Acad Dermatol 1997;37(1):8; with permission.)

or white lesions that may develop in the mouth, underarm, groin, or genitals. Other symptoms may include fever, malaise, weight loss, patchy alopecia, and ocular inflammation, and broad vasculitis.[19]

Diagnosis of syphilis requires testing with a nontreponemal test and a treponemal test. Darkfield examination is no longer recommended.[19] Penicillin G via different dosing regimens is the preferred agent for treating all stages of syphilis[18]; see **Table 3** for recommended treatment.

Table 3 Treatment of syphilis		
Stage of Syphilis	**Penicillin Treatment**	**Penicillin-Allergic Patients**
Primary, secondary, and early latent syphilis (no neurologic involvement)	Benzathine penicillin G, 2.4 million units IM, single dose	Doxycycline, 100 mg po bid × 2 wk Tetracycline, 500 mg po qid × 2 wk
Late latent or latent syphilis of unknown duration, no neurologic involvement	Benzathine penicillin G, 2.4 million units IM once per week for 3 wk	Doxycycline, 100 mg po bid × 28 d Tetracycline, 500 mg po qid × 28 d
Tertiary (late) syphilis without neurologic involvement	Benzathine penicillin G, 2.4 million units IM once per week × 3 wk	Consult infectious disease specialist
Neurosyphilis	Aqueous crystalline penicillin G, 3–4 million units IV q 4 h, or continuous infusion of total 18–24 million units per day, for 10–14 d Alternative: procaine penicillin, 2.4 million units IM daily, PLUS probenecid, 500 mg po qid, for 10–14 d	

Abbreviations: IM, intramuscularly; IV, intravenously.

Adapted from Workowski KA, Bolan GA, Centers for Disease Control and Prevention. Sexually transmitted diseases treatment guidelines, 2015. MMWR Recomm Rep 2015;64(RR-03):1–137.

Chancroid

Chancroid is a sexually transmitted infection caused by *Haemophilus ducreyi* with declining prevalence in the United States. Chancroid lesions are described as a tender papule that becomes a painful, undermined purulent ulcer; lesions may be solitary or multiple and are often associated with tender regional suppurative lymphadenopathy. Lesions typically present 3 to 10 days after transmission.[19] There are no Food and Drug Administration approved diagnostic tests for chancroid. A probable diagnosis is made if all the following criteria are met[18]:

1. Presence of one or more painful genital ulcers
2. The appearance of ulcers, and, if present, regional lymphadenopathy are typical for chancroid
3. The patient has no evidence of *T pallidum* infection at least 7 days after onset of ulcers
4. HSV testing on the ulcer exudate is negative

Treatment is curative of infection and is outlined in **Box 1**; patients should be examined 3 to 7 days after initiation of therapy, because successful treatment should result in symptomatic improvement within 3 days and objective improvement within 7 days. If no clinical improvement is evident, additional testing for HIV or other sexually transmitted infection should be performed.[19] Resolution of lymphadenopathy is slower and may require needle aspiration or incision and drainage.[18]

Scabies

Scabies infection caused by the mite *Sarcopetes scabiei* occurs via person-to-person transmission via passage of pregnant female mites; this may occur during sexual contact. Symptoms typically appear 2 to 6 weeks following infestation, and transmission may occur in the absence of symptoms. Symptoms include skin rash and itching caused by an allergic reaction to the mite proteins.[18] On examination, raised and serpiginous lines may appear on the skin, and the lesions may become secondarily infected.[18] Crusted scabies (ie, Norwegian scabies) is an aggressive infestation that occurs in immunodeficient, debilitated, or malnourished individuals, and is more easily transmissible than scabies. Diagnosis is made by microscopic examination of skin scrapings with demonstration of mites, mite eggs, or fecal matter.[19] Treatment involves topical therapy (permethrin 5% cream as first-line therapy, lindane 1% lotion or cream if one cannot tolerate other therapy) and oral regimens (ivermectin, 200 µg/kg by mouth). Crusted scabies should be treated with combination therapy with topical permethrin and oral ivermectin.[18]

Box 1
Treatment of chancroid

Azithromycin, 1 g po in a single dose

Ceftriaxone, 250 mg intramuscularly in a single dose

Ciprofloxacin, 500 mg po bid × 3 days

Erythromycin, base 500 mg po tid × 7 days

Adapted from Workowski KA, Bolan GA, Centers for Disease Control and Prevention. Sexually transmitted diseases treatment guidelines, 2015. MMWR Recomm Rep 2015;64(RR-03):1–137.

Molluscum Contagiosum

Molluscum contagiosum is a superficial skin infection caused by poxvirus. Transmission may occur via person-to-person contact but also via contaminated fomites, and may spread because of autoinoculation.[18] Lesions arise anywhere on the body including the genitalia, and are small, raised, firm papules with central umbillication, that are white, pink, or flesh-colored, with a waxy appearance. Lesions spontaneously disappear within 6 to 12 months but may take up to 4 years to resolve.[19] In immuno-compromised individuals, lesions may be more widespread in number and size; in HIV, low CD4 count is inversely proportional to the number of molluscum lesions.[18]

Diagnosis is made clinically. Lesions spontaneously resolve but treatment should be pursued for lesions arising in the anogenital region. Rapid treatment with cryotherapy, curettage, or laser therapy may be performed, or topical therapy with podophyllotoin cream, iodine and salicylic acid, potassium hydroxide, cantharidin, and imiquimod. In HIV-positive individuals, first treatment is to initiate highly active antiretroviral therapy.[18]

Balanitis and Balanoposthitis

Balanitis (inflammation of the glans penis; **Fig. 10**) and balanoposthitis (inflammation involving the foreskin) is commonly caused by bacterial or candida infection but may be caused by contact dermatitis.[9] Initial treatment includes lifestyle modifications including avoidance of irritating agents, improved hygiene, topical antibiotic or antifungal, or low-potency topical corticosteroid. Circumcision may be curative in recurrent balanoposthitis. If treatment fails, alternative diagnosis should be pursued.[9]

Cellulitis and Erysipelas

Cellulitis and erysipelas may occur on the genitalia and is commonly caused by gram-positive organisms. Etiology may be local infection or blood-borne infection.[9] Signs and symptoms include pain, erythema, warmth, and swelling. Erysipelas typically has a raised and distinct border at the interface with normal skin. Treatment with systemic antibiotics targeting *Streptococcus pyogenes* and *Staphylococcus aureus* according to local antimicrobial sensitivity patterns should be pursued, with marking

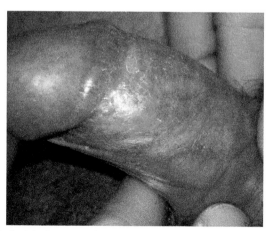

Fig. 10. Irritative balanitis. (*From* Andreassi L, Bilenchi R. Non-infectious inflammatory genital lesions. Clin Dermatol 2014;32(2):311; with permission.)

of the zone of involvement to allow monitoring for progression versus regression of the condition.[9]

Fournier Gangrene

Necrotizing fasciitis of the perineum, called Fournier gangrene, is a rare condition associated with a high mortality rate.[22] The condition occurs with a higher incidence in men and risk factors for development include diabetes mellitus, alcoholism, HIV, cancer, malnutrition, advanced age, recent genitourinary or anorectal instrumentation, and peripheral vascular disease.[9] The condition is characterized by rapid progression from signs and symptoms of cellulitis to clinically visible ischemia (**Fig. 11**). Patients often present with scrotal pain, swelling, and erythema, with systemic signs including fever, rigors, and tachycardia.[23] On examination, pain out of proportion to the visible extent of infection, purulent discharge, crepitus, tissue necrosis, foul odor, and edema may be present.[9,23] This condition is a surgical emergency and debridement combined with broad-spectrum antibiotics should not be delayed.

Hidradenitis Suppurativa

Hidradenitis suppurativa is a chronic inflammatory disease involving apocrine gland–bearing regions (axilla, groin, perianal, inframammary regions).[9] The condition is highly variable and ranges from mild cases with recurrent tender subcutaneous nodules, to more severe cases where deep abscesses, fibrosis, draining sinuses, and hypertrophic scars may develop (**Fig. 12**). In addition, serious complications may occur including hyperproteinemia, secondary amyloidosis, fistulae development, and development of SCC in regions of heavy scarring.[9] Typical presentation is with a painful nodule that flares or drains repeatedly in the same sites, despite incision and drainage and/or a short course of antibiotics.

Diagnosis is clinical. Severity of the condition is graded using the Hurley classification, which is also used to guide treatment.[24] Hurley grade II or III should be referred to specialists.[25] Mild disease may be treated with topical clindamycin 1% lotion applied twice a day, or oral tetracycline; alternative antibiotics, zinc, retinoids, cyclosporine, and hormone blockers (spironolactone and oral contraceptives in women, 5-alpha reductase inhibitors in men) may also be used.[9] Lifestyle modification, such as improvement in hygiene, weight loss, and efforts to minimize friction in affected areas, may also improve clinical course. Surgical management is sometimes necessary with

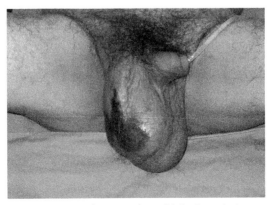

Fig. 11. Early Fournier gangrene. (*From* Kobayashi S. Fournier's gangrene. Am J Surg 2008;195(2):257; with permission.)

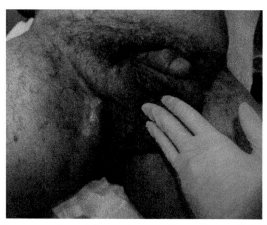

Fig. 12. Hidradenitis suppurativa of the perineum. (*From* Martorell A, García-Martínez FJ, Jiménez-Gallo D, et al. An update on hidradenitis suppurativa (part I): epidemiology, clinical aspects, and definition of disease severity. Actas Dermosifiliogr 2015;106(9):708; with permission.)

wide and deep excision of the affected regions. Simple incision and drainage of painful boils is not recommended because it does not prevent recurrence.[25]

NEOPLASTIC CONDITIONS

In men, the presence of foreskin is the greatest risk factor for developing penile malignancy. Phimosis and balanitis with poor personal and sexual hygiene increase risk for developing penile neoplasm. Rare cases of carcinoma of the penis have been reported in individuals circumcised at birth.[26] LS and LP may also predispose to development of neoplasm of the genitalia, as can HPV infection.[3]

Squamous Cell Carcinoma In Situ/Bowen Disease

SCC in situ is a full-thickness carcinoma that typically has an indolent course and rarely progresses to invasive disease. There are many names for this entity, including Bowen disease, erythroplasia of Queryat (when it occurs on mucosal surface of the penis), and penile or vulvar intraepithelial neoplasia. This condition is associated with HPV infection. The lesions of SCC in situ are sharply demarcated and usually solitary, with pink or red scaly plaques (**Fig. 13**), and may crust or ulcerate. Erythroplasia of Queryat occurs on the glans or inner foreskin with bright red shiny and nontender plaques (**Fig. 14**).[27] Lesions are typically asymptomatic but may be associated with pruritus, pain, bleeding, and difficulty retracting the foreskin.[3] It may be mistaken for basal cell carcinoma, eczema, or psoriasis. Diagnosis of the condition should be made by biopsy, and the affected areas should be surgically excised or ablated.

Bowenoid Papulosis

Bowenoid papulosis is a condition found on the penis and vulva, more commonly in young, sexually active patients. Lesions in this condition may be solitary or multiple papules that resemble flat warts with smooth, dark red or gray surfaces. Lesions may coalesce to form plaques or a verrucous surface.[9] In men, lesions typically involve the distal shaft or foreskin but may extend down the base of the penis and perianal region (**Fig. 15**); in women the condition may involve the whole vulva including the labia

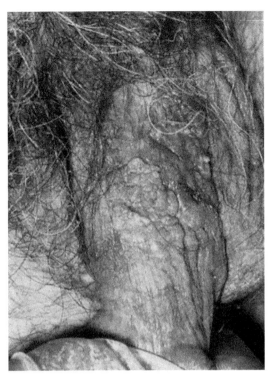

Fig. 13. Bowen disease of penile shaft. (*From* Bunker C. Skin conditions of the male genitalia. Medicine 2014;42(7):375; with permission.)

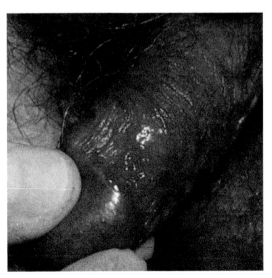

Fig. 14. Erythroplasia of Queryat. (*From* Bunker C. Skin conditions of the male genitalia. Medicine 2014;42(7):375; with permission.)

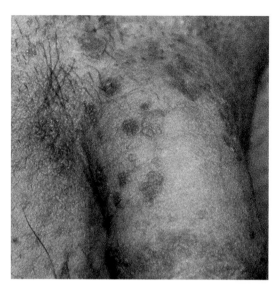

Fig. 15. Bowenoid papulosis of penile shaft. (*From* Kutlubay Z, Engin B, Zara T, et al. Anogenital malignancies and premalignancies: facts and controversies. Clin Dermatol 2013;31(4):369; with permission.)

majora and the perianal region.[9] Biopsy of the lesions should be performed and patients should be tested for HPV. Female partners of men with bowenoid papulosis are at increased risk for developing cervical neoplasia and should receive close follow-up.[28] Spontaneous resolution may occur but progression to invasive carcinoma has been reported so patients should be observed closely. Treatment includes local therapy with topical agents (5-fluorouracil, imiquimod) or ablation.[9]

Squamous Cell Carcinoma

SCC of the genitalia is a rare condition but is the most frequently encountered malignancy of the penis and vulva. Risk factors for development of SCC of the genitalia include chronic irritation; inflammation and scarring; tobacco exposure; LS or LP; HPV; HIV; presence of premalignant lesion; iatrogenic immunosuppression; radiotherapy or phototherapy; lupus; and in men, phimosis and uncircumcised state.[3,26,29] The relative risk for developing penile cancer in uncircumcised compared with those circumcised at birth is 3.2[3] and HPV DNA has been identified in nearly 15% to 71% of all cases of penile cancer.[26]

Lesions of SCC vary in morphology from erythematous plaques with induration, to more exophytic or verrucous lesions that can coalesce into an irregular shaped mass (**Fig. 16**). As the lesions increase in size, they may ulcerate, become necrotic, and bleed, with local tissue destruction.[30] Associated symptoms may precede development of visible tumor and include pruritus, irritation, pain, bleeding, and ulceration of the affected area. The patient should be assessed for inguinal lymphadenopathy, which may indicate metastatic disease. Diagnosis is made by biopsy and all patients with suspicious lesions should be referred to a urologist for biopsy and subsequent surgical therapy.

Verrucous Carcinoma (Buschke-Lowenstein Tumor)

Verrucous carcinoma is a low-grade variant of SCC with low metastatic potential but is locally aggressive and exophytic. When it occurs on the anogential mucosal surface,

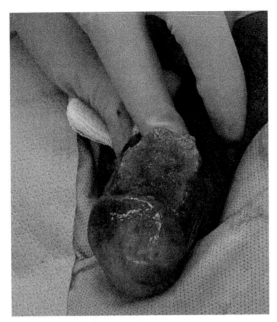

Fig. 16. Squamous cell carcinoma of the penis.

verrucous carcinoma is called Buschke-Lowenstein tumor. This condition represents about one-fourth of all penile tumors.[9] Like other penile cancers, this condition occurs most frequently in uncircumcised men on the glans or foreskin; in women, it may be located on the vulva, vagina, cervix, or anus. Lesions are exophytic, slow growing, and may have a fungating appearance and cause local destruction (**Fig. 17**).[29] Diagnosis is made by biopsy and therapy is local excision.

Kaposi Sarcoma

Kaposi sarcoma is a condition of endothelial origin associated with human herpesvirus 8 and may occur in immunocompetent or immunocompromised individuals. In immunocompetent patients, the genitalia are seldom involved. This is in contrast to

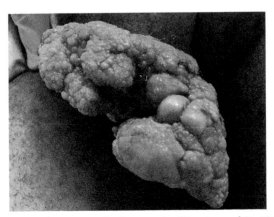

Fig. 17. Buschke-Lowenstein tumor of glans penis. (*Courtesy of* B. McArdle, DO, MBA, Chicago, IL.)

immunosuppressed individuals, specifically those with HIV/AIDS or solid organ transplant recipients, who may present initially with genital lesions. Extragenital manifestations are characterized by slow-growing, blue-red or violaceous pigmented macules; when present on the genitalia lesions are usually solitary and reddish purple or bluish nodules (**Fig. 18**).[9] Lesions frequently arise on the glans and may be associated with swelling, which can cause urethral obstruction and urinary retention.[31] Diagnosis is made by biopsy, and treatment of solitary lesions may include surgical excision, ablation, or intralesional chemotherapy. Radiotherapy may be used in extensive locoregional disease; for disseminated disease, systemic chemotherapy is the treatment of choice.[9] When the condition occurs in solid organ transplant recipients, modification or reduction in immunosuppression may lead to resolution without any additional intervention.[32]

Extramammary Paget Disease

Extramammary Paget disease is a rare dermatosis presenting with irritation, pruritus, or burning, with solitary or multiple red, scaly plaques. The condition occurs more frequently in women and may be present anywhere in the anogenital region. The condition is diagnosed histologically, but may be associated with another underlying malignancy in 10% to 30% of cases, so systematic evaluation for underlying carcinoma should be pursued.[9] When the condition is confined to the genitalia, it may be treated with wide excision, although radiotherapy and phototherapy or topical 5-fluorouracil or imiquimod may be used.[9,29]

MISCELLANEOUS BENIGN CONDITIONS
Angiokeratoma of Fordyce

Angiokeratomas of Fordyce are 1- to 2-mm red or purple smooth papules that arise because of vascular ectasias of dermal blood vessels. The lesions arise on the penis

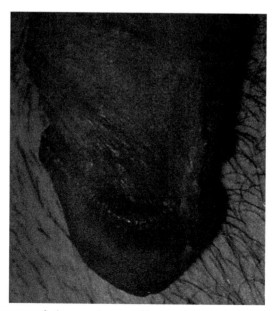

Fig. 18. Kaposi sarcoma of glans penis. (*From* Bunker C. Skin conditions of the male genitalia. Medicine 2014;42(7):376; with permission.)

and scrotum of adult men and may multiply. The condition is benign without systematic manifestations, but rarely may be associated with bleeding. Treatment is usually unnecessary but laser photocoagulation may be used in select cases.[33]

Pearly Penile Papules

Pearly penile papules are benign lesions found in up to 50% of men.[9] These lesions are typically asymptomatic and are skin-colored, dome-shaped, closely spaced 1- to 2-mm papules located circumferentially at the corona (**Fig. 19**). This condition is benign and not associated with HPV or cervical neoplasm in female partners. No treatment is required but if bothersome to the patient, cryotherapy or laser treatment can be pursued.[9]

Zoon Balanitis/Vulvitis

Zoon balanitis, also known as plasma cell balanitis, is a benign condition that arises in uncircumcised men usually after the third decade of life. The condition is caused by irritation from urine caused by a dysfunctional foreskin.[12] Lesions are located on the glans penis and foreskin, and are red-brown patches with a smooth, moist, shiny surface, with well-circumscribed borders (**Fig. 20**); shallow erosions may be present. This condition may rarely arise in women on the vulva and is associated with pain, pruritus, or bleeding.[16] Histologic diagnosis should be pursued to rule out SCC or extramammary Paget disease. Treatment of this condition in men is circumcision; in women or in men averse to surgery, topical steroids or calcineurin inhibitors may alleviate symptoms.[9]

Median Raphe Cyst

Median raphe cysts develop along the median line of the male genitalia from the anus to the external meatus. Most of these lesions occur on the penis and in the parameatal region. Lesions are generally present from birth but may not be noted until later in life; they are typically asymptomatic but may be excised surgically if bothersome.[34]

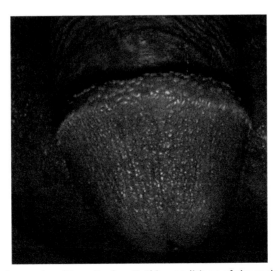

Fig. 19. Pink pearly papules. (*From* Bunker C. Skin conditions of the male genitalia. Medicine 2014;42(7):372; with permission.)

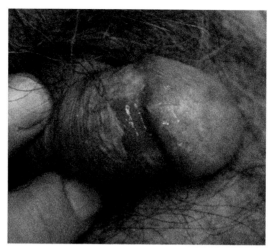

Fig. 20. Zoon balanitis. (*From* Andreassi L, Bilenchi R. Non-infectious inflammatory genital lesions. Clin Dermatol 2014;32(2):312; with permission.)

Epidermoid Cyst

Epidermoid or epidermal inclusion cysts are common and may be found anywhere on the body, including the anogenital region. Definitive therapy requires surgical excision of the entire cyst to prevent recurrence.[9]

Vitiligo

Vitiligo limited to the genitalia has been observed in less than 0.3% of the male population. When suspected, the condition should be differentiated form LS and postinflammatory hypopigmentation.[7] When diagnosed with vitiligo, all patients should be screened for autoimmune thyroid disease.[9]

REFERENCES

1. Farber EM, Bright RD, Nall ML. Psoriasis. A questionnaire survey of 2,144 patients. Arch Dermatol 1968;98(3):248–59.
2. Meeuwis KA, de Hullu JA, Massuger LF, et al. Genital psoriasis: a systematic literature review on this hidden skin disease. Acta Derm Venereol 2011;91(1):5–11.
3. Buechner SA. Common skin disorders of the penis. BJU Int 2002;90(5):498–506.
4. Kalb RE, Bagel J, Korman NJ, et al. Treatment of intertriginous psoriasis: from the Medical Board of the National Psoriasis Foundation. J Am Acad Dermatol 2009; 60(1):120–4.
5. Fisher BK, Margesson LJ. Genital skin disorders: diagnosis and treatment. St Louis (MO): Mosby; 1998.
6. Goldman BD. Common dermatoses of the male genitalia. Recognition of differences in genital rashes and lesions is essential and attainable. Postgrad Med 2000;108(4):89–91, 95–6.
7. Margolis D, Wein A. Color atlas of genital dermatology. In: Walsh P, editor. Campbell's urology, vol. 1. Philadelphia: Saunders; 2002. p. 731–42.
8. Gutiérrez-Pascual M, Vicente-Martín FJ, López-Estebaranz JL. Lichen sclerosus and squamous cell carcinoma. Actas Dermosifiliogr 2012;103(1):21–8.

9. Link RE, Rosen T. Cutaneous diseases of the external genitalia. In: Wein A, editor. Campbell's urology, Vol. 1. Philadelphia: Elsevier; 2016. p. 387–420.

10. Wojnarowska F, Cooper S. Anogenital (non-venereal) disease. In: Bolognia JL, Jorizzo JL, Schaeffer JV, editors. Dermatology, Vol. 1. Edinburgh (Scotland): Mosby; 2003. p. 1099–113.

11. English JC, Laws RA, Keough GC, et al. Dermatoses of the glans penis and prepuce. J Am Acad Dermatol 1997;37(1):1–24 [quiz: 25–6].

12. Shim TN, Ali I, Muneer A, et al. Benign male genital dermatoses. BMJ 2016;354: i4337.

13. Weston W. Erythema multiforme and Stevens-Johnson syndrome. In: Bolognia J, Jorizzo J, Rapini R, editors. Dermatology, vol. 1. Edinburgh (Scotland): Mosby; 2003. p. 313–21.

14. Tatnall FM, Schofield JK, Leigh IM. A double-blind, placebo-controlled trial of continuous acyclovir therapy in recurrent erythema multiforme. Br J Dermatol 1995;132(2):267–70.

15. Wu IB, Schwartz RA. Reiter's syndrome: the classic triad and more. J Am Acad Dermatol 2008;59(1):113–21.

16. Andreassi L, Bilenchi R. Non-infectious inflammatory genital lesions. Clin Dermatol 2014;32(2):307–14.

17. Sehgal VN, Pandhi D, Khurana A. Nonspecific genital ulcers. Clin Dermatol 2014; 32(2):259–74.

18. Workowski KA, Bolan GA, Centers for Disease Control and Prevention. Sexually transmitted diseases treatment guidelines, 2015. MMWR Recomm Rep 2015; 64(RR-03):1–137.

19. Pontari MA. Sexually transmitted diseases. In: Wein AJ, editor. Campbell's urology, vol. 1. Philadelphia: Elsevier; 2016. p. 372–86.

20. Basta-Juzbašić A, Čeović R. Chancroid, lymphogranuloma venereum, granuloma inguinale, genital herpes simplex infection, and molluscum contagiosum. Clin Dermatol 2014;32(2):290–8.

21. Ljubojevic S, Skerlev M. HPV-associated diseases. Clin Dermatol 2014;32(2): 227–34.

22. Kobayashi S. Fournier's gangrene. Am J Surg 2008;195(2):257–8.

23. Singh A, Ahmed K, Aydin A, et al. Fournier's gangrene. A clinical review. Arch Ital Urol Androl 2016;88(3):157–64.

24. Martorell A, García-Martínez FJ, Jiménez-Gallo D, et al. An update on hidradenitis suppurativa (part I): epidemiology, clinical aspects, and definition of disease severity. Actas Dermosifiliogr 2015;106(9):703–15.

25. Collier F, Smith RC, Morton CA. Diagnosis and management of hidradenitis suppurativa. BMJ 2013;346:f2121.

26. Micali G, Nasca MR, Innocenzi D, et al. Penile cancer. J Am Acad Dermatol 2006; 54(3):369–91 [quiz: 391–4].

27. Bunker C. Skin conditions of the male genitalia. Medicine 2014;42(7):372–7.

28. Rosemberg SK, Herman G, Elfont E. Sexually transmitted papilloma viral infection in the male. VII. Is cancer of penis sexually transmitted? Urology 1991;37(5): 437–40.

29. Kutlubay Z, Engin B, Zara T, et al. Anogenital malignancies and premalignancies: facts and controversies. Clin Dermatol 2013;31(4):362–73.

30. Pettaway CA, Crook JM, Pagliaro LC. Tumors of the penis. In: Wein A, editor. Campbell's urology, Vol. 1. Philadelphia: Elsevier; 2016. p. 847–78.

31. Swierzewski SJ, Wan J, Boffini A, et al. The management of meatal obstruction due to Kaposi's sarcoma of the glans penis. J Urol 1993;150(1):193–5.

32. Riva G, Luppi M, Barozzi P, et al. How I treat HHV8/KSHV-related diseases in posttransplant patients. Blood 2012;120(20):4150–9.
33. Occella C, Bleidl D, Rampini P, et al. Argon laser treatment of cutaneous multiple angiokeratomas. Dermatol Surg 1995;21(2):170–2.
34. Deliktas H, Sahin H, Celik OI, et al. Median raphe cyst of the penis. Urol J 2015; 12(4):2287–8.

Lower Urinary Tract Symptoms, Benign Prostatic Hyperplasia, and Urinary Retention

Omar Al Hussein Alawamlh, MD[1], Ramy Goueli, MD[2],
Richard K. Lee, MD, MBA*,[1]

KEYWORDS

- Voiding dysfunction • Lower urinary tract symptoms • Benign prostatic hyperplasia
- Acute urinary retention • Chronic urinary retention

KEY POINTS

- Lower urinary tract symptoms (LUTS) is a common set of urologic symptoms that can affect men of all ages, with a predilection for the elderly.
- Benign prostatic hyperplasia is the most common cause of voiding dysfunction, leading to higher prevalence of LUTS in the elderly.
- Managing a patient with LUTS starts with obtaining a thorough medical history and establishing symptom severity, followed by the appropriate utilization of diagnostic modalities.
- A variety of medical treatments exist for LUTS, which can be used either as monotherapy or in combination.

INTRODUCTION

Advancements in health care over the past several decades have significantly contributed to the increase in quality of life and life expectancy. It is projected that the elderly population in the United States will be 83.7 million in the year 2050, comprising about 21% of the entire population.[1] This change in demographics does not come without challenges, most notably an increase in the incidence and prevalence of chronic illnesses along with the associated economic burden.[2]

Conflicts of Interest: None.
Department of Urology, Weill Medical College of Cornell University, James Buchanan Brady Foundation, New York, NY, USA
[1] Present address: 425 East 61st Street, New York, NY 10065.
[2] Present address: 525 East 68th Street, STAR 9, New York, NY 10065.
* Corresponding author.
E-mail address: ril9010@med.cornell.edu

It is well known that advanced age is associated with a higher likelihood of morbidity, including urologic conditions such as lower urinary tract symptoms (LUTS) and benign prostatic hyperplasia (BPH).[3,4] One may assume that the prevalence of LUTS and BPH will significantly rise with increasing age. This increase warrants a more active role by primary care physicians (PCPs) in both the diagnosis and management of patients presenting with those conditions because PCPs typically are the first point of medical contact.[5]

VOIDING DYSFUNCTION

Voiding dysfunction is abnormal, slow, and/or incomplete micturition as defined by the International Continence Society (ICS) and the International Urogynecological Association.[6] The different types of voiding dysfunction, however, are described by the term LUTS.[7] LUTS are divided into 3 groups of symptoms (storage, voiding, and postmicturition) according to the ICS (**Box 1**).[8] It is estimated that by the year 2018, 2.3 billion people will be affected by at least 1 of the LUTS.[9]

VOIDING DYSFUNCTION AND BENIGN PROSTATIC HYPERPLASIA

Prostatic hyperplasia is a phenomenon that affects more than 70% of men aged 60 to 69 years in the United States.[10] Several mechanisms have been proposed to explain the causes behind the development of this nonmalignant growth. Some investigators looked at modifiable factors, such as obesity, as a cause of metabolic derangements, whereas others considered the role of inflammation. Perhaps the most popular proposed mechanism is the effect of androgens on the prostate gland.[11–13]

Box 1
The 3 groups of lower urinary tract symptoms

Storage symptoms
- Daytime frequency
- Nocturia
- Urgency
- Different types of incontinence
- Enuresis
- Abnormal bladder sensation

Voiding symptoms
- Slow or intermittent stream
- Splitting or spraying
- Hesitancy
- Straining
- Terminal dribble

Postmicturition symptoms
- Feeling of incomplete emptying
- Postmicturition dribble

Data from Abrams P, Cardozo L, Fall M, et al. The standardisation of terminology of lower urinary tract function: report from the Standardisation Sub-committee of the International Continence Society. Neurourol Urodyn 2002;21(2):167–78.

BPH is considered the most common cause that leads to LUTS in men.[14] BPH promotes bladder outlet obstruction (BOO), which then gives rise to LUTS via 2 components:

1. A dynamic obstruction component characterized by smooth muscle hyperplasia
2. A static component consisting of the enlargement of the prostate gland driven by the excessive growth of stromal and epithelial elements.

LUTS that results from BOO is also complicated by the detrusor's response to obstruction, which can manifest as impaired contractility or overactivity.[15,16]

BENIGN PROSTATIC HYPERPLASIA AND URINARY RETENTION

Urinary retention is a fairly common complication of BPH. Estimates show that 10% of men in their seventies and one-third of men in their eighties will experience acute urinary retention (AUR) within the next 5 years.[17]

Acute Urinary Retention

AUR is a sudden unexpected inability to pass urine that is usually associated with pain.[18] Acute retention is regarded as an emergency requiring urgent medical attention. Patients usually present with lower abdominal pain and swelling (palpable pelvic mass that is dull to percussion), and either the frank inability to pass urine or the ability to pass only a small amount.[19]

AUR can either occur spontaneously or secondary to a precipitating event. Spontaneous AUR represents almost all cases and is most commonly associated with BPH, in which it serves as a sign of progression. Precipitated AUR, however, follows a triggering factor, such as a surgical procedure (pain, anesthesia, or immobility), excessive fluid intake (eg, alcohol), a urinary tract infection (UTI), medications with sympathomimetic or anticholinergic effects, or neuropathic causes (diabetic cystopathy). Distinguishing between the 2 types of AUR is relevant because BPH surgery is required more often in cases of spontaneous AUR.[17,19]

CHRONIC URINARY RETENTION

The ICS defines chronic urinary retention (CUR) as a "non-painful bladder, which remains palpable or percussable after the patient has passed urine. Such patients may be incontinent."[8] Patients with CUR may complain of increased urinary frequency, hesitancy, poor urinary flow, nocturnal incontinence, or may even be asymptomatic.[20] The literature varies in its criteria for diagnosis of CUR, with multiple sources using postvoid volumes ranging between 300 to 500 mL as their cutoff.[19,21] CUR may occur in young or elderly patients, and can be independent of prostatic volume.[22]

This condition can be divided into high-pressure and low-pressure CUR, referring to the detrusor pressures generated either during filling or micturition. High-pressure CUR accounts for most cases of CUR and is associated with BOO; it often leads to the development of hydronephrosis and resultant renal failure from the backward pressure generated. In contrast, patients with low-pressure CUR have a very compliant bladder and retain a large volume without the development of hydronephrosis or renal failure.[19,22]

DIAGNOSIS OF VOIDING DYSFUNCTION

For basic management of BPH-related LUTS, the American Urological Association (AUA) classifies diagnostic tests into recommended or optional, in which a recommended test should be had by every patient, whereas an optional test is performed for select patients and is generally carried out by a urologist. A review of the recommended tests follows.

History and Patient-Specific Questionnaires

Obtaining a thorough patient history is a key element with any patient presenting with LUTS. In the initial work-up of LUTS, the symptoms must be identified and the degree of severity established. BPH-associated symptoms are best quantified using the AUA Symptom Index and the International Prostate Symptom Score. The AUA describes the 2 indices as self-administered questionnaires that assess the severity of both storage and voiding symptoms. Another survey instrument is the Overactive Bladder Questionnaire. Additionally, AUA guidelines recommend the use of frequency volume charts in patients with nocturia as the dominant symptom.

Physical Examination

A physical examination includes assessing the abdominal and genital regions for abnormalities. Particular attention should be given to suprapubic distension and tenderness or neurologic (sensory and motor) dysfunction. A critical component of the examination is the digital rectal examination (DRE) that evaluates prostate size, consistency, tenderness, and surface, in addition to sphincter tone.

Laboratory Testing

Despite its importance, DRE must be concomitantly used with other diagnostic tools. One such tool, which provides more accuracy in assessing prostate volume and can correlate with symptom progression, is the prostate-specific antigen (PSA) test.[23] Specifically, serum PSA has been shown to be a strong predictor of prostatic growth. However, testing serum PSA to diagnose prostate cancer (PCa) in men with LUTS should be discussed with the patient, including false-positive or false-negative results, as well as potential overdiagnosis and treatment of PCa.[24,25] Additional laboratory tests should be performed at the discretion of the provider, although the AUA recommends against checking creatinine in the initial diagnosis of LUTS secondary to BPH.

Urinalysis

Urinalysis (UA) is another recommended test used to assess LUTS. Dipstick tests are able to detect hematuria, proteinuria, pyuria, ketonuria, and glucosuria. Abnormalities in dipstick tests indicate the need to examine the urinary sediment and perform a culture.[26] UA can provide guidance in both determining the cause of LUTS and directing further testing.

DIFFERENTIAL DIAGNOSIS

The differential for LUTS in men is incredibly broad and relies on the diligence of the clinician to obtain a good history, and physical and symptom-directed diagnostic evaluations (**Table 1**).

Infectious Cause

In patients who have a sudden onset of dysuria, increased frequency, urgency, and foul smelling or discolored urine, an infectious cause should be considered. On UA, the presence of either positive leukocyte esterase or nitrates, yields a sensitivity of 81% and a specificity of 77% for diagnosing a UTI with greater than 100,000 colony-forming units.[27] If the urine culture is negative with ongoing LUTS, despite a

Table 1
Differential diagnosis for lower urinary tract symptoms

	Differential Diagnosis
Infectious	UTI • Bacterial • Parasitic • Viral • Fungal
Obstruction	BPH Bladder neck contracture Urethral stricture
Inflammation	Interstitial cystitis or bladder pain syndrome Foreign body (bladder calculus, ureteral stent, urethral catheter) Vesicoenteric fistulas
Neoplastic	Urothelial carcinoma Locally invasive PCa Metastatic disease Extrinsic pelvic mass
Metabolic	Diabetes mellitus
Medication Induced	Diuretics Chemo-immunotherapy (ie, cyclophosphamide and intravesical therapeutics)
Neurologic	Multiple sclerosis Normal pressure hydrocephalus Stroke or cerebrovascular accident Parkinson disease Cauda equina syndrome Tethered cord syndrome Spinal shock or spinal cord injuries Pelvic surgery

positive UA, then one should consider atypical infectious causes, including mycoplasma or ureaplasma infections that are difficult to culture. Additionally, consider urinary tuberculosis or schistosomiasis in patients who have a history of travel to an endemic area or have known risk factors or contact exposures.[28,29] Finally, for patients who are sexually active, gonococcal and nongonococcal urethritis should be on the differential diagnosis.[30]

Obstruction

Patients who present with a history of LUTS, including nocturia, increased frequency, postvoid dribbling, and a sensation of incomplete emptying with no known infectious cause, should be considered for an obstructive cause.[31] A bladder neck contracture should be considered in any patient who has undergone a transurethral procedure, most commonly including transurethral resection of the prostate. Although advanced BPH can present with obstructive symptoms, it can be distinguished from PCa by the presence of an abnormal PSA and/or DRE.[32] A stricture of the urethra should be considered in patients with history of trauma, gonococcal urethritis, urethral instrumentation or surgery, and penile or pelvic radiation.[33,34]

Inflammation

Inflammation in the absence of infection that can lead to LUTS may arise from a foreign body (bladder stone, Foley catheter, or ureteral stent), vesicoenteric fistulae, prior pelvic radiation, interstitial cystitis or bladder pain syndrome. A vesicoenteric fistula should be considered in select patients with risk factors and recurrent multiple organism UTIs, and/or pneumaturia or fecaluria.[26]

Neoplasm

Locally advanced PCa was previously discussed as a potential obstructive cause of LUTS. Additional possible neoplastic causes for LUTS in men are urothelial carcinoma, extrinsic pelvic mass, or metastatic disease. Urothelial carcinoma is more common in men and should be highly considered in patients with known risk factors (smoking, chronic cystitis, or chemical or radiation exposure) and either microscopic or gross hematuria on evaluation. These patients should warrant a prompt referral to a urologist.[35,36]

Metabolic

Patients who complain of LUTS related to polyuria and urinary frequency should undergo evaluation for diabetes mellitus because this can present with polyuria and polydipsia. Patients with diabetes mellitus should work to achieve tight glycemic control to minimize urinary symptoms and limit microvascular insults to the kidneys.[37]

Medication-Induced

There are 2 major classes of medications that can precipitate LUTS, specifically diuretics and chemoimmunotherapy (ie, cyclophosphamide). Diuretics will cause increased urination, which is particularly bothersome when taken before bed, thus affecting the patient's quality of life. Cyclophosphamide increases the risk for both hemorrhagic cystitis and associated bladder cancer, therefore warranting further workup from a urologist.

Neurologic

Neurologic conditions that can cause LUTS include multiple sclerosis, normal pressure hydrocephalus, stroke, Parkinson disease, cauda equina syndrome, tethered cord, and spinal shock, as well as prior pelvic surgery with manipulation of the sacral plexus.[38,39] The presentation of LUTS with associated neurologic dysfunction requires further investigation by a specialist. The use of pressure-flow studies may be helpful in this population.

TREATMENT

The treatment of LUTS largely depends on the likely causes of the patient's symptoms and level of bother. Treatment options should include lifestyle modifications; behavioral modifications; and, when necessary, pharmacotherapy. The AUA recommends addressing all 3 aspects in creating a treatment plan.

Watchful Waiting

Men whose urinary symptoms are not bothersome to their lives may be candidates for watchful waiting or active surveillance. In these patients, the AUA recommends annual reassessment of symptoms, including a medical history and physical examination; an evaluation of symptom severity; and, in appropriate men, PSA measurement.[26,40] Watchful waiting should also include lifestyle and behavioral modifications, such as avoiding caffeine, alcohol, and spicy and acidic food.[37] Clinicians can specifically address bothersome nocturia by recommending decreased evening fluid intake and avoidance of diuretics before sleep.[41] Additionally, treatment of a patient's underlying disease (diabetes, obstructive sleep apnea, or edema) can also improve symptoms.

Medical Therapy

For men who are significantly bothered by their LUTS, the AUA recommends that risk and benefits of treatment of LUTS secondary to BPH should be discussed with patients before starting any and all treatments, with the following available options.

Phytotherapy

Phytotherapeutic agents include saw palmetto, African plum tree, stinging nettle, pumpkin seed, African star grass, and rye grass pollen. Those agents are claimed to benefit patients with LUTS related to BPH; however, due to the paucity of available data, the AUA currently does not recommend their use.[42]

Alpha-Blockers

Alpha-blockers work through the antagonism of alpha-1 adrenergic receptors, which causes a relaxation of the smooth muscle in the prostate and bladder neck. Alpha-blockers differ in their selectivity and, thus, differ in their dosing and side effect profile.[43] Terazosin, doxazosin, and alfuzosin are nonselective alpha-blockers, whereas tamsulosin and silodosin are alpha-1A selective blockers. Terazosin; immediate release doxazosin; and, occasionally, tamsulosin will require dose titration based on symptoms, whereas the others will not require titration. These medications have all been shown to have equal clinical significance and can be tailored to a patient's individual needs.[44] The AUA recognizes that older, generic alpha-blockers remain a reasonable choice but require dose titration and blood pressure monitoring. The long-term use and safety of alpha-blockers was partly demonstrated in the Medical Therapy of Prostatic Symptoms (MTOPS) study.[45] Use of alpha-blockers was shown to have long-term symptom improvement but had no effect on progression to AUR or the need for surgery. Improvement in urinary symptoms can happen within a couple of days of starting the medication but may take 1 to 3 months for maximal improvement.[46]

All alpha-blockers can cause variable levels of fatigue, nasal congestion, orthostatic hypotension, and retrograde ejaculation. Silodosin and tamsulosin have the highest rate of retrograde ejaculation with 28% and 18% of patients experiencing this adverse effect, respectively. Tamsulosin, silodosin, extended release doxazosin, and alfuzosin have been shown to cause less dizziness and orthostatic hypotension than their counterparts.[43] Floppy iris syndrome can occur with the continued use of any alpha-blocker during cataract surgery, in which the AUA recommends against the initiation of alpha-blockers in men planning to undergo cataract surgery.

5-Alpha Reductase Inhibitors

The inhibition of 5-alpha reductase blocks the conversion of testosterone to dihydrotestosterone, the reduction of which has been shown to reduce prostate volume by 25%, decrease total PSA by 50%, and reduce the risk of AUR and the need for surgical BPH management.[47] There are 2 medications available, finasteride, a type 2 5-alpha reductase inhibitor (ARI), and dutasteride, a type 1 and 2 5-ARI.

The benefit and efficacy of 5-ARIs was demonstrated in the Proscar (Finasteride) Long-term Efficacy and Safety Study (PLESS), which showed an improvement in urinary symptoms and flow rates in select patients taking this medication.[48] The 5-ARI arm of the MTOPS and Combination Avodart and Tamsulosin (CombAT) trial both confirmed improvement in voiding symptoms, as well as a decrease BPH progression and a lower need for surgical BPH treatment.[45] Because these studies focused on patients with larger prostates (>30 g), the AUA recommends against the use of 5-ARIs in men with LUTS without demonstrable prostatic enlargement. The adverse effects of 5-ARIs include decreased volume of ejaculate; impotence; decreased libido; and, rarely, breast and nipple tenderness. After starting 5-ARIs, patients will need to wait 6 to 9 months before noticing a full effect of the medication.

Phosphodiesterase 5 Inhibitors

Tadalafil (Cialis) is the only phosphodiesterase 5 (PDE5) inhibitor approved by the US Food and Drug Administration for treatment of BPH-related LUTS. Although it's exact mechanism of action in BPH-related disease is unknown, its use has been shown to improve erectile dysfunction, voiding symptoms, and quality of life in men with LUTS related to BPH, although no change was seen in objective voiding parameters.[49]

After starting tadalafil, the effect may be noted within a week but may take up to 2 months for a full effect. Like other PDE5 inhibitors, patients are at risk for headaches and flushing; and, less commonly, nasal congestion, back pain, diplopia, impaired color vision, and priapism. PDE5 inhibitors should be used with caution in patients taking alpha-blockers and are contraindicated in patients taking nitrates.[50]

Antimuscarinics

Anticholinergic medications can be useful in treating the associated overactive bladder related to BOO from BPH.[51] These medications have been shown to be an effective adjunctive treatment of management of storage symptoms. The AUA recommends that, before starting these medications, obtain a postvoid residual assessment because caution is advised when it is greater than 250 mL.[52,53] The adverse effects of these medications include dry mouth; constipation; blurry vision; headache; dizziness; and, rarely, cognitive impairment and AUR.

Combination Therapy

Several studies have shown the improved efficacy of combining alpha-blockers and 5-ARIs in select patients. According to the AUA, this combination is a viable option for patients with LUTS associated with BPH diagnosed via PSA, DRE, or volume measurement. Two paramount studies were the MTOPS trial and the CombAT trial, which focused mainly on men with larger glands (>30 g) and higher serum PSA levels (PSA >1.5 ng/mL). Both studies showed combination therapy, compared with either agent alone, prevented BPH progression, and improved individual voiding symptoms and voiding parameters.[45,54]

In select patients, the combination of alpha-blockers and anticholinergics has also been studied. In men with predominant storage or irritative voiding symptoms related to BPH, this combination has been shown to lead to greater improvement in symptoms and quality of life than either agent alone.[55,56]

MANAGEMENT

Patient follow-up depends on the therapies initiated. Patients started on alpha-blockers or PDE5 inhibitors should be reevaluated in 2 to 4 weeks, whereas patients started on 5-ARIs can be seen in 3 months to ensure enough time is given for treatment effect. Following reevaluation, if the patient is satisfied, they can transition to yearly follow-up. As mentioned, follow-up should consist of history and physical, a validated voiding symptom questionnaire, and a PSA.[31]

Patients who have undergone basic therapies with no benefit warrant a referral to a urologist. Additionally, patients who present with complicated LUTS, defined as voiding symptoms combined with an abnormal PSA, abnormal DRE, hematuria, a palpable bladder, upper tract dysfunction, or neurologic disease, also warrant referral to a urologist for further management.

REFERENCES

1. Ortman JM, Velkoff VA, Hogan H. An aging nation: the older population in the United States. Current Population Report. Suitland (ML): United States Census Bureau; 2014. p. 1–28.
2. Pritchard D, Petrilla A, Hallinan S, et al. What contributes most to high health care costs? Health care spending in high resource patients. J Manag Care Spec Pharm 2016;22(2):102–9.
3. Coyne KS, Sexton CC, Bell JA, et al. The prevalence of lower urinary tract symptoms (LUTS) and overactive bladder (OAB) by racial/ethnic group and age: results from OAB-POLL. Neurourol Urodyn 2013;32(3):230–7.
4. Wei JT, Calhoun E, Jacobsen SJ. Urologic diseases in America project: benign prostatic hyperplasia. J Urol 2005;173(4):1256–61.
5. Miner MM. Primary care physician versus urologist: how does their medical management of LUTS associated with BPH differ? Curr Urol Rep 2009;10(4):254–60.
6. Chen P-C, Wang C-C. Managing voiding dysfunction in young men. Urol Sci 2013;24(3):78–83.
7. Chaikin DC, Blaivas JG. Voiding dysfunction: definitions. Curr Opin Urol 2001; 11(4):395–8.
8. Abrams P, Cardozo L, Fall M, et al. The standardisation of terminology of lower urinary tract function: report from the Standardisation Sub-committee of the International Continence Society. Neurourol Urodyn 2002;21(2):167–78.
9. Irwin DE, Kopp ZS, Agatep B, et al. Worldwide prevalence estimates of lower urinary tract symptoms, overactive bladder, urinary incontinence and bladder outlet obstruction. BJU Int 2011;108(7):1132–8.
10. Parsons JK, Kashefi C. Physical activity, benign prostatic hyperplasia, and lower urinary tract symptoms. Eur Urol 2008;53(6):1228–35.
11. Kristal AR, Arnold KB, Schenk JM, et al. Race/ethnicity, obesity, health related behaviors and the risk of symptomatic benign prostatic hyperplasia: results from the prostate cancer prevention trial. J Urol 2007;177(4):1395–400 [quiz: 1591].
12. Chughtai B, Lee R, Te A, et al. Role of inflammation in benign prostatic hyperplasia. Rev Urol 2011;13(3):147–50.
13. Carson C 3rd, Rittmaster R. The role of dihydrotestosterone in benign prostatic hyperplasia. Urology 2003;61(4 Suppl 1):2–7.
14. Parsons JK. Benign prostatic hyperplasia and male lower urinary tract symptoms: epidemiology and risk factors. Curr Bladder Dysfunct Rep 2010;5(4):212–8.
15. Scofield S, Kaplan SA. Voiding dysfunction in men: pathophysiology and risk factors. Int J Impot Res 2008;20(Suppl 3):S2–10.
16. Lepor H. Pathophysiology of lower urinary tract symptoms in the aging male population. Rev Urol 2005;7(Suppl 7):S3–11.
17. Fitzpatrick JM, Kirby RS. Management of acute urinary retention. BJU Int 2006; 97(Suppl 2):16–20 [discussion: 21–2].
18. Emberton M, Anson K. Acute urinary retention in men: an age old problem. BMJ 1999;318(7188):921–5.

19. Kalejaiye O, Speakman MJ. Management of acute and chronic retention in men. Eur Urol Suppl 2009;8(6):523–9.
20. Speakman MJ, Cheng X. Management of the complications of BPH/BOO. Indian J Urol 2014;30(2):208–13.
21. Negro CL, Muir GH. Chronic urinary retention in men: how we define it, and how does it affect treatment outcome. BJU Int 2012;110(11):1590–4.
22. George NJ, O'Reilly PH, Barnard RJ, et al. High pressure chronic retention. BMJ 1983;286(6380):1780–3.
23. Tanguay S, Awde M, Brock G, et al. Diagnosis and management of benign prostatic hyperplasia in primary care. Can Urol Assoc J 2009;3(3 Suppl 2):S92–100.
24. Roehrborn CG, McConnell J, Bonilla J, et al. Serum prostate specific antigen is a strong predictor of future prostate growth in men with benign prostatic hyperplasia. PROSCAR long-term efficacy and safety study. J Urol 2000;163(1):13–20.
25. Heidenreich A, Bastian PJ, Bellmunt J, et al. EAU guidelines on prostate cancer. Part 1: screening, diagnosis, and local treatment with curative intent-update 2013. Eur Urol 2014;65(1):124–37.
26. Abrams P, Chapple C, Khoury S, et al. Evaluation and treatment of lower urinary tract symptoms in older men. J Urol 2009;181(4):1779–87.
27. St John A, Boyd JC, Lowes AJ, et al. The use of urinary dipstick tests to exclude urinary tract infection: a systematic review of the literature. Am J Clin Pathol 2006; 126(3):428–36.
28. Matthews SJ, Lancaster JW. Urinary tract infections in the elderly population. Am J Geriatr Pharmacother 2011;9(5):286–309.
29. Sourial MW, Brimo F, Horn R, et al. Genitourinary tuberculosis in North America: a rare clinical entity. Can Urol Assoc J 2015;9(7–8):E484–9.
30. Barbee LA, Khosropour CM, Dombrowski JC, et al. An estimate of the proportion of symptomatic gonococcal, chlamydial and non-gonococcal non-chlamydial urethritis attributable to oral sex among men who have sex with men: a case-control study. Sex Transm Infect 2016;92(2):155–60.
31. Roehrborn CG. Male lower urinary tract symptoms (LUTS) and benign prostatic hyperplasia (BPH). Med Clin North Am 2011;95(1):87–100.
32. Crain DS, Amling CL, Kane CJ. Palliative transurethral prostate resection for bladder outlet obstruction in patients with locally advanced prostate cancer. J Urol 2004;171(2 Pt 1):668–71.
33. Lumen N, Hoebeke P, Willemsen P, et al. Etiology of urethral stricture disease in the 21st century. J Urol 2009;182(3):983–7.
34. Angermeier KW, Rourke KF, Dubey D, et al. SIU/ICUD consultation on urethral strictures: evaluation and follow-up. Urology 2014;83(3 Suppl):S8–17.
35. Babjuk M, Bohle A, Burger M, et al. EAU guidelines on non-muscle-invasive urothelial carcinoma of the bladder: update 2016. Eur Urol 2017;71(3):447–61.
36. Woldu SL, Bagrodia A, Lotan Y. Guideline of guidelines: non-muscle-invasive bladder cancer. BJU Int 2017;119(3):371–80.
37. Bradley CS, Erickson BA, Messersmith EE, et al. Evidence of the Impact of Diet, Fluid Intake, Caffeine, Alcohol and Tobacco on Lower Urinary Tract Symptoms: A Systematic Review. The Journal of urology 2017;198(5):1010–20.
38. Winge K. Lower urinary tract dysfunction in patients with parkinsonism and other neurodegenerative disorders. Handb Clin Neurol 2015;130:335–56.
39. Madersbacher H. The various types of neurogenic bladder dysfunction: an update of current therapeutic concepts. Paraplegia 1990;28(4):217–29.
40. Kaplan SA. AUA Guidelines and their impact on the management of BPH: an update. Rev Urol 2004;6(Suppl 9):S46–52.

41. Gacci M, Corona G, Sebastianelli A, et al. Male lower urinary tract symptoms and cardiovascular events: a systematic review and meta-analysis. Eur Urol 2016; 70(5):788–96.
42. Dedhia RC, McVary KT. Phytotherapy for lower urinary tract symptoms secondary to benign prostatic hyperplasia. J Urol 2008;179(6):2119–25.
43. Roehrborn CG, Schwinn DA. Alpha1-adrenergic receptors and their inhibitors in lower urinary tract symptoms and benign prostatic hyperplasia. J Urol 2004; 171(3):1029–35.
44. Roehrborn CG. Efficacy of alpha-adrenergic receptor blockers in the treatment of male lower urinary tract symptoms. Rev Urol 2009;11(Suppl 1):S1–8.
45. McConnell JD, Roehrborn CG, Bautista OM, et al. The long-term effect of doxazosin, finasteride, and combination therapy on the clinical progression of benign prostatic hyperplasia. N Engl J Med 2003;349(25):2387–98.
46. Marks LS, Gittelman MC, Hill LA, et al. Rapid efficacy of the highly selective alpha1A-adrenoceptor antagonist silodosin in men with signs and symptoms of benign prostatic hyperplasia: pooled results of 2 phase 3 studies. J Urol 2009; 181(6):2634–40.
47. Kaplan SA, Roehrborn CG, McConnell JD, et al. Long-term treatment with finasteride results in a clinically significant reduction in total prostate volume compared to placebo over the full range of baseline prostate sizes in men enrolled in the MTOPS trial. J Urol 2008;180(3):1030–2 [discussion: 1032–3].
48. Bruskewitz R, Girman CJ, Fowler J, et al. Effect of finasteride on bother and other health-related quality of life aspects associated with benign prostatic hyperplasia. PLESS Study Group. Proscar long-term efficacy and safety study. Urology 1999;54(4):670–8.
49. Dmochowski R, Roehrborn C, Klise S, et al. Urodynamic effects of once daily tadalafil in men with lower urinary tract symptoms secondary to clinical benign prostatic hyperplasia: a randomized, placebo controlled 12-week clinical trial. J Urol 2010;183(3):1092–7.
50. Chapple CR. Monotherapy with α-blocker or phosphodiesterase 5 inhibitor for lower urinary tract symptoms? Eur Urol 2012;61(5):926–7.
51. Gacci M, Sebastianelli A, Salvi M, et al. Tolterodine in the treatment of male LUTS. Curr Urol Rep 2015;16(9):60.
52. Athanasopoulos A, Chapple C, Fowler C, et al. The role of antimuscarinics in the management of men with symptoms of overactive bladder associated with concomitant bladder outlet obstruction: an update. Eur Urol 2011;60(1): 94–105.
53. Kaplan SA, Roehrborn CG, Abrams P, et al. Antimuscarinics for treatment of storage lower urinary tract symptoms in men: a systematic review. Int J Clin Pract 2011;65(4):487–507.
54. Montorsi F, Roehrborn C, Garcia-Penit J, et al. The effects of dutasteride or tamsulosin alone and in combination on storage and voiding symptoms in men with lower urinary tract symptoms (LUTS) and benign prostatic hyperplasia (BPH): 4-year data from the Combination of Avodart and Tamsulosin (CombAT) study. BJU Int 2011;107(9):1426–31.
55. Athanasopoulos A, Gyftopoulos K, Giannitsas K, et al. Combination treatment with an alpha-blocker plus an anticholinergic for bladder outlet obstruction: a prospective, randomized, controlled study. J Urol 2003;169(6):2253–6.
56. Filson CP, Hollingsworth JM, Clemens JQ, et al. The efficacy and safety of combined therapy with alpha-blockers and anticholinergics for men with benign prostatic hyperplasia: a meta-analysis. J Urol 2013;190(6):2153–60.

Female Voiding Dysfunction and Urinary Incontinence

Amanda Vo, MD, Stephanie J. Kielb, MD*

KEYWORDS

- Overactive bladder (OAB) • Urge urinary incontinence (UUI)
- Stress urinary incontinence (SUI) • Vesicovaginal fistula (VVF)
- Ureterovaginal fistula (UVF)

KEY POINTS

- Urinary continence relies on coordination of the autonomic and somatic nervous systems, in addition to normal lower urinary tract support and sphincter function.
- Overactive bladder may be treated in a stepwise fashion with behavioral therapies, pharmacologic management, and procedural options.
- Stress urinary incontinence is most effectively treated with minimally invasive surgical techniques that reinforce urethral support.
- Urogenital fistulas, although more common in developing countries than in the United States, are extremely distressful to patients and repair often requires larger reconstructive surgery.

NORMAL URINARY CONTINENCE AND VOIDING

The lower urinary tract (LUT) has 2 main functions, low-pressure storage of urine, then consciously controlled, coordinated emptying. This involves coordination of the autonomic and somatic nervous systems. Coordination occurs at the pontine micturition center and the cerebral cortex provides inhibition. Disease states affecting the cortex such as stroke or Parkinson's disease can, therefore, cause of loss of inhibition, with urinary urgency, frequency, and at times urge incontinence. Neurologic disease below the pontine micturition center can cause a variety of LUT complications, including coordination issues which may put upper tract (renal) function at risk; the details of such conditions are complex and are not discussed further in this review.

Disclosures: The authors have no disclosures to report.
Department of Urology, Northwestern University Feinberg School of Medicine, 303 East Chicago Avenue, Tarry 16-703, Chicago, IL 60611, USA
* Corresponding author.
E-mail address: stephanie.kielb@nm.org

Med Clin N Am 102 (2018) 313–324
https://doi.org/10.1016/j.mcna.2017.10.006
0025-7125/18/© 2017 Elsevier Inc. All rights reserved.

Urinary continence depends on normal LUT support as well as normal sphincter function, both internal and external. The involuntary internal sphincter at the bladder neck may be affected by previous surgery. The external sphincter in the distal urethra is controlled by voluntary muscle contraction, normally ensuring continence if the internal sphincter is compromised. Continence is achieved when the urethra maintains a pressure greater than the bladder pressure.

Pelvic floor musculature is responsible for supporting the bladder neck and proximal urethra. Weakened support of these structures may result in stress urinary incontinence (SUI).[1] As the bladder fills, the "guarding reflex" inhibits the parasympathetic nervous system and activates the sympathetic nervous system, reducing detrusor tone and increasing sphincter tone. When capacity is reached, sensory nerves detect detrusor distension and signal the spinal cord to suppress the guarding reflex. The voiding reflex can then be activated, which stimulates the parasympathetic nervous system and inhibits the sympathetic nervous system, thereby leading to bladder contraction and sphincter relaxation. The voiding reflex is usually under voluntary control by the central nervous system, but if the central nervous system is unable to suppress the voiding reflex, involuntary voiding occurs when the bladder becomes full ("reflex voiding").[2]

Lower Urinary Health Across the Lifespan in Women

LUT symptoms (LUTS) in childhood may be predictive of overactive bladder (OAB) in adults. Risk factors for LUTS in children include obesity, holding of urine, and constipation. The prevalence of LUTS increases with age, particularly in the reproductive years. Pregnancy and vaginal delivery stretch pelvic muscles, which can affect innervation and connective tissue support of the bladder and urethra.[3]

As menopause is reached, the rate of LUTS and urinary incontinence increases. The onset of symptoms may be attributable to age. Hormones may also play a role, but there is limited understanding of this mechanism. Fifty percent of women over the age of 65 in the community have urinary incontinence, and rates increase to more than 70% for those in long-term care facilities.[4]

Urodynamics

Urodynamics (UDS) is the dynamic study of the transport, storage, and emptying of urine. UDS include various tests, such as postvoid residual (the amount of urine in the bladder after urination), uroflowmetry (measuring flow rate over time), cystometry (measuring bladder pressure and volume), videourodynamics (simultaneous fluoroscopy), and urethral function tests (measuring outlet competence).[5]

The clinical usefulness of UDS is not well-defined, but lends valuable information in the appropriate setting. According to the American Urological Association, UDS are useful in the following situations: to identify factors contributing to LUT dysfunction and assess their relevance; to predict the consequences of LUT dysfunction on the upper tracts; to predict the consequences and outcomes of therapeutic intervention; to confirm and/or understand the effects of interventional techniques; and to investigate the reasons for failure of a treatment.[5]

Because performing UDS is not without risks (ie, risk of infection with catheter placement, risk of radiation with fluoroscopy), clinicians often contemplate whether the information potentially gained from UDS outweighs the risks. In uncomplicated cases, physicians may choose conservative treatment before performing invasive testing.

OVERACTIVE BLADDER

OAB is a clinical diagnosis defined by the International Continence Society as the presence of "urinary urgency, usually accompanied by frequency and nocturia, with or without urgency urinary incontinence (UUI), in the absence of a urinary tract infection (UTI) or other obvious pathology."[6] Although OAB is usually idiopathic, it is associated with bladder inflammation, chronic bladder outlet obstruction, pregnancy, vaginal childbirth, postmenopausal status, obesity, and older age.[7] Notably, OAB is more prevalent in women (12.8%) than in men (10.8%).[8] Neurologic disease such as stroke, Parkinson's disease, transverse myelitis, and cord injuries may also manifest with OAB-like symptoms.

Epidemiology and Impact

The incidence of OAB varies by the definition used, but in population-based studies, rates range from 9% to 47%. OAB increases steadily with age, and is more common in the frail elderly, with rates as high as 9 times as great in patients aged 65 to 74 compared with those aged 18 to 24.[9–11]

OAB has been shown to have a negative impact on quality of life and can result in increased morbidity and mortality. Symptoms can be highly bothersome to patients, negatively affecting sleep, work productivity, and overall health-related quality of life.[9,12] Women with symptoms of OAB report frequent awakening at night to void, leading to poor sleep quality and feelings of fatigue.[13] Additionally, symptoms of OAB can lead to anxiety, depression, and social isolation for fear of urinary incontinence.[14]

Consequences are even greater in the elderly population given their increased chronic comorbidities.[15] One-fourth of falls occur at night and more than one-half of these are related to toilet visits.[16] A common and serious repercussion of falls is hip fractures, which can lead to postoperative cardiac complications, urinary tract infections, pressure ulcers, and pneumonia.[17] In-hospital mortality after a hip fracture in the elderly reaches almost 5%, and all-cause mortality within 3 months is 5 to 8 times greater in this population compared with controls.[18] In the long term, hip fractures also negatively affect patients' functional status, ability to complete activities of daily living, and overall health-related quality of life.[19]

In addition to individual impact, consequences of OAB can be seen within society. The economic consequences of OAB are significant, with annual costs estimated to be more than $12 billion annually in the United States. This figure includes direct costs related to treating OAB, the treatment of associated conditions as described previously, and the indirect costs from loss of productivity. On average, approximately $410 is spent for each female patient with OAB.[20] A study by Coyne and colleagues[12] found that patients with OAB were more likely to be unemployed compared with those without symptoms (9.0% compared with 7.7%), and those with OAB were also more likely to change jobs and retire early. Of patients who were employed, 26% reported always worrying about interrupting work with frequent trips to the bathroom.

Initial Evaluation: Patient History, Symptoms, and Physical Examination

A diagnosis of OAB is given when urinary frequency (daytime and nighttime) and urgency, with urgency incontinence (OAB-wet) or without urgency incontinence (OAB-dry) is self-reported as bothersome. Urgency is defined as "a sudden, compelling desire to pass urine which is difficult to defer."[21] Nocturia associated with OAB is often characterized by small volume voids, in contrast with the normal or large volumes present in nocturnal polyuria, which is associated with other comorbidities such as sleep disturbances, and vascular and/or cardiac disease.[22]

The initial workup of a patient for OAB includes a thorough history to assess for symptoms and their degree of bother. Comorbid conditions should also be reviewed as well as medications that may have an impact, such as diuretics. A fluid intake and voiding diary may also be obtained to better objectively measure voiding frequency and leakage episodes, and to assess whether excessive fluid consumption or caffeine use may be contributing to the patient's symptoms.

A physical examination should be performed on each patient, including an abdominal examination, pelvic examination, and lower extremity examination to assess for edema and possible comorbid condition. If a neurologic condition is suspected a basic neurologic examination, including a lower extremity assessment, should be included.

Diagnostic testing and imaging
In addition to complete history and physical examination, evaluation of OAB should include a urinalysis to rule out infection and hematuria. UDS, cystoscopy, and diagnostic renal and bladder ultrasound examination should not be used in the initial workup of a patient with OAB and normal urinalysis. Obtaining a postvoid residual is left at the clinician's discretion and is usually recommended in patients with a neurologic condition or history of genitourinary surgery.[22]

Management goals
The first step in managing OAB is patient education of normal urinary tract function, counseling on the risks and benefits of available treatment, and patient–provider agreement on treatment goals. Some patients may deny further treatment and accept their current voiding habits. If patients are significantly bothered by their symptoms, the primary goal is to lessen symptoms and optimize quality of life.[22]

First-line treatment: behavioral therapies
All patients with OAB who are interested in treatment should be offered behavioral therapies, which are noninvasive and are associated with very minimal adverse events. Therapies include bladder training (timed voiding, relaxation techniques, incremental voiding) and behavioral training (pelvic floor muscle training). Weight loss, reduction of fluid intake, treatment of constipation, and avoiding bladder irritants such as caffeine and alcohol have also shown to reduce bothersome OAB symptoms.

Second-line treatment: pharmacologic management
Behavioral therapies are often used in combination with drug therapies to optimize symptom control and quality of life. Antimuscarinics decrease OAB symptoms, because the detrusor muscle of the bladder is innervated with muscarinic receptors. The most bothersome side effects include dry mouth and constipation, but can also lead to blurred vision, urinary retention, and impaired cognitive function. There is no evidence for differential efficacy across medications, although pharmacologically they vary in muscarinic receptor affinity and selectivity and in ability to cross the blood–brain barrier. The choice of medication should be determined by the patient's history of antimuscarinic use, comorbidities, and other medications. Efficacy for anticholinergics range from 15.1% to 23.6%, depending on type and dose.[23] Rates of side effects also differ, with 4.9% to 12.1% of patients reporting constipation and 23.7% to 61.4% reporting dry mouth.[22] Of note, 51.3% of patients do not refill anticholinergic prescriptions after 2 years or less of use, owing to either loss of efficacy or bothersome side effects.[24] Mirabegron, a β_3-adrenoceptor agonist, has also been shown to be effective in reducing OAB symptoms of urgency, nocturia, and incontinence. Potential side effects include nasal congestion and hypertension, and there is also a black box warning regarding angioedema.[25]

Third-line treatment: surgical management

For patients whose symptoms are still not adequately controlled with behavioral modifications and a trial of pharmacologic treatment, clinicians may counsel patients on procedural options. Third-line treatments include intradetrusor onabotulinumtoxin A, peripheral tibial nerve stimulation, and sacral neuromodulation.

Onabotulinumtoxin A injection into the detrusor is done cystoscopically in the office under local anesthesia or light sedation, taking only 15 minutes. It is approved by the US Food and Drug Administration for both neurogenic and idiopathic urge leakage, urgency, and frequency. Effects last 3 to 6 months, and there are typically no systemic side effects. However, short-term adverse effects such as urinary tract infection, acute urinary retention, and incomplete voiding with an increased postvoid residual should be discussed with patients.

Peripheral tibial nerve stimulation is delivered via a 34-G needle electrode inserted above the medial malleolus once weekly for 12 weeks with maintenance therapy once monthly thereafter. Impulses travel from the ankle along the posterior tibial nerve to the sacral nerves, which innervate the detrusor muscle. Although the exact mechanism of action is not completely understood, it is thought to interrupt abnormal reflex arcs that may affect bladder dysfunction.[26]

Sacral neuromodulation may also be used as third-line treatment for patients with refractory symptoms. Sacral neuromodulation involves an implantable device that consists of a lead and a stimulator device that delivers a low level electrical stimulation to the S3 sacral nerve root or the pudendal nerve. It is placed in 2 stages; the first as a test to evaluate efficacy, where the wire is connected to an external stimulating, and the second involving implantation of the permanent device. The mechanism of action is also not fully understood, but is thought to activate somatic afferent axons that modulate sensory processing and the micturition reflex pathways in the spinal cord. Infection of the sacral neuromodulating system occurs in 3% to 10% of patients, requiring explantation with the possibility to undergo reimplantation at a later date.[27] Patients with a sacral neuromodulation implant have restrictions regarding MRI, with the most recent version allowing only MRI of the head and no other areas of the body.[28]

STRESS URINARY INCONTINENCE

SUI is the involuntary leakage of urine owing to increased abdominal pressure, which can be caused by activities such as sneezing, coughing, exercise, lifting, and position change.[29] SUI results from the weakening of the pelvic floor musculature and subsequent weakening of the urinary sphincter, which allow bladder pressure to exceed urethral pressure. Pure SUI is not preceded by urge; if the patient also complains of urgency, the term mixed urinary incontinence is used.

Risk factors for SUI include female gender, pregnancy, vaginal childbirth, hysterectomy, high-impact activities such as running or jumping over many years, pelvic organ prolapse, obesity, smoking, and older age. One study found each 5-unit increase in body mass index is associated with a 20% to 70% increased risk of urinary incontinence, with a stronger association of increasing weight with SUI than urge urinary incontinence.[30] Up to 80% of trampolinists have reported SUI[31] and up to 80% of patients with pelvic organ prolapse also have SUI.[32]

Epidemiology and Impact

The prevalence of SUI in the overall female population ranges from 15% to 37%.[33] Like urge urinary incontinence, SUI can negatively impact quality of life. Women with SUI also have lower overall sexual function, lower frequency of sexual intercourse, less satisfaction, and higher avoidance of sex, which in turn may lead to partner dissatisfaction and relationship stress.[34] Although SUI does have a significant impact on quality of life, overall, urge symptoms were generally associated with more impairment compared with stress symptoms.[35]

SUI can have a large impact on costs to both patients and society. On a per-patient basis, patients with SUI had direct costs that were 134%, or $5642, more than those for their controls. In terms of indirect workplace expenses, each employee with SUI is estimated to have $4208 in indirect costs.[36]

Initial evaluation: patient history, symptoms, and physical examination

SUI is a clinical diagnosis characterized by leakage of urine with increased intraabdominal pressure (coughing, sneezing, laughing, physical exertion). A thorough patient history should be taken and may include a questionnaire for leakage of urine with the aforementioned activities.

A complete physical examination including a pelvic examination should also be performed. SUI often coexists with pelvic organ prolapse, because they both are caused by pelvic floor dysfunction. A pelvic examination can also rule out urethral or pelvic masses that may cause mass effect on the bladder, exacerbating symptoms of SUI. Pooling of urine in the vagina should prompt evaluation for a urinary tract fistula.

A urinary stress test consists of having a patient with a full bladder perform a Valsalva maneuver or cough. The test can be performed in the standing or dorsal lithotomy position while assessing the urethra for leakage. A false negative may result from a small bladder volume or from patient inhibition. Assessment of urethral hypermobility (Q-tip test) often does not aid in diagnosis, and is no longer used routinely.

Diagnostic Testing and Imaging

Additional diagnostic testing is usually not necessary for women with uncomplicated SUI and a positive cough stress test result. If women have a history of prior continence surgery, prior pelvic radiation, neurogenic LUT dysfunction (ie, spinal cord injury, multiple sclerosis), or the diagnosis of SUI is not clear, additional evaluation with urodynamic studies may be warranted.[29]

Management Goals

Similar to the treatment of urge urinary incontinence, the first step of managing SUI is a discussion with the patient involving expectations as well as risks and benefits of each therapy available. Should the patient and provider decide to pursue treatment, options range from conservative to surgical approaches.

Nonsurgical, Conservative Therapies

Patients who are mildly symptomatic or patients who do not want immediate surgical intervention may opt for conservative measures to treat SUI. These include continence pessaries, vaginal inserts, and pelvic floor physical therapy. Behavioral modifications, such as weight loss and dietary changes to reduce consumption of alcohol, caffeine, and carbonated beverages, may also decrease symptoms.[37]

There is no pharmacologic therapy approved by the US Food and Drug Administration for SUI in the United States. Duloxetine, a selective serotonin reuptake inhibitor, is approved for treating SUI in Europe, but is still under investigation in the United States owing to potential adverse effects on mental health.[38]

Surgical Treatment

Surgical options are available for patients whose symptoms are not adequately controlled with conservative therapy. In a randomized study comparing efficacy of surgery with physiotherapy, approximately 50% of women in the physiotherapy group crossed over to the surgery group owing to inadequately controlled symptoms.[39] The main categories of surgical intervention include injection of bulking agents, slings, and colposuspension. Physicians should advise patients that surgical management may cause urinary retention, requiring intermittent catheterization or reoperation.[29]

The least invasive surgical option for SUI is the use of urethral bulking agents, although few long-term data exist. Urethral bulking agents are endoscopically injected into the submucosa of the mid urethra, providing increased sphincter pressure to improve continence.[40] This is typically done in the office with local anesthesia and may be recommended for elderly patients, patients with an increased risk of anesthetic complications, and patients who are reluctant to undergo a more invasive procedure.[29] Efficacy rates for urethral bulking agents range from 40% to 80% depending on the definition of success used.[41] It is important to counsel patients that repeat injections may be required for continued effect, with some studies citing injections as often as every 3 months.[41]

The placement of a midurethral synthetic sling (MUS) is widely used for SUI with data exceeding 15 years of follow-up. The advent of the MUS has had a significant impact on SUI treatment because it can be performed in less than an hour as an outpatient procedure with low morbidity. The sling involves the passage of a small strip of tape through either the retropubic or obturator space, with entry or exit points in the abdomen or groin, to provide additional support to the urethra. Midurethral slings can be placed via a retropubic, transobturator, or single incision approach. Both retropubic RMUS and transobturator MUS have been shown to have success rates between 43% and 92% and short-term analyses have found the 2 approaches to have equivalent safety profiles.[42] Although there have been safety warnings issued by the US Food and Drug Administration about the use of mesh for transvaginal pelvic organ prolapse, there are no concerns regarding the use of mesh for MUS procedures.[43]

Pubovaginal slings (PVS) involve the placement of autologous fascia lata or rectus fascia beneath the urethra to provide additional support. A PVS is an option for patients who decline implantation of synthetic materials, although it does have the added morbidity of fascial harvest, which include longer operating time, bleeding, and infection.[44] A PVS has been shown to have high efficacy with rates between 87% and 92% with a follow-up of 15 years.[45]

Colposuspension is a suture-only surgery that suspends and stabilizes the urethra to replace the urethrovesical junction and proximal urethra intraabdominally. Colposuspension has been largely replaced by MUS, and is primarily performed on patients who are undergoing concomitant open or laparoscopic or robotic surgery, such as a hysterectomy.[29] Colposuspension has similar rates of efficacy compared with MUS,[46] although it carries a higher retreatment rate compared with autologous PVS.[47]

VESICOVAGINAL AND URETEROVAGINAL FISTULAS

Fistulas of the urogenital tract are abnormal connections between the female genital tract and the bladder, urethra, or ureters. Risk factors for the formation of a vesicovaginal fistula (VVF) include history of pelvic radiation, cesarean delivery, endometriosis, previous pelvic surgery, pelvic inflammatory disease, vasculopathy, tobacco use, retained pessary, and use of vaginal mesh.[48] Fistula formation may appear years after radiation (ie, radiation for cervical, vaginal, or endometrial cancer) has been completed.[49]

Epidemiology and Impact

In the United States and other developed countries, the majority of VVF are a result of injury to the LUT during benign gynecologic surgery.[50] In developing countries, VVF are often a complication of obstructed labor during childbirth.[51]

The symptoms of a urogenital fistula are very distressing to patients. The continuous urinary incontinence excoriates adjacent genital areas, produces painful rashes, and results in an offensive odor. Consequences tend to be even greater in developing countries because obstructed labor often results in perinatal loss of the infant. Social constructs in developing countries also lead to ostracizing of women with VVFs, because the condition is considered a punishment from God. Women are often deserted by their husbands after diagnosis, and are not allowed to prepare food or participate in social events or religious ceremonies.[52]

Initial Evaluation: Patient History, Symptoms, and Physical Examination

Signs of VVF or ureterovaginal fistula (UVF) include gross hematuria, urinoma formation, and painless urinary incontinence. The pattern of urinary incontinence is often predictive of the type of fistula present. Constant incontinence with no voluntary voids is more characteristic of VVF, whereas constant incontinence in addition to voids is predictive of UVF; intermittent incontinence with positional changes indicates a small fistula.

Evaluation of a VVF or UVF involves a thorough physical examination, including a pelvic examination, to assess for location of the fistula, size, and quality of vaginal tissue surrounding the tract. Small fistulas may be difficult to visualize, and dye tests may be needed for further evaluation. Endoscopic evaluation of the urethra, bladder, and vagina should be performed to identify the relationship of the fistula to the ureteral orifices and bladder neck. Biopsy of the fistulous tract should be also be considered to rule out malignancy.[53] Retrograde pyelograms may also be considered to assess ureteral anatomy.[54]

Treatment of Fistulas

Treatment of fistulas may include prolonged catheterization of 4 to 8 weeks for urinary diversion, which may lead to resolution of very small (<5 mm) fistulas.[55] Minimally invasive therapies for urogenital fistulas have been shown to be successful, including injection of cynanoacrylic glue fibrin glue, and fulguration, although the sample sizes are small and follow-up limited.[56–61]

Surgical management of VVF was traditionally delayed for 3 months after diagnosis to allow for reduced tissue edema and inflammation,[62] but studies have shown that expedited surgical management is beneficial and reduces patient suffering.[63,64] VVFs may be repaired with either a vaginal or abdominal approach with success rates for both reaching nearly 100%.[18] Vaginal approaches are used for 32% to 100% of repairs, depending on institution and surgeon preferences.[62,65,66] Transvaginal approaches are generally favored over transabdominal approaches, given the avoidance of an abdominal procedure with improved pain control and recovery time.[67,68] The Martius graft, or labial fibrofatty tissue graft, is commonly used to reinforce repair of fistulas high in the vaginal vault. Abdominal approaches are usually reserved for recurrent or complex fistulas.[62] Indications for an abdominal approach include involvement of the ureteral orifice, need for bladder augmentation, vaginal stenosis, and uterine or cervical involvement. These approaches may use interposition of omentum between the bladder and the vagina, and are often performed laparoscopically or with robot assistance, especially if patients require concomitant procedures.[69]

Repair of UVFs are typically distal and involve excision of the fistula with surgical reimplantation of the ureter into the bladder, though other techniques may be used for fistulas with more proximal ureteral involvement.[70]

SUMMARY

The initial evaluation of women with voiding dysfunction or incontinence begins with a thorough history and physical examination, including a pelvic examination. Urodynamic studies are usually not indicated for uncomplicated cases. The provider and patient should discuss goals of management to set a realistic course that meets expectations. Conservative management of OAB includes behavioral therapies as well as pharmacologic treatment. SUI and urogenital fistulas are best treated with surgical intervention.

REFERENCES

1. DeLancey JOL. Anatomy and physiology of urinary continence. Clin Obstet Gynecol 1990;33(2):298.
2. de Groat WC, Griffiths D, Yoshimura N. Neural control of the lower urinary tract. Compr Physiol 2015;5(1):327–96.
3. Losada L, Amundsen CL, Ashton-Miller J, et al. Expert panel recommendations on lower urinary tract health of women across their life span. J Womens Health (Larchmt) 2016;25(11):1086.
4. Bettez M, Tu LM, Carlson K, et al. 2012 update: guidelines for adult urinary incontinence collaborative consensus document for the Canadian Urological Association. Can Urol Assoc J 2012;6(5):354.
5. Winters JC, Dmochowski RR, Goldman HB, et al. Urodynamic studies in adults: AUA/SUFU guideline. J Urol 2012;188(6):2464.
6. Haylen BT, de Ridder D, Freeman RM, et al. An International Urogynecological Association (IUGA)/International Continence Society (ICS) joint report on the terminology for female pelvic floor dysfunction. Neurourol Urodyn 2010;29(1):4–20.
7. de Boer TA, Slieker-ten Hove MCP, Burger CW, et al. The prevalence and risk factors of overactive bladder symptoms and its relation to pelvic organ prolapse symptoms in a general female population. Int Urogynecol J 2011;22(5):569–75.
8. Irwin DE, Milsom I, Hunskaar S, et al. Population-based survey of urinary incontinence, overactive bladder, and other lower urinary tract symptoms in five countries: results of the EPIC study. Eur Urol 2006;50(6):1306.
9. Sexton CC, Coyne KS, Thompson C, et al. Prevalence and effect on health-related quality of life of overactive bladder in older Americans: results from the epidemiology of lower urinary tract symptoms study. J Am Geriatr Soc 2011; 59(8):1465–70.
10. Stewart W, Van Rooyen J, Cundiff G, et al. Prevalence and burden of overactive bladder in the United States. World J Urol 2003;20(6):327–36.
11. Coyne KS, Sexton CC, Vats V, et al. National community prevalence of overactive bladder in the United States stratified by sex and age. Urology 2011;77(5): 1081–7.
12. Coyne KS, Sexton CC, Thompson CL, et al. Impact of overactive bladder on work productivity. Urology 2012;80(1):97–103.
13. Newman DK, Koochaki PE. Characteristics and impact of interrupted sleep in women with overactive bladder. Urol Nurs 2011;31(5):304–12.

14. Milsom I, Kaplan SA, Coyne KS, et al. Effect of bothersome overactive bladder symptoms on health-related quality of life, anxiety, depression, and treatment seeking in the United States: results from EpiLUTS. Urology 2012;80(1):90–6.

15. Asplund R. Hip fractures, nocturia, and nocturnal polyuria in the elderly. Arch Gerontol Geriatr 2006;43(3):319–26.

16. Jensen J, Lundin-Olsson L, Nyberg L, et al. Falls among frail older people in residential care. Scand J Public Health 2002;30(1):54–61.

17. Beaupre LA, Cinats JG, Senthilselvan A, et al. Reduced morbidity for elderly patients with a hip fracture after implementation of a perioperative evidence-based clinical pathway. Qual Saf Health Care 2006;15(5):375.

18. Orces CH. In-hospital hip fracture mortality trends in older adults: the national hospital discharge survey, 1988–2007. J Am Geriatr Soc 2013;61(12):2248.

19. Zidén L, Kreuter M, Frändin K. Long-term effects of home rehabilitation after hip fracture – 1-year follow-up of functioning, balance confidence, and health-related quality of life in elderly people. Disabil Rehabil 2010;32(1):18–32.

20. Teh-Wei H, Wagner TH. Health-related consequences of overactive bladder: an economic perspective. BJU Int 2005;96:43–5.

21. Van Kerrebroeck P, Abrams P, Chaikin D, et al. The standardization of terminology in nocturia: report from the standardization subcommittee of the International Continence Society. BJU Int 2002;90:11–5.

22. Gormley EA, Lightner DJ, Faraday M, et al. Diagnosis and treatment of overactive bladder (non-neurogenic) in adults: AUA/SUFU guideline amendment. J Urol 2015;193(5):1572–80.

23. Anderson RU, MacDiarmid S, Kell S, et al. Effectiveness and tolerability of extended-release oxybutynin vs extended-release tolterodine in women with or without prior anticholinergic treatment for overactive bladder. Int Urogynecol J Pelvic Floor Dysfunct 2006;17(5):502–11.

24. Chancellor MB, Migliaccio-Walle K, Bramley TJ, et al. Long-term patterns of use and treatment failure with anticholinergic agents for overactive bladder. Clin Ther 2013;35(11):1744–51.

25. Myrbetriq. Northbrook (IL): Astellas Pharma US, Inc; 2015.

26. Peters KM, MacDiarmid SA, Wooldridge LS, et al. Randomized trial of percutaneous tibial nerve stimulation versus extended-release tolterodine: results from the overactive bladder innovative therapy trial. J Urol 2009;182(3):1055–61.

27. Lee C, Pizarro-Berdichevsky J, Clifton MM, et al. Sacral neuromodulation implant infection: risk factors and prevention. Curr Urol Rep 2017;18(2):16.

28. MRI guidelines for InterStim therapy neurostimulation systems. Minneapolis (MN): Medtronic, Inc; 2012.

29. Kobashi KC, Albo ME, Dmochowski RR, et al. Surgical treatment of female stress urinary incontinence: AUA/SUFU guideline. J Urol 2017;198(4):875–83.

30. Subak LL, Richter HE, Hunskaar S. Obesity and urinary incontinence: epidemiology and clinical research update. J Urol 2009;182(6, Supplement):S2–7.

31. Eliasson K, Larsson T, Mattsson E. Prevalence of stress incontinence in nulliparous elite trampolinists. Scand J Med Sci Sports 2002;12(2):106–10.

32. Richardson DA, Bent AE, Ostergard DR. The effect of uterovaginal prolapse on urethrovesical pressure dynamics. Am J Obstet Gynecol 1983;146(8):901–5.

33. Bø K, Sundgot-Borgen J. Are former female elite athletes more likely to experience urinary incontinence later in life than non-athletes? Scand J Med Sci Sports 2010;20(1):100–4.

34. Lim R, Liong ML, Leong WS, et al. Effect of stress urinary incontinence on the sexual function of couples and the quality of life of patients. J Urol 2016;196(1): 153–8.

35. Hunskaar S, Vinsnes A. The quality of life in women with urinary incontinence as measured by the sickness impact profile. J Am Geriatr Soc 1991;39(4):378–82.

36. Birnbaum HG, Leong SA, Oster EF, et al. Cost of stress urinary incontinence: a claims data analysis. Pharmacoeconomics 2004;22(2):95–105.

37. Dallosso HM, McGrother CW, Matthews RJ, et al. The association of diet and other lifestyle factors with overactive bladder and stress incontinence: a longitudinal study in women. BJU Int 2003;92(1):69–77.

38. Maund E, Guski LS, Gøtzsche PC. Considering benefits and harms of duloxetine for treatment of stress urinary incontinence: a meta-analysis of clinical study reports. CMAJ 2017;189(5):E194–203.

39. Labrie J, Berghmans BLCM, Fischer K, et al. Surgery versus physiotherapy for stress urinary incontinence. N Engl J Med 2013;369(12):1124–33.

40. Klarskov N, Lose G. Urethral injection therapy: what is the mechanism of action? Neurourol Urodyn 2008;27(8):789–92.

41. Matsuoka PK, Locali RF, Pacetta AM, et al. The efficacy and safety of urethral injection therapy for urinary incontinence in women: a systematic review. Clinics (Sao Paulo) 2016;71:94–100.

42. Ford AA, Rogerson L, Cody JD, et al. Mid-urethral sling operations for stress urinary incontinence in women. Cochrane Database Syst Rev 2017;(7):CD006375.

43. Clemons JL, Weinstein M, Guess MK, et al. Impact of the 2011 FDA transvaginal mesh safety update on AUGS members' use of synthetic mesh and biologic grafts in pelvic reconstructive surgery. Female Pelvic Med Reconstr Surg 2013; 19(4):191–8.

44. Bang S-L, Belal M. Autologous pubovaginal slings: back to the future or a lost art? Res Rep Urol 2016;8:11–20.

45. Athanasopoulos A, Gyftopoulos K, McGuire EJ. Efficacy and preoperative prognostic factors of autologous fascia rectus sling for treatment of female stress urinary incontinence. Urology 2011;78(5):1034–8.

46. Drahoradova P, Martan A, Svabik K, et al. Longitudinal trends with Improvement in quality of life after TVT, TVT O and Burch colposuspension procedures. Med Sci Monit 2011;17(2):CR67–72.

47. Albo ME, Richter HE, Brubaker L, et al. Burch colposuspension versus fascial sling to reduce urinary stress incontinence. N Engl J Med 2007;356(21):2143–55.

48. Tancer ML. Observations on prevention and management of vesicovaginal fistula after total hysterectomy. Surg Gynecol Obstet 1992;175(6):501–6.

49. Pushkar DY, Dyakov VV, Kasyan GR. Management of radiation-induced vesicovaginal fistula. Eur Urol 2009;55(1):131–8.

50. Bai SW, Huh EH, Jung DJ, et al. Urinary tract injuries during pelvic surgery: incidence rates and predisposing factors. Int Urogynecol J Pelvic Floor Dysfunct 2006;17(4):360–4.

51. Wall LL, Karshima JA, Kirschner C, et al. The obstetric vesicovaginal fistula: characteristics of 899 patients from Jos, Nigeria. Am J Obstet Gynecol 2004;190(4): 1011–9.

52. Ahmed S, Holtz SA. Social and economic consequences of obstetric fistula: life changed forever? Int J Gynaecol Obstet 2007;99:S10–5.

53. Narayanan P, Nobbenhuis M, Reynolds KM, et al. Fistulas in malignant gynecologic disease: etiology, imaging, and management. Radiographics 2009;29(4): 1073–83.

54. Chou MT, Wang CJ, Lien RC. Prophylactic ureteral catheterization in gynecologic surgery: a 12-year randomized trial in a community hospital. Int Urogynecol J Pelvic Floor Dysfunct 2009;20(6):689–93.
55. Bazi T. Spontaneous closure of vesicovaginal fistulas after bladder drainage alone: review of the evidence. Int Urogynecol J 2007;18(3):329–33.
56. Sawant A, Kasat G, Kumar V. Cyanoacrylate injection in management of recurrent vesicovaginal fistula: our experience. Indian J Urol 2016;32(4):323–5.
57. Muto G, D'Urso L, Castelli E, et al. Cyanoacrylic glue: a minimally invasive nonsurgical first line approach for the treatment of some urinary fistulas. J Urol 2005; 174(6):2239–43.
58. Shirvan MK, Alamdari DH, Ghoreifi A. A novel method for iatrogenic vesicovaginal fistula treatment: autologous platelet rich plasma injection and platelet rich fibrin glue interposition. J Urol 2013;189(6):2125–9.
59. D'Arcy FT, Jaffry S. The treatment of vesicovaginal fistula by endoscopic injection of fibrin glue. Surgeon 2010;8(3):174–6.
60. Shah SJ. Role of day care vesicovaginal fistula fulguration in small vesicovaginal fistula. J Endourol 2010;24(10):1659–60.
61. Stovsky MD, Ignatoff JM, Blum MD, et al. Use of electrocoagulation in the treatment of vesicovaginal fistulas. J Urol 1994;152(5 Pt 1):1443–4.
62. Angioli R, Penalver M, Muzii L, et al. Guidelines of how to manage vesicovaginal fistula. Crit Rev Oncol Hematol 2003;48(3):295–304.
63. Badenoch DF, Tiptaft RC, Thakar DR, et al. Early repair of accidental injury to the ureter or bladder following gynaecological surgery. Br J Urol 1987;59(6):516–8.
64. Margolis T, Mercer LJ. Vesicovaginal fistula. Obstet Gynecol Surv 1994;49(12): 840–7.
65. Zambon JP, Batezini NSS, Pinto ERS, et al. Do we need new surgical techniques to repair vesico-vaginal fistulas? Int Urogynecol J 2010;21(3):337–42.
66. Bodner-Adler B, Hanzal E, Pablik E, et al. Management of vesicovaginal fistulas (VVFs) in women following benign gynaecologic surgery: a systematic review and meta-analysis. PLoS One 2017;12(2):e0171554.
67. Cohen BL, Gousse AE. Current techniques for vesicovaginal fistula repair: surgical pearls to optimize cure rate. Curr Urol Rep 2007;8(5):413–8.
68. Eilber KS, Kavaler E, RodríGuez LV, et al. Ten-year experience with transvaginal vesicovaginal fistula repair using tissue interposition. J Urol 2003;169(3):1033–6.
69. Ezzat M, Ezzat MM, Tran VQ, et al. Repair of giant vesicovaginal fistulas. J Urol 2009;181(3):1184–8.
70. Papanikolaou A, Tsolakidis D, Theodoulidis V, et al. Surgery for ureteral repair after gynaecological procedures: a single tertiary centre experience. Arch Gynecol Obstet 2013;287(5):947–50.

Penile and Urethral Reconstructive Surgery

Jonathan E. Kiechle, MD[a], Nathan Chertack, BS[b],
Christopher M. Gonzalez, MD, MBA[a],*

KEYWORDS

- Urethral stricture • Urethral diseases • Reconstructive surgical procedures
- Urethral sphincters

KEY POINTS

- Penile and urethral reconstructive surgical procedures are used to treat a variety of urologic diagnoses.
- Urethral stricture disease can lead to progressive lower urinary tract symptoms and may require multiple surgical procedures to improve patient's symptoms.
- Male stress urinary incontinence is associated with intrinsic sphincter deficiency oftentimes associated with radical prostatectomy.
- Men suffering from urethral stricture disease and stress urinary incontinence should be referred to a urologist because multiple treatment options exist to improve their quality of life.

INTRODUCTION

Penile and urethral reconstructive surgery is a broad area of urologic care that encompasses the surgical treatment of urethral stricture disease and voiding dysfunction, erectile dysfunction (ED), urologic issues after cancer treatment, and many other diseases of the male external genitalia and lower urinary tract. This article discusses various surgical options for the treatment of urethral stricture disease and male stress urinary incontinence (SUI).

A urethral stricture begins as a scar within the corpus spongiosum surrounding the anterior urethra (urethral meatus, fossa navicularis, penile urethra, bulbar urethra). Contraction of this scarred tissue results in narrowing of the urethral lumen and can lead to lower urinary tract symptoms (**Fig. 1**). A bladder neck contracture (BNC) or urethral stenosis refers to narrowing of the bladder neck or posterior urethra

Disclosures: None of the authors have any disclosures or conflicts of interest.
[a] Urology Institute, University Hospitals Cleveland Medical Center, Case Western Reserve University School of Medicine, 11100 Euclid Avenue, Cleveland, OH 44106, USA; [b] Case Western Reserve University School of Medicine, 11100 Euclid Avenue, Cleveland, OH 44106, USA
* Corresponding author. Urology Institute, University Hospitals Cleveland Medical Center, Case Western Reserve University School of Medicine, 11100 Euclid Avenue, Cleveland, OH 44106.
E-mail address: Christopher.Gonzalez@UHhospitals.org

Med Clin N Am 102 (2018) 325–335
https://doi.org/10.1016/j.mcna.2017.10.007
0025-7125/18/© 2017 Elsevier Inc. All rights reserved.

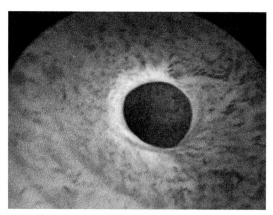

Fig. 1. Cystoscopic view of urethral stricture.

(membranous urethra, prostatic urethra) respectively usually as a result of prior surgical intervention or pelvic trauma. Urethral strictures and BNCs both present significant treatment challenges for urologists and can necessitate multiple surgical procedures to keep patients voiding without substantial difficulty. These procedures vary from endoscopic dilation of the urethra to formal urethral repair requiring excision of the stricture or the use of autologous grafts for urethral augmentation.

The incidence of urethral stricture disease is not well defined, but a recent analysis of Medicare data found the prevalence of male urethral stricture disease to be 0.9%.[1] Many underlying conditions can lead to the development of urethral strictures, including pelvic trauma, lichen sclerosis, previous lower urinary tract instrumentation, and sexually transmitted infections. Unfortunately, for many patients, it is not possible to determine the underlying cause of their stricture disease because the factor inciting the development of spongiofibrosis may occur many years before the onset of lower urinary tract symptoms.

Male SUI is associated with intrinsic sphincter deficiency and can occur following radical prostatectomy or may be associated with pelvic trauma, congenital conditions, and other surgical procedures. A recent meta-analysis of incontinence outcomes following robotic radical prostatectomy reported an overall incidence of SUI of 4% to 31% at 12 months following surgery.[2] The treatment of male SUI following radical prostatectomy is also highly variable, ranging from observation to the use of external clamps to the implantation of prosthetic devices to improve continence.

URETHRAL DILATION AND DIRECT VISION INTERNAL URETHROTOMY
Indications/Contraindications

Urethral dilation and direct vision internal urethrotomy (DVIU) offer minimally invasive approaches to the management of urethral stricture disease in appropriately selected patients. Dilation may be the procedure of choice for patients who cannot safely undergo general anesthesia, have limited life expectancy, or present emergently in acute urinary retention. However, the repeated use of urethral dilation is contraindicated in patients appropriate for urethroplasty who present with recurrent stricture disease.[3]

DVIU may be considered in patients with symptomatic bulbar urethral strictures less than 2 cm in length.[3] DVIU is not recommended for strictures in the penile urethra, and repeated treatment with DVIU following an initial recurrence is unlikely to provide durable long-term success.[4,5] Importantly, both urethral dilation and DVIU are less technically demanding than open urethroplasty, and neither endoscopic approach appears to offer an advantage over the other.

Patient Preparation

Patient preparation for urethral reconstruction involves a history and physical examination and diagnostic testing to determine the full extent of the patient's stricture disease. The history and physical examination focus on the patient's lower urinary tract symptoms and include an International Prostate Symptom Score questionnaire to objectively measure the patient's urinary symptoms. A thorough surgical history is taken to determine if the patient has had prior surgery on the lower urinary tract.

Diagnostic testing may include a urinalysis, post–void residual, retrograde urethrogram (RUG), voiding cystogram (VCUG), ultrasound, and cystoscopy. An RUG allows for anatomic evaluation of the urethra, whereas a VCUG provides both anatomic and functional information about the lower urinary tract (**Fig. 2**). Ultrasound has also been shown to allow accurate determination of total stricture length through assessment of the extent of spongiofibrosis.[6]

Approach

Urethral dilation is generally performed by passing sequentially larger caliber dilators past the point of stricture within the urethra. The goal of dilation is to widen the scar without causing more significant scarring. There are numerous techniques available for urethral dilation, including urethral sounds, filiforms and followers, and dilating balloons.

DVIU is performed by visually identifying the area of stricture with a cystoscope and incising the scar tissue. The goal of DVIU is to cut the urethral scar, leading to healing by secondary intention so that the urethral lumen remains wider than before surgery. If the urethra reepithelializes before significant wound contraction the urethra will remain patent. However, if significant and rapid wound contraction occurs, the stricture will recur.

Various instruments have been used for DVIU, including "cold" knives without energy, knives using cutting current, and various types of laser fibers. There are no definitive data proving the benefit of one technique over another; however, in general, a cold knife should be used within the urethra, whereas a hot or cold knife can be

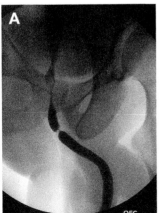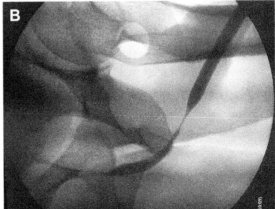

Fig. 2. (A, B) Retrograde urethrogram.

used within the prostate or bladder neck. In addition, significant debate exists about where the DVIU incision should be made. The classic DVIU involves a single incision at the 12 o'clock position, but multiple variations exist without definitive evidence proving the efficacy of a specific technique.

Postprocedure Care

Patients will have a urinary catheter placed following the procedure to drain the bladder postoperatively. Although historically the catheter was often left in situ for an extended period to force the urethra to heal around the lumen of the catheter, it is now accepted that the catheter can be safely removed after 72 hours.[3,7] Some patients may be started on regimens of self-catheterization following catheter removal because there is evidence that postoperative self-catheterization can improve long-term patency rates.[8] Finally, patients require follow-up to evaluate for stricture recurrence because urethral dilation and DVIU have high rates of stricture recurrence.

Reducing Complications

Complications of urethral dilation and DVIU include bleeding secondary to aggressive tearing of scar tissue, urinary tract infection, urethral perforation, and rectal injury. Patients are given a dose of antibiotics periprocedurally to help reduce the risk of urinary tract infection.[9] The risk of urethral perforation and rectal injury can be reduced by endoscopically passing a wire into the bladder and dilating over the wire.

DVIU can also lead to de novo ED. Reported rates of ED following DVIU range from 2.2% to 10.6%.[10] The risk of ED following DVIU increases with long, dense strictures as post-DVIU ED is thought to occur secondary to injury to the corpora cavernosa during the scar incision, leading to veno-occlusive dysfunction. Limiting the use of DVIU to relatively short strictures in the bulbar urethra may limit the development of post-DVIU ED.

Outcomes and Evidence

Outcomes data following DVIU and dilation are hampered by the lack of prospective, randomized trials and the varying definitions of surgical success used in different studies. A randomized study from a single surgeon including 210 patients found no difference in the rate of stricture recurrence between DVIU and dilation. About 60% of patients who underwent DVIU or dilation for strictures less than 2 cm remained stricture free with a maximal follow-up of 48 months. However, for strictures longer than 4 cm, the stricture recurrence rate by 12 months was 80%, and for strictures between 2 cm and 4 cm, patients initially did well with a recurrence rate of 50% at 1 year, but this success rate decreased to 25% by 48 months.[11]

A recent retrospective study of 128 patients found similar success rates, defined by avoiding recurrent stricture, for patients treated with DVIU. Patients were followed for a median of 16 months with an overall success rate following DVIU of 51.3%. Median time to recurrence was 6 months, and repeat DVIU was found to be a risk factor for recurrence on univariate and multivariate analysis.[12]

URETHROPLASTY
Indications/Contraindications

Urethroplasty refers to the formal open repair of the strictured urethra by either excising the stricture and primarily anastomosing the ends of the urethra (excision and primary anastomosis [EPA]) or performing a substitution urethroplasty with autologous flap or graft tissue. Indications for EPA include a relatively short stricture or stenosis in the bulbar or membranous urethra, respectively, that can be completely excised and repaired with a tension-free anastomosis. Contraindications to EPA include stricture in the penile urethra because EPA in the penile urethra can lead to penile curvature. Indications for substitution urethroplasty include long-segment bulbar urethral stricture, urethral stricture in the penile urethra, and panurethral stricture.

Patient Preparation

As with urethral dilation or DVIU, a full history and physical examination are required as is diagnostic testing to determine the full extent of the patient's stricture disease. If substitution urethroplasty is considered, physical examination of potential donor sites, including the foreskin (if present) and buccal (cheek) mucosa, should be performed.

It is generally recommended that patients with an indwelling urethral catheter or who perform intermittent catheterization have a period of urethral rest before undergoing urethroplasty. For patients with severe strictures who are unable to void or are catheter dependent, a suprapubic tube is placed to keep the urethra free of instrumentation in the weeks leading up to urethroplasty. At least 4 weeks of urethral rest is preferred, and some urologists recommend 3 months of rest before urethroplasty.[13]

Approach

Urethroplasty can be performed through a penile, penoscrotal, or perineal incision depending on the location and length of the strictured urethra. As previously mentioned, substitution urethroplasty uses autologous flaps or grafts to repair the urethra. A flap refers to a piece of tissue that is transferred to a new location with its vascular supply intact. Alternatively, a graft is a piece of tissue that has been excised and transferred to a recipient bed without its prior vascular supply. Therefore, a graft must develop a new vascular supply from its recipient bed through a process known as "take."

Take has 2 phases with each phase lasting about 48 hours. The first step of take is known as imbibition, and during this phase, the graft maintains itself by absorbing nutrients from the underlying recipient bed. The second step is known as inosculation, and during this phase, a new microcirculation develops in the grafted tissue. Both recipient bed and graft tissue characteristics influence the success of this process and the ultimate survival of the grafted tissue.

Donor flaps for urethral reconstruction are generally taken from penile skin, prepuce, or deepithelialized scrotal skin. It is imperative that non–hair-bearing skin be used for urethral reconstruction because the presence of hair in the urethra can cause urinary stone formation, recurrent urinary tract infections, and lower urinary tract symptoms.[14]

A wide variety of different grafts have been used for urethral reconstruction, including full-thickness skin, bladder mucosa, rectal mucosa, and a variety of mucosal tissue from the oral cavity. Currently, the buccal mucosal graft (BMG) is the most commonly used graft tissue for substitution urethroplasty. BMGs are hairless and durable, have hidden donor sites, and are associated with minimal postoperative morbidity.[15,16] BMGs are harvested from the inner cheek, being careful to avoid Stensen duct, the drainage site of the parotid gland.

Urethroplasty is usually performed as a 1-stage procedure whether an EPA or substitution urethroplasty is performed. However, for extremely long segment, recurrent, or panurethral strictures, a 2-stage urethroplasty may be required. Two-stage urethroplasty involves temporarily moving the urethral meatus proximally while allowing the distal urethral plate to heal. After 3 to 6 months, the second stage of the repair is performed with the distal urethra retubularized and the meatus reconstructed in the orthotopic anatomic position. Two-stage urethroplasty can be performed using local skin or BMG as the tissue used to create the neourethra.

Postprocedure Care

Postprocedural care varies based on the location and length of the stricture. Invariably, patients will have a urethral catheter to facilitate healing. The urethral catheter may be capped, with the urine drained via a suprapubic tube, or may be kept to gravity drainage based on the location of the stricture. If a BMG was harvested, patients may be advised to use a chlorhexidine-based mouthwash in the immediate postoperative period. Urinary catheters are generally kept in place for 14 to 21 days, and repeat RUG may be performed before catheter removal to ensure that there is no urine leak at the repair site.[7]

Reducing Complications

Complications following urethroplasty vary based on the location of the urethral stricture and the urethroplasty technique used for repair. Penile curvature, or chordee, is possible following EPA if a long-segment stricture is repaired without adequate mobilization of the urethra. Performing adequate urethral mobilization and limiting the use of EPA to strictures of appropriate length limit the risk of post-EPA penile curvature.

Worsening erectile function has also been reported following urethroplasty. In an early report of ED following urethroplasty, EPA was associated with a 5% risk of subjective ED, and substitution urethroplasty was associated with a 0.9% risk of the same.[17] A recent meta-analysis reported a 1% risk of ED following urethroplasty.[18] It is thought that ED develops following urethroplasty secondary to surgical injury to the nerves and/or vascular supply to the penis. Injury to these anatomic structures is most likely during bulbar urethroplasty, and strictures in the bulbar urethra are associated with higher rates of postoperative ED than strictures in the other segments of the anterior urethra.[19] There is significant debate in the urologic community about how to limit the risk of permanent ED following bulbar urethroplasty, and this topic remains an active area of research.

Substitution urethroplasty is also associated with recurrent stricture, the formation of urethral diverticula, and the development of urethrocutaneous fistulae.[20,21] Recurrent stricture can occur regardless of the graft material used, the length of the stricture repaired, and the location of the original stricture. Urethral diverticula formation is associated with grafts placed on the ventral surface of the urethra (mostly in the penile urethra) because there is less native supportive tissue overlying the ventral urethra, compared with the dorsal urethra, to prevent the development of excessive laxity in the graft over time.[22] Similarly, a urethrocutaneous fistula can develop with ventrally placed grafts because the graft is anatomically closer to the skin, increasing the risk of fistula formation.[20] Placing the graft in a dorsal position on the urethra can help limit this complication but is more technically challenging.

Outcomes

Interpreting outcome data following urethroplasty is challenging, because the definition of success is not standardized across published series. However, many studies use the surrogate marker of not requiring further surgical procedures or instrumentation to maintain a patent urethra as a success. Reported success rates for substitution urethroplasty are generally higher than 80% with similar success rates for many different surgical techniques.[23] Reported success rates following EPA are also high, with success rates greater than 90%.[24] A recent retrospective analysis of greater than 500 patients who underwent bulbar urethroplasty (EPA or substitution urethroplasty) reported an overall success rate of 93% with a mean follow-up of 65 months. On multivariate analysis, patients with longer strictures, increased Charlson Comorbidity Index scores, obesity, and infectious strictures were more likely to fail urethroplasty.[25] Stricture-free rates following substitution urethroplasty may not be as durable as outcomes following EPA.[26] However, there is also the possibility that preoperative characteristics have led to these long-term differences, because more complex, longer strictures generally require substitution urethroplasty rather than EPA.

ARTIFICIAL URINARY SPHINCTER IMPLANTATION
Indications/Contraindications

An artificial urinary sphincter (AUS) is an implantable device that consists of an inflatable cuff that surrounds the urethra and acts as an artificial sphincter, a pump that is placed in the scrotum for operation by the patient, and a pressure-regulating balloon implanted in the submuscular abdominal wall or in the prevesical space. The device is indicated for the treatment of moderate to severe male SUI.

As described previously, male SUI is associated with intrinsic sphincter deficiency and often presents following radical prostatectomy. There is some debate about the appropriate time following radical prostatectomy to offer an AUS to patients, but many urologists would consider offering a continence procedure for patients with significant stress incontinence as soon as 6 months after prostatectomy.[27] Absolute contraindications to AUS implant include a noncompliant or poorly compliant bladder that would put the kidneys at risk of permanent damage with high urinary storage pressures in the bladder. Relative contraindications for implantation include recurrent BNCs and concurrent history of bladder cancer because these patients may require future transurethral surgeries. An additional relative contraindication is poor manual dexterity in the patient as the patient may not be able to operate the scrotal pump to deflate the urethral cuff and empty the bladder.

Patient Preparation

A thorough history and physical examination are required before proceeding with AUS implantation. The history should focus on relevant issues, including when urinary incontinence occurs (stress maneuvers vs urge incontinence), onset of symptoms, number of pads per day, and a voiding diary. As with urethral stricture disease, additional diagnostic testing may be required, including a urinalysis and urine culture, cystoscopy to evaluate for BNC, a post–void residual to ensure that patients are not in overflow incontinence, and potentially formal urodynamics if the patient presents with symptoms of mixed urinary incontinence.

Approach

The AUS can be implanted using a perineal or penoscrotal incision.[28] In the standard AUS implant, the cuff is placed around the proximal bulbar urethra; the pressure-regulating balloon is placed below the fascia of the rectus abdominis muscle, and the pump is placed in a dependent position in the anterior scrotum with the activation button facing out for easy manipulation by the patient. Urethral cuffs of various sizes exist, and the surgeon measures the urethral diameter, without a catheter in the urethra, using a measuring device to determine the appropriate cuff. The pressure-regulating balloon is filled with isotonic saline or contrast depending on surgeon preference. Following placement of the components, appropriate connections are made, and the incision or incisions are closed in multiple layers. Some surgeons perform cystoscopy before closure to identify proper coaptation of the urethra with the cuff inflated. Variations on this classic technique exist for more complex patients, including placing the urethral cuff around the bladder neck, implanting 2 urethral cuffs simultaneously, or placing the cuff in a transcorporal position that incorporates some of the tissue of the corpora cavernosa in the lumen of the urethral cuff.

Postprocedure Care

Patients are generally discharged within 24 hours of surgery. The AUS is deactivated using the scrotal pump in the operating room and is not reactivated for 4 to 6 weeks following the procedure.[29] During this period of postoperative healing, patients will continue to experience SUI as they did preoperatively. After 6 weeks, the patient returns to the office for a postoperative visit; the pump is activated, and the patient is taught how to cycle the device to urinate.

Reducing Complications

Complications following AUS implantation include urinary retention, urethral erosion, urethral atrophy, device infection, and device malfunction.[30–32] Postoperative urinary retention is usually self-limited and can be managed by placing a small-caliber urethral catheter after ensuring that the cuff is deactivated. Urethral erosion occurs when the cuff erodes into the urethra. Erosion requires urgent explantation of all device components because the device is considered infected following urethral erosion. A urethral catheter or suprapubic tube is placed following explantation to facilitate urethral healing. Reimplantation of a new AUS is possible after the urethral erosion has healed completely. A new location on the urethra should be selected for cuff placement. The incidence of urethral erosion can be limited by ensuring that the cuff is deactivated during the perioperative period and by avoiding periods of prolonged urethral catheterization.[29,33,34]

Urethral atrophy tends to present with worsening incontinence in patients with long-standing, previously functional devices. Atrophy occurs because of chronic compression from the urethral cuff. Treatment involves removing and replacing the cuff in a new location, adding a second, or tandem, cuff to the system, or removing and replacing the cuff with a smaller cuff in the same location.[30,35]

Device infection, as with any prosthetic implant, is a devastating complication necessitating urgent explantation and potentially leading to sepsis. Reported infection rates for de novo AUS implantation range from 1% to 3%.[32,36] Current devices are coated with antibiotics at the time of manufacture to try to decrease the infection rate. However, a recent single-institution, retrospective study found no difference in the rate of AUS infections since the introduction of the antibiotic coating.[37] Patients are generally kept on postoperative antibiotics for 3 to 7 days following implantation to try to limit postoperative infection.

Device malfunction can occur if any of the device components develop a leak or if the tubing becomes kinked preventing free flow of fluid through the device. In a recent single-institution, retrospective study of greater than 1000 patients who underwent AUS implantation, 12% of devices developed a mechanical failure with a median follow-up of 4.1 years.[38]

Reported Outcomes

Data regarding functional outcomes following AUS implantation are limited by the retrospective nature of most published studies and the lack of standardization defining success across the literature. Success following AUS implantation is commonly defined as continence (often meaning patients are using 0–1 pads per day) or improved quality of life. A recent systematic review of AUS literature reported an overall "continence" rate of 79% from 7 studies, including 262 patients. Pooling data that included 326 patients, the same review reported an overall dry (no pads) rate of 42.5%.[39]

Male urinary incontinence can significantly affect quality of life because patients alter their lifestyle to avoid activities that lead to incontinence. In a prospective study of 40 patients (mean follow-up 53.4 months) who underwent AUS implantation, all patients described their preoperative quality of life as bad or horrible. The patients also reported that their incontinence was significantly impacting their quality of life. Following implantation, the 36 patients who achieved continence with the AUS reported their quality of life as good and were satisfied with the procedure, and their incontinence was no longer dramatically affecting their quality of life. Overall pad usage decreased from 4 pads per day preoperatively to 0.62 pads per day postoperatively.[40]

SUMMARY

Urethral reconstructive surgery is used to treat a broad range of urologic diagnoses. Although urethral stricture disease and male SUI do not represent life-threatening conditions, they are life altering. Severe stricture disease can lead to painful episodes of acute urinary retention and can require multiple surgical interventions. Severe SUI can cause men to significantly limit their activities because they try to avoid actions that will precipitate episodes of incontinence. Men suffering from urethral stricture disease and SUI should be referred to a urologist because multiple treatment options exist to improve their quality of life.

REFERENCES

1. Anger JT, Buckley JC, Santucci RA, et al. Trends in stricture management among male Medicare beneficiaries: underuse of urethroplasty? Urology 2011;77(2): 481–5.
2. Ficarra V, Novara G, Rosen RC, et al. Systematic review and meta-analysis of studies reporting urinary continence recovery after robot-assisted radical prostatectomy. Eur Urol 2012;62(3):405–17.
3. Wessells H, Angermeier KW, Elliot SP, et al. Male urethral stricture—American Urological Association guideline 2016. 2016:1–34.
4. Pansadoro V, Emiliozzi P. Internal urethrotomy in the management of anterior urethral strictures: long-term followup. J Urol 1996;156(1):73–5.
5. Zehri AA, Ather MH, Afshan Q. Predictors of recurrence of urethral stricture disease following optical urethrotomy. Int J Surg 2009;7(4):361–4.
6. Morey AF, McAninch JW. Role of preoperative sonourethrogram in bulbar urethral reconstruction. J Urol 2005;158(4):1376–9.
7. Al-Qudah HS, Cavalcanti AG, Santucci RA. Early catheter removal after anterior anastomotic (3 days) and ventral buccal mucosal onlay (7 days) urethroplasty. Int Braz J Urol 2005;31(5):459–64.
8. Kjaergaard B, Walter S, Bartholin J, et al. Prevention of urethral stricture recurrence using clean intermittent self-catheterization. BJU Int 1994;73(6):692–5.
9. Wolf JS Jr, Bennett CJ, Dmochowski RM, et al. Urologic surgery antimicrobial prophylaxis—American Urological Association best practice statement. 2013:1–48.
10. Schneider T, Sperling H, Lümmen G, et al. [Sachse internal urethrotomy. Is erectile dysfuction a possible complication?]. Urologe A 2001;40(1):38–41 [in German].

11. Steenkamp JW, Heyns CF, de Kock MLS. Internal urethrotomy versus dilation as treatment for male urethral strictures: a prospective, randomized comparison. J Urol 1997;157(1):98–101.

12. Kluth LA, Ernst L, Vetterlein MW, et al. Direct vision internal urethrotomy for short anterior urethral strictures and beyond: success rates, predictors of treatment failure and recurrence management. Urology 2017;106:210–5.

13. Terlecki RP, Steele MC, Valadez C, et al. Urethral rest: role and rationale in preparation for anterior urethroplasty. Urology 2011;77(6):1477–81.

14. Barbagli G, De Angelis M, Palminteri E, et al. Failed hypospadias repair presenting in adults. Eur Urol 2006;49(5):887–95.

15. Sharma AK, Chandrashekar R, Keshavamurthy R, et al. Lingual versus buccal mucosa graft urethroplasty for anterior urethral stricture: a prospective comparative analysis. Int J Urol 2013;20(12):1199–203.

16. Kamp S, Knoll T, Osman M, et al. Donor-site morbidity in buccal mucosa urethroplasty: lower lip or inner cheek? BJU Int 2005;96(4):619–23.

17. Mundy AR. Results and complications of urethroplasty and its future. BJU Int 1993;71(3):322–5.

18. Blaschko SD, Sanford MT, Cinman NM, et al. De novo erectile dysfunction after anterior urethroplasty: a systematic review and meta-analysis. BJU Int 2013;112(5):655–63.

19. Erickson BA, Granieri MA, Meeks JJ, et al. Prospective analysis of erectile dysfunction after anterior urethroplasty: incidence and recovery of function. J Urol 2010;183(2):657–61.

20. Fichtner J, Filipas D, Fisch M, et al. Long-term outcome of ventral buccal mucosa onlay graft urethroplasty for urethral stricture repair. Urology 2004;64(4):648–50.

21. Andrich DE, Leach CJ, Mundy AR. The Barbagli procedure gives the best results for patch urethroplasty of the bulbar urethra. BJU Int 2001;88(4):385–9.

22. Bhargava S, Chapple CR. Buccal mucosal urethroplasty: is it the new gold standard? BJU Int 2004;93(9):1191–3.

23. Chapple C, Andrich D, Atala A, et al. SIU/ICUD consultation on urethral strictures: the management of anterior urethral stricture disease using substitution urethroplasty. Urology 2014;83(3):S31–47.

24. Santucci RA, Mario LA, Aninch JWMC. Anastomotic urethroplasty for bulbar urethral stricture: analysis of 168 patients. J Urol 2002;167(4):1715–9.

25. Chapman D, Kinnaird A, Rourke K. Independent predictors of stricture recurrence following urethroplasty for isolated bulbar urethral strictures. J Urol 2017;198(5):1107–12.

26. Andrich DE, Dunglison N, Greenwell TJ, et al. The long-term results of urethroplasty. J Urol 2003;170(1):90–2.

27. Vickers AJ, Kent M, Mulhall J, et al. Counseling the post-radical prostatectomy patients about functional recovery: high predictiveness of current status. Urology 2014;84(1):158–63.

28. Wilson SK, Delk JR II, Henry GD, et al. New surgical technique for sphincter urinary control system using upper transverse scrotal incision. J Urol 2003;169(1):261–4.

29. Furlow WL, Barrett DM. The artificial urinary sphincter: experience with the AS 800 pump-control assembly for single-stage primary deactivation and activation—a preliminary report. Mayo Clin Proc 1985;60(4):255–8.

30. Raj GV, Peterson AC, Toh KL, et al. Outcomes following revisions and secondary implantation of the artificial urinary sphincter. J Urol 2005;173(4):1242–5.

31. Montague DK. The artificial urinary sphincter (AS 800): experience in 166 consecutive patients. J Urol 1992;147(2):380–2.

32. Montague DK, Angermeier KW. Postprostatectomy urinary incontinence: the case for artificial urinary sphincter implantation. Urology 2000;55(1):2–4.

33. Motley RC, Barrett DM. Artificial urinary sphincter cuff erosion. Experience with reimplantation in 38 patients. Urology 1990;35(3):215–8.

34. Seideman CA, Zhao LC, Hudak SJ, et al. Is prolonged catheterization a risk factor for artificial urinary sphincter cuff erosion? Urology 2013;82(4):943–7.

35. Saffarian A, Walsh K, Walsh IK, et al. Urethral atrophy after artificial urinary sphincter placement: is cuff downsizing effective? J Urol 2003;169(2):567–9.

36. Kowalczyk JJ, Spicer DL, Mulcahy JJ. Long-term experience with the double-cuff AMS 800 artificial urinary sphincter. Urology 1996;47(6):895–7.

37. de Cógáin MR, Elliott DS. The impact of an antibiotic coating on the artificial urinary sphincter infection rate. J Urol 2013;190(1):113–7.

38. Linder BJ, Rivera ME, Ziegelmann MJ, et al. Long-term outcomes following artificial urinary sphincter placement: an analysis of 1082 cases at Mayo Clinic. Urology 2015;86(3):602–7.

39. Van der Aa F, Drake MJ, Kasyan GR, et al, Young Academic Urologists Functional Urology Group. The artificial urinary sphincter after a quarter of a century: a critical systematic review of its use in male non-neurogenic incontinence. Eur Urol 2013;63(4):681–9.

40. Trigo Rocha F, Gomes CM, Mitre AI, et al. A prospective study evaluating the efficacy of the artificial sphincter AMS 800 for the treatment of postradical prostatectomy urinary incontinence and the correlation between preoperative urodynamic and surgical outcomes. Urology 2008;71(1):85–9.

Male Infertility Diagnosis and Treatment in the Era of In Vitro Fertilization and Intracytoplasmic Sperm Injection

Michael M. Pan, MD[a],*, Mark S. Hockenberry, MD[b],
Edgar W. Kirby, MD[b], Larry I. Lipshultz, MD[b]

KEYWORDS

- Male - Fertility - IVF - ICSI - Men's health

KEY POINTS

- Evaluation of male factor infertility is often being overlooked.
- Improvement in male factors can improve overall health and pregnancy and live birth rates for both natural and assisted reproduction.
- All couples undergoing a fertility evaluation should have a comprehensive male assessment.

INTRODUCTION

Each year more than seven million couples worldwide seek evaluation for the inability to conceive a child, a problem that affects approximately 15% of couples.[1,2] Among these couples, a male factor contributing to infertility is present in up to half, and one-third of these cases can be attributed to a male factor alone. However, 27% of these men are never evaluated and examined as the potential cause for infertility.[1,3] Both the American Urologic Association and the American Society for Reproductive Medicine recommend the routine and concurrent evaluation of the man in an infertile relationship because many of these couples are offered assisted reproductive technologies (ARTs) without any evaluation of the male partner.[2]

Since the advent of ARTs leading to the birth of Louise Brown, the first child born using in vitro fertilization (IVF), in 1978, the utilization of this procedure has exploded. More than 7 million ART cycles were performed between 2004 and 2013, resulting in

[a] Scott Department of Urology, Baylor College of Medicine, 6624 Fannin Street #1700, Houston, TX 77030, USA; [b] Scott Department of Urology, Center for Reproductive Medicine and Surgery, Baylor College of Medicine, 6624 Fannin Street #1700, Houston, TX 77030, USA
* Corresponding author.
E-mail address: pan@bcm.edu

Med Clin N Am 102 (2018) 337–347
https://doi.org/10.1016/j.mcna.2017.10.008
0025-7125/18/© 2017 Elsevier Inc. All rights reserved.
medical.theclinics.com

more than 1.5 million live births.[4] With this dramatic increase in use of ARTs, techniques aimed to increase successful outcomes have also been developed, progressing from conventional incubation of sperm with oocytes to the now widely used intracytoplasmic sperm injection (ICSI). The refinement of this technique has not only increased the options available to infertile couples with severe male factor but also has improved success rates. Current ART live birth rates range from 55% to 90%, depending on number of cycles completed, use of donor versus autologous oocyte, age of autologous donor, and use fresh versus thawed embryos.[5] These techniques require very few sperm (10–20 sperm cells) and even severely oligospermic men can successfully provide enough sperm to be used.[6] Many of these men may not be offered a full evaluation because they are able to provide an adequate sample to be used for ART. However, a large body of literature shows that treatment of underlying causes of male infertility, such as varicocele, can significantly increase natural pregnancy rates, as well as success rates with ARTs.[7] In addition, male infertility is associated with other comorbid conditions, such as diabetes mellitus, cardiovascular disease, genitourinary malignancy, and genetic abnormalities.[8–11] As many as 6% of men undergoing a fertility evaluation may have a previously undiagnosed medical condition and recent studies have shown an increased mortality among those men with decreased fertility potential.[8,12]

ARTs are also not without their own risks, which can include high cost, compounded with each cycle, and the possibility of multiple gestations and promulgation of genetic defects. High costs for ARTs can often be prohibitive, particularly if multiple cycles are needed to achieve a live birth. The cost of per single IVF cycle is approximately $12,400 and the cost per delivery is approximately $56,000.[13] These costs do not include those associated with multiple births and subsequent childcare or hospitalization costs. Additional risks include an increased chance of birth defects because many of the techniques bypass the natural barriers to abnormal genetic replication.[14,15]

More than ever, the full evaluation and treatment of the male partner remains a key component in the care of an infertile couple. Attempting ARTs with poor quality or quantity of sperm can lead to decreased success rates and increased cost and morbidity. Many infertile men may have a reversible medical condition and would benefit from comprehensive evaluation. Optimizing the male factor evaluation represents a fundamental step in the management of the infertile couple.

EVALUATION
History

The initial evaluation of the male partner of an infertile couple should start with a careful history and physical examination, with particular focus on sexual and pregnancy history, current therapies, childhood diseases, and current medical or surgical issues. Male erectile dysfunction is a common and treatable comorbidity of primary or secondary infertility and should be treated whenever possible. Any history of diseases associated with the testicles, such as testicular torsion, trauma, tumors, varicoceles, or cryptorchidism, should be elucidated. It is well known that even if unilateral, these processes can often have a bilateral effect on the testes and impair fertility.[16] Detailed history of prior medical and surgical issues, such as injuries to the pelvis or retroperitoneum, can affect any of the nerves, blood vessels, and structures vital to the production and transportation of sperm. Prior surgeries, such as a transurethral resection of the prostate, can result in retrograde ejaculation or obstruction of the ejaculatory ducts and decreased sperm counts. Herniorrhaphy, particularly with mesh, can also potentially affect fertility if the vas deferens or the blood supply to the testicle is affected. Additionally, propylene mesh can cause desmoplastic reactions, resulting in obstruction of the vas deferens.[17] Any history of prior cancers and treatments with chemotherapeutic agents and/or radiation may also have a profound effect on sperm production because many of these agents are gonadotoxins.[18] Any patient undergoing chemotherapy or radiation therapy should be offered sperm banking before initiation of therapy due to the potentially harmful and often irreversible effects of these treatments.[18]

Physical Examination

A detailed physical examination of the man can provide insights into many disease processes responsible for infertility. Examination of the chest for abnormal breast development should raise concern for possible hormone imbalance or congenital syndromes, such as Klinefelter syndrome. The male genitalia should be carefully examined, with particular attention paid to the urethral meatus, testes, and paratesticular structures. Meatal location is an important anatomic consideration because any ectopic position may affect the effective delivery of sperm. Hypospadias is a common abnormality of the urethral meatus and occurs in approximately 1 in 300 men.[19] The urethra in a man with hypospadias may occur at any location along the ventrum of the penis to the penoscrotal junction and rarely in the perineum. Frequently, those patients with severe hypospadias will have been already evaluated by a urologist at a young age for reconstruction. However, if newly discovered, hypospadias should prompt urologic referral for potential surgical correction.

The testes typically measure approximately 6 cm in length and 4 cm in width, with a volume of approximately 20 mL, and should be firm and rubbery in consistency.[19] Small, soft testes should raise concern for integrity of the germinal epithelium or hypogonadism, and any firm lesions within the testicle should be promptly imaged with ultrasonography and referred for urologic evaluation for possible malignancy. This diagnostic procedure is especially important because infertile men are at increased risk of having testicular germ cell cancers.[11]

The epididymis lies posterior and superior to the testicle and should be examined carefully as well, noting any abnormalities, including cysts, masses, or induration. The vas deferens can be palpated within the spermatic cord rising superiorly from the testicle and can be differentiated from the surrounding vessels as a rigid tubular structure; any absence should be noted and should raise suspicion for vasal agenesis or congenital bilateral absence of the vas deferens.[19] The spermatic cord should also be carefully examined for any varicocele because the incidence of varicoceles is significantly higher in infertile men, as many as 37% compared with 20% in fertile men.[20,21] Varicoceles can be palpated as spongy prominent vessels in the spermatic cord and should be examined in the supine and standing positions. Asking the patient to perform Valsalva maneuvers can aid in the diagnosis and should cause increase in size and turgidity of the vessels. Further attention should be paid to the presence of any abdominal and inguinal scars because scarring and inflammatory responses in these areas can lead to ductal obstructions. A digital rectal examination to examine the prostate gland, noting any nodules or irregularities, can also provide information regarding presence of prostate infections, malignancy, or other anatomic sources of obstruction, particularly because infertile men are also associated with a higher risk of seminal vesicle cysts and high-grade prostatic malignancies.[10]

Hormonal Evaluation

In all patients, especially if an abnormality on history of physical examination suggests possible hormonal imbalance, evaluation should include a quantitation of the hypothalamic-pituitary-gonadal hormones, including luteinizing hormone (LH) and follicle-stimulating hormone (FSH), which are released episodically in response to pulsatile secretion of the hypothalamic gonadotropin-releasing hormone. Testosterone then acts on the hypothalamus and anterior pituitary to inhibit further production and creates a negative feedback loop to regulate the production of additional testosterone. FSH acts on Sertoli cells in the testis in combination with testosterone to stimulate sperm cell production. Inhibin, reflecting an intact germinal epithelium and Sertoli cell interaction, then acts on the anterior pituitary to inhibit further FSH production, creating a separate negative feedback loop. Any derangement in these pathways can lead to abnormalities in sperm production, as seen in **Table 1**. Elevation in the serum prolactin level can hinder proper gonadotropin secretion and should raise suspicions for a possible pituitary adenoma. Further diagnostic testing and MRI of the brain is indicated. Treatment in patients with hormonal abnormalities (see later discussion) should be targeted at normalizing these pathways.

Semen Analysis

A mainstay of the initial evaluation for male factor infertility is the semen analysis. When possible, 2 semen samples should be collected about 1 month apart to rule out transient fluctuations in sperm parameters.[2] These samples should be collected after 2 to 5 days of abstinence from ejaculation to ensure optimal quality of sperm for analysis.[2] The World Health Organization (WHO) guidelines for ranges for normal semen parameters can be found in **Table 2**.[22] The first step in interpreting semen parameters starts with semen volume. Low semen volumes can be caused by improper collection, short abstinence, ejaculatory duct obstruction, hypogonadism, or congenital bilateral absence of the vas deferens.[23] In patients with low semen volumes, a postejaculatory urine should be obtained, tested for fructose, and examined microscopically for sperm. A positive finding of many sperm in the postejaculate urine suggests a component of retrograde ejaculation. If a significant number of sperm is seen in the postejaculatory urine, it can be centrifuged, resuspended, and subsequently analyzed as a semen specimen.

A significantly decreased sperm count (density) can be divided into 2 broad categories: obstructive and nonobstructive oligospermia or azoospermia. Obstruction can occur at any point from the testis to the urethra and can include causes such as vasal obstruction from inflammation, prior transurethral resection of prostatic tissue, occluded ejaculatory ducts, and urethral strictures, among others. Hormonal evaluation in these patients typically will be within normal limits and imaging with scrotal and transrectal ultrasound can be considered to better evaluate for potential causes of obstruction. An important cause of oligospermia and azoospermia is

Table 1
Hormonal profile of common conditions related to male infertility

	Testosterone	FSH	LH
Hypogonadotropic hypogonadism (hypothalamic or pituitary abnormality)	Low	Low	Low
Hypergonadotropic hypogonadism (primary testicular failure)	Low	High	High
Impaired spermatogenesis	Normal	High	Normal
Androgen resistance	High	Normal	High
Exogenous testosterone use	High	Low	Low

Table 2
World Health Organization semen analysis reference values

Parameter	Lower Limit of Reference Range
Semen volume	1.5 mL
Total sperm	39 million
Sperm concentration	15 million/mL
Total motility	40%
Forward progression	32%
Sperm morphology	4% normal forms
Peroxidase-positive leukocytes	<1 million/mL

Adapted from World Health Organization (WHO). WHO laboratory manual for the examination and processing of human semen. 5th edition. Geneva (Switzerland): World Health Organization; 2010; with permission.

congenital bilateral absence of the vas deferens, which is associated with a mutation in the cystic fibrosis transmembrane conductance regulator gene and is considered a genital form of cystic fibrosis.[24] Physical examination will typically reveal bilateral absent vasa deferentia. In cases with unilateral vasal agenesis, additional imaging will sometimes reveal concurrent ipsilateral renal agenesis. If positive for abnormal cystic fibrosis regulator genes, patients should be referred for genetic counseling. Nonobstructive oligospermia or azoospermia will typically show abnormal hormone production and may be related to hypogonadism or genetic abnormalities. Initial genetic evaluation includes a karyotype to rule out genetic disorders, such as Klinefelter syndrome, as well as Y chromosome analysis. Y-chromosome microdeletions occur in approximately 10% to 15% of men with severe oligospermia and azoospermia, and may be hereditary.[2,25] These patients should also receive counseling regarding their reproductive potential, as well as any possible effects on their future offspring.

Additional semen testing includes evaluation of sperm morphology and function, looking at the head, body, and tail for any defects or abnormalities. The most recent 2010 WHO criteria for semen parameters now lists the normal range for morphology as being greater than 4%, which mirrors findings in 1988 by Kruger and colleagues[26] that called for adoption of a strict morphology criterion of greater than 4% normal forms.[27] Further testing includes evaluation for pyospermia because white blood cells are major sources of reactive oxygen species (oxidants), which can cause direct damage to sperm by lipid peroxidation and DNA damage.[28,29] Elevated reactive oxygen species in the semen impair sperm motility and morphology, embryo development, and decrease the rate of pregnancy.[30] The hypoosmotic swelling test can be used to determine whether nonmotile sperm are viable based on which sperm have intact cell membranes.[2] Finally, the presence of antisperm antibodies can reduce pregnancy rates and can be seen after ductal obstruction, prior genital infection, trauma, or after vasectomy.[2,31]

Imaging

Although complex imaging modalities exist to precisely delineate the anatomy of the ejaculatory tract, the mainstay of imaging for infertility evaluation is the use of ultrasonography. Scrotal ultrasound provides objective measurements for each testicle, and can show abnormalities in the size, consistency, and location of the testicles. Any solid mass within the testicle should increase concerns for possible malignancy, which requires surgical intervention. Particularly useful is the ability of duplex ultrasonography to detect the presence of varicoceles. Radiographic criteria for diagnosis of a varicocele consists of veins in the pampiniform plexus that measure greater than 3 mm in diameter in combination with a reversal of blood flow. The traditional grading system, however, is based on office evaluation. Additional paratesticular abnormalities may also be discovered during sonographic evaluation, including epididymal abnormalities and hydroceles. Often, a scrotal ultrasound can also be used to assist in identifying a nonpalpable vas deferens before an expensive genetic workup is pursued.

A transrectal ultrasound is important to evaluate the prostate and seminal vesicles, particularly if there is concern for ejaculatory duct obstruction. Frequently, the seminal vesicles will be dilated owing to obstruction of the ejaculatory ducts as they pass through the prostate, causing reflux into the seminal vesicles. If a partial duct obstruction is present, the seminal vesicles may not be enlarged. Transrectal aspiration of enlarged seminal vesicles under ultrasound guidance can be performed to confirm that viable sperm exists within the dilated seminal vesicles. If the aspirate contains greater than 3 to 5 sperm per every high-power field, ejaculatory duct obstruction is considered very likely and the patient should undergo resection of the ejaculatory ducts to relieve the obstruction.

TREATMENT
Medical

Treatment of male infertility should be approached in a multimodal fashion. Conservative measures, such as smoking and alcohol cessation, avoidance of laptop and hot tub use, and improvement in overall health should be heavily counseled. Common lubricants, including saliva and commercial over-the-counter lubricants, should be avoided because they can impair sperm motility. Intercourse is typically recommended to occur every 48 hours beginning 2 days before expected ovulation.

Sex hormone abnormalities should be addressed if discovered. Depressed LH and FSH from secondary hypogonadism can be treated with oral clomiphene citrate (off-label use), which acts to increase these endogenous hormones to stimulate sperm and testosterone production.[32–34] Direct administration of human chorionic gonadotropin (hCG) and FSH may need to be considered. Administration of exogenous testosterone often has deleterious effects on sperm production and should be ceased whenever possible.[35,36] Recovery of testosterone-suppressed spermatogenesis has been shown to be possible with the use of high-dose hCG and clomiphene. Primary testicular failure as marked by elevated FSH and LH levels, and low serum testosterone levels, may not respond to exogenous hormonal stimulation. If there is concern for abnormal spermatogenesis, such as with primary testicular failure or androgen resistance, biopsy and either testicular or epididymal sperm extraction procedures may be required.

Surgical

Surgical management for infertility is varied and is tailored to the patient. Particularly important is the correction of any varicocele present. Varicoceles result in increased intratesticular temperatures, which can subsequently affect sperm production by decreasing testosterone synthesis, altering the function and morphology of sperm-supporting Sertoli cells, and damaging germinal cell membranes, amino acid transport, and protein biosynthesis.[37] Men with varicoceles frequently have lower testosterone levels than those without varicoceles, and surgical correction can result in significant improvement in serum testosterone in 70% of these men.[38] Compared with normal controls, men with varicoceles also show a significantly higher quantity of reactive oxygen species in their semen samples, which can affect cell membranes and cell function.[39] Surgical correction of varicoceles can be accomplished with different approaches, including laparoscopic, microsurgical, and percutaneous radiographic approaches. Microsurgical procedures with an inguinal or subinguinal approach have the lowest rates of recurrence and involve an outpatient procedure to ligate affected veins of the spermatic cord.[40]

A recent metaanalysis showed significant improvements in semen quality in 70% of men and an increase in overall pregnancy rate by 3 to 6 months after varicocelectomy, with enough improvement in motile sperm in the ejaculate to avoid further invasive procedures, such as testicular and epididymal surgical extraction to harvest viable sperm.[41] Varicocele repair not only improves semen parameters, such as density, motility, and normal forms, but also reduces sperm damage and can benefit those patients already committed to the use of ARTs for conception.[42–44] Varicocele repair improved fertilization from 28% to 43% and increased pregnancy rates from 18% to 64% in patients who had previously failed IVF. Patients undergoing ICSI after varicocele repair showed not only improved sperm count and motility but also increased clinical pregnancy rates from 48% to 73%, and live birth rates from 37% to 51%.[45,46] Ligation of these dilated spermatic veins has also been reported to improve pregnancy rates per cycle, live births per cycle, and live births per couple with less invasive and costly ARTs.[47] In fact, after varicocele repair, a significant number of couples can experience a shift in their ART to less costly and invasive procedures, moving from ICSI to IVF, IVF to intrauterine insemination (IUI), or from IUI to spontaneous pregnancy.[48] Consequently, the sum of literature regarding varicocelectomy shows that any varicocele, if discovered, should be surgically addressed, even if the couple is considering pursuing ARTs.

Additional surgical techniques for the infertile male focus on relieving obstruction in the ductal system. Stenosis or other obstruction at the level of the vas deferens can be corrected by excising the offending segment and performing a vasovasostomy to reconnect the ends of the vas deferens. Obstructions at the level of the ejaculatory ducts can be managed endoscopically by transurethral resection of the ejaculatory ducts (TURED) to open the stenotic or obstructed ducts. TURED improves semen quality in 38% to 60% of men and increases the pregnancy rate by 22% to 31% in couples with men with ejaculatory duct obstruction.[49]

Finally, if no sperm can be found in the ejaculate and the remainder of the workup remains unremarkable, the patient can be taken to the operating room for a testis biopsy with or without sperm harvesting. Under general anesthesia, the testicle is incised and the seminiferous tubules examined for the presence of any sperm. Any viable sperm found can be immediately sent for banking or for ART cycles. Additional samples can be collected and sent for pathologic testing for evaluation for possible dysfunctional abnormalities.

Assisted Reproductive Technologies

ARTs remain an option for those couples who are unable to achieve a pregnancy through natural means. Current techniques include delivery of sperm cells to the uterus through IUI, the least expensive and least invasive option for assisted reproduction. Conventional IVF involves extraction of sperm and oocytes, which are then coincubated. Fertilized embryos are then transferred into the uterine lining. Finally, ICSI can be performed in which the sperm cell is injected directly into the oocyte using a micropipette. In cases with azoospermia or cryptozoospermia in which no viable sperm can be obtained from the ejaculate, testicular or epididymal sperm extraction can be performed to provide a pathologic diagnosis of testicular and epididymal tissue and/or obtain an adequate sperm sample that can be banked or used directly for concurrent IVF.

Cost is almost always an important consideration for couples undergoing assisted reproduction and can range anywhere from a few hundred dollars for IUI to tens of thousands of dollars for a single IVF-ICSI cycle.[4] Given that the total ART success rate is approximately 55% after 3 cycles and up to 85% after 8 cycles, multiple cycles are often needed before successful delivery of a child.[5]

Both IVF and IVF-ICSI are also associated with risks. IVF and IVF-ICSI have increased rates of congenital defects compared with natural pregnancies but no difference is seen between the 2 modalities.[50] The most common congenital malformations are anencephaly and limb abnormalities.[50] IVF-ICSI is also associated with an increased risk of sex chromosomal and imprinting disorders, such as Angelman and Prader-Willi syndromes.[14,15] Patients should be counseled regarding these risks, as well as the potential costs associated with performing these procedures.

FUTURE CONSIDERATIONS AND SUMMARY

The diagnosis and treatment of infertility remains a prominent concern among affected couples. The advent of ARTs has given infertile couples more options for conceiving children. However, much of the evaluation and treatment of infertility is focused on the female partner, with many men never receiving any evaluation despite a significant contribution of the male factor to infertility. A careful history and examination of the male partner should be performed in every infertile couple, and should include hormonal evaluation and semen analysis. Hormonal abnormalities can be treated medically, and the importance of diagnosis and surgical correction of varicoceles cannot be overstated. Varicocelectomy has been shown in multiple studies to not only improve semen parameters but, more importantly, live birth rates both naturally and with ARTs, as well as to reduce the invasiveness and complexity of the ARTs required for successful conception. Other surgical options are aimed at relieving points of semen obstruction. Even in the era of increased utilization of ARTs, the evaluation and treatment of the man is a critical aspect for effective infertility care.

REFERENCES

1. Eisenberg ML, Lathi RB, Baker VL, et al. Frequency of the male infertility evaluation: data from the national survey of family growth. J Urol 2013;189(3):1030–4.
2. Male Infertility Best Practice Policy Committee of the American Urological AssociationPractice Committee of the American Society for Reproductive Medicine. Report on optimal evaluation of the infertile male. Fertil Steril 2006;86(5 Suppl 1):S202–9.
3. Thonneau P, Marchand S, Tallec A, et al. Incidence and main causes of infertility in a resident population (1,850,000) of three French regions (1988-1989). Hum Reprod 1991;6(6):811–6.
4. Connolly MP, Hoorens S, Chambers GM. The costs and consequences of assisted reproductive technology: an economic perspective. Hum Reprod Update 2010;16(6):603–13.
5. Luke B, Brown MB, Wantman E, et al. Cumulative birth rates with linked assisted reproductive technology cycles. New Engl J Med 2012;366(26):2483–91.
6. Hockenberry MS, Lipshultz LI. Lack of male factor evaluation and opportunities lost. Fertil Sterility 2016;106(6):1326–7.
7. Kirby EW, Wiener LE, Rajanahally S, et al. Undergoing varicocele repair before assisted reproduction improves pregnancy rate and live birth rate in azoospermic

and oligospermic men with a varicocele: a systematic review and meta-analysis. Fertil Sterility 2016;106(6):1338–43.

8. Kolettis PN, Sabanegh ES. Significant medical pathology discovered during a male infertility evaluation. J Urol 2001;166(1):178–80.

9. Eisenberg ML, Li S, Behr B, et al. Relationship between semen production and medical comorbidity. Fertil Sterility 2015;103(1):66–71.

10. Walsh TJ. Male reproductive health and prostate cancer risk. Curr Opin Urol 2011;21(6):506–13.

11. Walsh TJ, Croughan MS, Schembri M, et al. Increased risk of testicular germ cell cancer among infertile men. Arch Intern Med 2009;169(4):351–6.

12. Eisenberg ML, Park Y, Hollenbeck AR, et al. Fatherhood and the risk of cardiovascular mortality in the NIH-AARP diet and health study. Hum Reprod 2011;26(12): 3479–85.

13. Lindgren MC, Ross LS. Reproductive health care delivery. Urol Clin North Am 2014;41(1):205–11.

14. Devroey P, Van Steirteghem A. A review of ten years experience of ICSI. Hum Reprod Update 2004;10(1):19–28.

15. Bonduelle M, Wennerholm UB, Loft A, et al. A multi-centre cohort study of the physical health of 5-year-old children conceived after intracytoplasmic sperm injection, in vitro fertilization and natural conception. Hum Reprod 2005;20(2): 413–9.

16. Hendry WF. Testicular, epididymal and vasal injuries. BJU Int 2000;86(3):344–8.

17. Shin D, Lipshultz LI, Goldstein M, et al. Herniorrhaphy with polypropylene mesh causing inguinal vasal obstruction: a preventable cause of obstructive azoospermia. Ann Surg 2005;241(4):553–8.

18. Wyns C. Male fertility preservation before gonadotoxic therapies. Facts Views Vis ObGyn 2010;2(2):88–108.

19. McDougal WS, Wein AJ, Kavoussi LR, et al. Campbell-Walsh urology 11th edition review. Philadelphia: Elsevier; 2015.

20. Pryor JL, Howards SS. Varicocele. Urol Clin North Am 1987;14(3):499–513.

21. Fretz PC, Sandlow JI. Varicocele: current concepts in pathophysiology, diagnosis, and treatment. Urol Clin North Am 2002;29(4):921–37.

22. World Health Organization (WHO). WHO laboratory manual for the examination and processing of human semen. 5th edition. Geneva (Switzerland): World Health Organization; 2010.

23. Cooper TG, Noonan E, von Eckardstein S, et al. World Health Organization reference values for human semen characteristics. Hum Reprod Update 2010;16(3): 231–45.

24. Anguiano A, Oates RD, Amos JA, et al. Congenital bilateral absence of the vas deferens. A primarily genital form of cystic fibrosis. Jama 1992;267(13):1794–7.

25. Pryor JL, Kent-First M, Muallem A, et al. Microdeletions in the Y chromosome of infertile men. New Engl J Med 1997;336(8):534–9.

26. Kruger TF, Acosta AA, Simmons KF, et al. Predictive value of abnormal sperm morphology in in vitro fertilization. Fertil Sterility 1988;49(1):112–7.

27. Menkveld R. Clinical significance of the low normal sperm morphology value as proposed in the fifth edition of the WHO laboratory manual for the examination and processing of human semen. Asian J Androl 2010;12(1):47–58.

28. Kessopoulou E, Tomlinson MJ, Barratt CL, et al. Origin of reactive oxygen species in human semen: spermatozoa or leucocytes? J Reprod Fertil 1992;94(2): 463–70.

29. RJ A. Bruce Stewart Lectureship. ASRM Annual Meeting. October 18-22, 1997.

30. Zorn B, Vidmar G, Meden-Vrtovec H. Seminal reactive oxygen species as predictors of fertilization, embryo quality and pregnancy rates after conventional in vitro fertilization and intracytoplasmic sperm injection. Int J Androl 2003; 26(5):279–85.

31. Ayvaliotis B, Bronson R, Rosenfeld D, et al. Conception rates in couples where autoimmunity to sperm is detected. Fertil Sterility 1985;43(5):739–42.

32. Rodriguez KM, Pastuszak AW, Lipshultz LI. Enclomiphene citrate for the treatment of secondary male hypogonadism. Expert Opin Pharmacother 2016; 17(11):1561–7.

33. Roth LW, Ryan AR, Meacham RB. Clomiphene citrate in the management of male infertility. Semin Reprod Med 2013;31(4):245–50.

34. Willets AE, Corbo JM, Brown JN. Clomiphene for the treatment of male infertility. Reprod Sci 2013;20(7):739–44.

35. Moss JL, Crosnoe LE, Kim ED. Effect of rejuvenation hormones on spermatogenesis. Fertil sterility 2013;99(7):1814–20.

36. de Souza GL, Hallak J. Anabolic steroids and male infertility: a comprehensive review. BJU Int 2011;108(11):1860–5.

37. Saypol DC, Howards SS, Turner TT, et al. Influence of surgically induced varicocele on testicular blood flow, temperature, and histology in adult rats and dogs. J Clin Invest 1981;68(1):39–45.

38. Tanrikut C, Goldstein M, Rosoff JS, et al. Varicocele as a risk factor for androgen deficiency and effect of repair. BJU Int 2011;108(9):1480–4.

39. Hendin BN, Kolettis PN, Sharma RK, et al. Varicocele is associated with elevated spermatozoal reactive oxygen species production and diminished seminal plasma antioxidant capacity. J Urol 1999;161(6):1831–4.

40. Cayan S, Shavakhabov S, Kadioglu A. Treatment of palpable varicocele in infertile men: a meta-analysis to define the best technique. J Androl 2009;30(1): 33–40.

41. Richardson I, Grotas AB, Nagler HM. Outcomes of varicocelectomy treatment: an updated critical analysis. Urol Clin North America 2008;35(2):191–209, viii.

42. Reichart M, Eltes F, Soffer Y, et al. Sperm ultramorphology as a pathophysiological indicator of spermatogenesis in males suffering from varicocele. Andrologia 2000;32(3):139–45.

43. Schatte EC, Hirshberg SJ, Fallick ML, et al. Varicocelectomy improves sperm strict morphology and motility. J Urol 1998;160(4):1338–40.

44. Scott RT Jr, Oehninger SC, Menkveld R, et al. Critical assessment of sperm morphology before and after double wash swim-up preparation for in vitro fertilization. Arch Androl 1989;23(2):125–9.

45. Ashkenazi J, Dicker D, Feldberg D, et al. The impact of spermatic vein ligation on the male factor in in vitro fertilization-embryo transfer and its relation to testosterone levels before and after operation. Fertil Sterility 1989;51(3):471–4.

46. Esteves SC, Oliveira FV, Bertolla RP. Clinical outcome of intracytoplasmic sperm injection in infertile men with treated and untreated clinical varicocele. J Urol 2010;184(4):1442–6.

47. Daitch JA, Bedaiwy MA, Pasqualotto EB, et al. Varicocelectomy improves intrauterine insemination success rates in men with varicocele. J Urol 2001;165(5): 1510–3.

48. Cayan S, Erdemir F, Ozbey I, et al. Can varicocelectomy significantly change the way couples use assisted reproductive technologies? J Urol 2002;167(4): 1749–52.

49. Popken G, Wetterauer U, Schultze-Seemann W, et al. Transurethral resection of cystic and non-cystic ejaculatory duct obstructions. Int J Androl 1998;21(4): 196–200.
50. Sala P, Ferrero S, Buffi D, et al. Congenital defects in assisted reproductive technology pregnancies. Minerva Ginecologica 2011;63(3):227–35.

Sexual Dysfunction
Behavioral, Medical, and Surgical Treatment

Nelson Bennett Jr, MD

KEYWORDS

- Sexual dysfunction • Erectile dysfunction • Phosphodiesterase inhibitors
- Penile prosthesis

KEY POINTS

- Follow a stepwise approach for evaluation and management of erectile dysfunction. Low-risk simple interventions initially, followed by more complex and invasive options.
- Improvements of modifiable risk factors should occur at every stage of evaluation and management of sexual dysfunction.
- Referral to a sexual medicine specialist should be considered after failure of oral medications.

INTRODUCTION

When considering the initiation of erectile dysfunction (ED) treatment of a patient, a complete medical history and physical should be completed. Contraindications to sexual dysfunction treatments, oral medications, surgical interventions, and behavioral modifications should be noted. Cardiac reserve should be assessed according to Princeton III criteria. A stepwise approach for evaluation and management of ED, as per Esposito and colleagues,[1] is still valid. The simplest and lowest-risk interventions are completed first, followed by increasingly complex and invasive options (**Fig. 1**).

NONPHARMACOLOGIC TREATMENT OPTIONS

Because ED is often a manifestation of generalized vascular disease, it makes sense in theory and has been shown in practice that lifestyle modifications that improve cardiovascular health may also improve erectile function. When ED is identified,

Disclosure: The author is a consultant for Endo Pharmaceuticals, Boston Scientific, Inc, and Coloplast, Inc.
Department of Urology, Northwestern University Feinberg School of Medicine, Galter Pavilion Suite: 20-150, 675 North Saint Clair Street, Chicago, IL 60611, USA
E-mail address: Nelson.Bennett@nm.org

Med Clin N Am 102 (2018) 349–360
https://doi.org/10.1016/j.mcna.2017.10.010
0025-7125/18/© 2017 Elsevier Inc. All rights reserved.

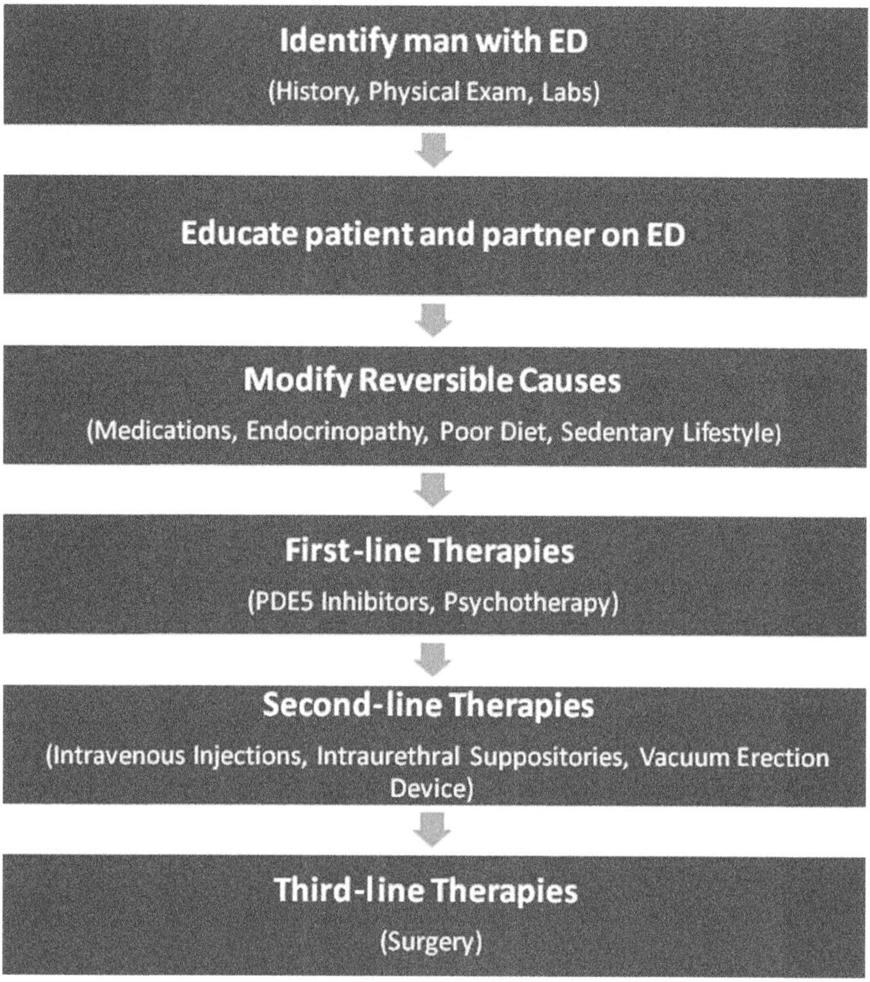

Identify man with ED

(History, Physical Exam, Labs)

Educate patient and partner on ED

Modify Reversible Causes

(Medications, Endocrinopathy, Poor Diet, Sedentary Lifestyle)

First-line Therapies

(PDE5 Inhibitors, Psychotherapy)

Second-line Therapies

(Intravenous Injections, Intraurethral Suppositories, Vacuum Erection Device)

Third-line Therapies

(Surgery)

Fig. 1. Algorithm for ED management. PDE5, phosphodiesterase type 5. (*Adapted from* The process of care model for evaluation and treatment of erectile dysfunction. The process of care consensus panel. Int J Impot Res 1999;11(2):62; with permission.)

interventions to optimize the patient's cardiovascular health should be considered. Eliminating, managing, or minimizing risk factors for cardiovascular disease may also improve erectile health and function. Evidence from the Massachusetts Male Aging Study indicates that lifestyle changes are most effective for prevention/resolution of ED when they are started before age 50 years; it may be hypothesized that lifestyle interventions in later life may be too late to reverse penile vascular disease.[2]

Diet

Animal and human studies have shown that obesity is a significant independent risk factor for ED.[3] Obesity may contribute to ED through a variety of mechanisms, including the presence of proinflammatory molecules (C-reactive protein, free radicals) and alterations of hormone levels, such as testosterone deficiency. Obesity and the metabolic syndrome (the combination of central obesity, insulin resistance, high blood pressure, and increased lipid levels) are associated with many sexual problems, including ED and low sexual desire.[3]

Improving diet quality and matching the number of calories consumed to caloric expenditures is the most reliable means of preventing and treating obesity. Weight loss has been shown to produce significant improvements in erectile function among obese men. A series of studies from Italy have evaluated the relationship between diet and ED. It was noted that men on a Mediterranean diet (rich in polyunsaturated oils, fish, and fresh produce, and light in processed foods, saturated fats, dairy, and red meat) had lower rates of ED than those on a more typical Western diet.[4]

Exercise and Physical Activity

There is an inverse relationship between ED and physical activity. Men who engage in regular vigorous physical activity have greatly reduced rates of ED.[5,6] Physical activity is associated with reductions in vascular comorbidities known to be associated with ED risk (high blood pressure, glucose intolerance). Several studies have quantified the impact of exercise on ED.

A unique Austrian study examined city workers and categorized their activity into numbers of kilojoules expended per week in their recreation and other active pursuits.[7] This categorization was done using the Paffenbarger score, which measures activity in kilojoules per week for both work (walking, climbing stairs) and recreation. It was determined that the prevalence of ED, especially severe ED, decreased with every incremental increase (in increments of 500–1000 kJ/wk) in energy expenditure.[7]

The aforementioned study by Esposito and colleagues[4] also showed the role of increased physical activity in recovery of erectile function. Note that, in the aforementioned study on the Mediterranean diet, physical activity was an important component of the lifestyle intervention.

Medication Adjustment

More than 200 medications have been implicated in the pathogenesis of ED. Antihypertensives have been clearly linked to ED, particularly nonspecific β-blockers and thiazide diuretics.[7,8] Other common medications associated with ED include antiandrogens, antidepressants (especially selective serotonin reuptake inhibitor agents), and other psychotropics. When these medications are identified as a potentially significant contributor to ED, cessation should be considered if possible; if the medication is essential, substitution with a different agent in the same class may be worthwhile. However, robust evidence supporting the efficacy of medication adjustment is lacking. Changes in medications should be coordinated with the patient's prescribing health providers to minimize risk of ceasing essential medications.

Tobacco, Alcohol, and Marijuana Use

Multiple case-controlled trials have shown a dose-related association between tobacco use and ED.[9,10] Curiously, alcohol may have either positive or negative effects on erectile function, depending on how much is consumed. With smaller amounts (typically up to 2 normal-volume beverages), there may be improved erection and libido, likely caused by suppression of anxiety (reduction in adrenaline levels). Increased amounts of alcohol are known to produce central nervous system sedation, decreased libido, and transient ED.[11] Chronic alcohol abuse may result in liver dysfunction, decreased testosterone and increased estrogen levels, and alcoholic polyneuropathy, all of which may affect erectile function negatively.

Habitual marijuana use may contribute to sexual difficulties and has been linked to orgasmic function.[12] Marijuana use has also been shown to be associated with an increased number of sexual partners in both men and women. Presumably, this is the result of a lowering of inhibition among chronic marijuana users.

PHARMACOLOGIC TREATMENT OPTIONS
Over-the-Counter and Herbal Supplements

Supplements, nutriceuticals, and other over-the-counter agents for ED are a robust industry with minimal regulation. Common nutriceutical agents used for ED include L-arginine, ginseng, yohimbine, horny goat weed, and *Ginkgo biloba*. Efficacy of these herbal formulations is variable and is often of low quality. Manufacturers may make claims of efficacy using carefully coded language that does not promise to treat or prevent a specific condition or disease.

Arginine

L-Arginine is a semiessential or conditionally essential amino acid that is abundant in dairy, meat, seafood, grains, and legumes. L-Arginine is a precursor in the production of nitric oxide, which is the essential vasodilatory compound that facilitates erectogenic action.[13] A prospective randomized, double-blind, placebo-controlled study of men taking 5 g of L-arginine per day concluded that a third of the men in the trial experienced enhanced sexual function, but this effect was seen only in men with abnormal nitric oxide metabolism.[14] Other studies have found that men using L-arginine had significant improvements in sexual function without side effects.

Ginseng

Korean red ginseng is thought to stimulate erectile function either through promotion of the nitric oxide system or its saponin content.[15,16] In a 2002 double-blind, placebo-controlled, crossover study, Hong and colleagues[16] reported that mean International Index of Erectile Function scores were significantly higher in patients treated with Korean red ginseng (900 mg, 3 times daily) than in those who received placebo.

Horny goat weed

Horny goat weed is a naturally occurring plant of the *Epimedium* genus that may enhance erectile function, as well as producing aphrodisiac effects. The active component is icariin, which has phosphodiesterase type 5 inhibitor (PDE5i)–like activities.[17,18] Icariin also has been linked to an increase in the circulating levels of testosterone.[19] In many Western countries, horny goat weed has been marketed as natural Viagra.

Ginkgo biloba

Ginkgo has been purported to increase circulation and is thought to improve memory, global cognitive function, and ED. *Ginkgo* extracts may improve sexual function by enhancing blood flow to the brain, as well as to the penis. However, the positive cognitive benefits of this supplement have not been realized and the benefits to sexual functioning have been questioned.[20–23] Three randomized placebo-controlled trials have not found significant increases in sexual function with *Ginkgo* extracts.[24–26]

Phosphodiesterase Type 5 Inhibitors

The introduction of orally bioavailable pharmacotherapy for ED revolutionized sexual medicine and improved the lives of millions of men and their partners. PDE5i's have shown efficacy for ED of any cause, including psychogenic (when used in conjunction with psychosexual counseling).

Mechanism/pharmacokinetics

Phosphodiesterase type 5 (PDE5) is the predominant phosphodiesterase enzyme in the penis.[27] PDE5 hydrolyzes cyclic guanosine monophosphate (cGMP) to the inactive form 1'-guanosine monophosphate. cGMP is a key regulator of calcium hemostasis and smooth muscle contraction in the penile vasculature; hence, depletion of cGMP by the action of PDE5 tends to oppose penile erection.[28] PDE5i's are competitive inhibitors of PDE5 by binding to the catalytic domain and hence promote high levels of cGMP in the penile vasculature.[29]

Sildenafil and vardenafil are pyrimidine compounds. Peak absorption for each is approximately 30 to 60 minutes.[30–32] The serum half-life of these drugs is 3 to 5 hours.[30,31] Tissue levels are likely to remain high after serum levels decline; this drives the observation that many men experience benefit from these drugs up to 12 hours after administration.[33,34] Absorption of these drugs is slowed by dietary lipids and hence they should not be taken after a meal, particularly one high in fat content. Some authorities suggest ingestion of these agents in a preprandial fashion (1–2 hours before a meal).

Tadalafil is structurally distinct from vardenafil and sildenafil.[35] Peak absorption of this drug occurs between 2 and 4 hours, with a half-life of 17.5 hours. Tadalafil absorption is not affected by food intake.[35] Tadalafil is the only PDE5i that is currently approved as a daily dose (as opposed to on-demand) treatment of ED.[36,37] Daily tadalafil has also shown efficacy in the management of lower urinary tract symptoms from benign prostatic enlargement.

Avanafil is an amino-heterocyclic compound that is structurally distinct from other approved PDE5i's.[38,39] Peak absorption occurs in 20 to 30 minutes and half-life is about 6 hours.[40]

Optimization of use

In all studies published to date, each PDE5i has shown a superior erectile response rate compared with placebo.[41,42] Typically, success rates with first-time prescription are 60% to 75%.[34,36,41] It is clear that some men prefer one drug versus another; the rationale for preference may related to tolerability, efficacy, or economic concerns.[43] Some men who fail one PDE5i may have a better response to another; a trial of an alternative PDE5i should be considered before advancing to second-line therapies.[43] It is essential that PDE5i administration be coupled with sexual stimulation.[44] Some men who receive a PDE5i from a nonspecialist do not receive instructions on the time and arousal requirements for maximal efficacy. A patient who presents to the urologist with failure of a PDE5i should have a thorough evaluation of how the drug failed. It is recommended that men use the drug at maximum dose at least 4 times per acceptable protocol before declaring the drug a failure. Up to 50% of PDE5i failures may be salvaged with reeducation.[45]

Contraindications

The only strict contraindication to use of a PDE5i is concurrent use of nitrate-containing medications (eg, sublingual nitroglycerin, isosorbide mononitrate or dinitrate).[46] Concurrent use of nitrates and PDE5i may lead to life-threatening hypotension. Relative contraindications to PDE5i therapy include use of α-blocking medications for hypertension or lower urinary tract symptoms because there is concern that combined treatment may predispose men to orthostatic hypotension.[46] Patients on stable α-blocker therapy are advised to commence a PDE5i at one-quarter maximum dose; dosage increases can be made as tolerated/indicated. α-Blockers and PDE5i should be taken at least 4 hours apart. Vardenafil is not recommended in men with congenital QT syndrome and men taking class IA or III antiarrhythmics (amiodarone, sotalol, quinidine).[46]

Adverse events

The most common adverse events associated with this class of medications include headache, facial flushing, dyspepsia/heartburn, nasal congestion, visual changes, and myalgia.[42] The incidence of these effects ranges from 1% to 16%.[42] Tadalafil and avanafil have the lowest incidence of visual disturbances. Tadalafil has significant association with myalgia. Priapism theoretically may be caused by any ED drug; however, the rate of priapism with PDE5i is close to zero.[47] Of course, the risk of priapism may be amplified in men who combine PDE5i's with other drugs (prescription or recreational).

In the mid-2000s there was concern that PDE5i's were associated with an increased risk of nonarteritic ischemic optic neuropathy (NAION), a cause of irreversible unilateral blindness. Reviews of databases have to date have failed to show a significantly increased risk of NAION in men using PDE5i's compared with the general population.[48] Consultation with an ophthalmologist before use of a PDE5i may be prudent if the patient has vision concerns.

Vacuum Erection Device

The vacuum erection device (VED) is a mechanical device used to generate a negative pressure environment around the penis to produce erection. The VED is coupled with a rubberized constriction device, deployed at the base of the penis, which prevents venous outflow, producing and maintaining an erection. There are a variety of models available, ranging from simple cylinders with hand-driven pumps to complex electronic vacuum systems. VEDs are now nonprescription and may be purchased over-the-counter. Devices of low quality typically do not possess a pop-off valve to limit the risk of overpressurization.[49]

VEDs may lead to petechiae formation or hematoma if the device is overpressurized. Ecchymosis or even skin necrosis may also occur at the site of the constriction band if left on for too long a time. It is recommended that the rubberized band be applied for no longer than 30 minutes.[50] Men taking anticoagulants are at increased risk of bruising and/or petechiae. Depending on tightness of the ring, disruption of ejaculation may occur; this may lead to pain with ejaculation, personal or partner distress, and potentially (although rarely) disruption of planned fertility.[51]

Intraurethral Suppository

The medicated urethral system for erections (MUSE) is an intraurethral suppository of prostaglandin-E_1 (PGE_1) that is administered via the urethral meatus. The suppository dissolves, leading to PGE_1 diffusion across the urethra and into the corpus spongiosum, and from there into the corpora cavernosa via collateral vessels. PGE_1 increases intracellular levels of cyclic AMP (cAMP) in smooth muscle cells, leading to penile erection.

Administration of the first dose of the medication should occur in the office to monitor the patient for hypotension (2% incidence at maximum dose).

Penile pain is reported by 32% of patients using PGE_1. Urethral burning is reported in up 12% of patients, minor urethral bleeding and irritation in 5%, and testicular pain in 5% of men. Also, 6% of female sexual partners reported vaginal burning/itching compared with 1% in a matched placebo group. Priapism is possible with MUSE but the incidence seems to be low. Rarely, patients experience dizziness, presumably from hypotension caused by systemic absorption of the PGE_1.

Intracavernosal (Penile) Injection Therapy

Intracavernosal injection (ICI), originally introduced in 1982, involves the process of injecting a vasoactive agent (or combination of agents) directly into the corpora cavernosa. This injection results in penile erection by relaxation of vascular smooth muscle and increased arterial flow into the penis. The injection is performed via a 29-gauge to 31-gauge needle.

The single most commonly used agent is PGE_1, which is a direct cAMP stimulator. Use of PGE_1 as monotherapy by penile injection is US Food and Drug Administration (FDA) approved. Two other agents are commonly used in erectogenic therapy; these agents are not FDA approved for this indication but are widely used. Papaverine is a nonspecific phosphodiesterase inhibitor and increases intracellular levels of both cAMP and cGMP. Phenotolamine is an alpha1-adrenergic receptor blocker that reduces sympathetic tone in the penis, thereby opposing vasoconstriction. Compounds that contain 2 of these 3 erectogenic agents (most commonly papaverine and phentolamine) are commonly called bimix, whereas compounds containing all 3 of the agents are called trimix. Note that there is no standard formulation of bimix or trimix; each pharmacy may produce a solution that differs markedly in concentrations so it is essential to be familiar with the specific contents of a given solution.

Adverse events/side effects/contraindications

The most common side effect is penile pain. Up to 30% of men using PGE_1 report penile pain. Continued use of PGE_1 may ultimately decrease the incidence of penile pain. Alternatively, discontinuation of the PGE_1 and substitution with another intractable agent may abrogate penile discomfort. Commonly patients have ecchymosis following the injection. They are reminded to hold direct pressure on the injection site for 60 seconds after the injection to minimize this cosmetic issue. Rarely, a hematoma forms after injection (3%); this is thought to result from injury to a superficial penile vein. Gentle compression ameliorates this issue.

Potentially, the most serious event that occurs after penile injections is priapism. In studies evaluating the safety of alprostadil, priapism was found in only 4% of the study population.[52] If a patient has an erection lasting more than 4 hours, urgent medical intervention is necessary. Priapism can be prevented by education and close monitoring of patients.

Men who are needlephobic and those who are unable to perform the injection procedure should not be prescribed ICI therapy. Patients with Peyronie disease should be carefully monitored because penile scarring may make injection technically difficult. Patients with a short or buried penis, large pannus, poor vision, and poor manual dexterity are advised to have a partner perform the injection. Being on anticoagulation is not a contraindication to penile injection therapy.

SURGICAL TREATMENT OPTIONS

A penile implant (also known as penile prosthesis) is a device that is surgically implanted into the corpora cavernosa. Penile implants are used in patients who:

1. Have failed nonsurgical management of ED
2. Are not candidates for nonsurgical management, or
3. Cannot tolerate nonsurgical management or find it unpalatable

Noninflatable Implants (Malleable or Semirigid)

The most mechanically simple device uses 2 flexible rods, which are surgically inserted into each corporal body. Examples of malleable implants include the American Medical Systems Spectra and the Coloplast Genesis implants. These cylinders remain rigid but can be bent downward or upward. For men who need penile turgidity for the application of a condom catheter, these devices may be beneficial.

If used in spinal cord injured patients, the implanter and patient need to be aware of the potential for distal perforation caused by the constant pressure on the glans and distal penile skin. Although the device allows the man to have a functional erection for sexual activity, there is no flaccid state once implanted.

Two-Piece Inflatable Implant

There is currently only a single type of 2-piece device (Ambicor, American Medical Systems). This device consists of 2 inflatable cylinders and a pump, which resides in the scrotum. The device allows a fully rigid erection; however, in the flaccid state, the penis has some degree of tumescence because the device is prefilled (given the absence of a reservoir). The fluid reservoir resides in the proximal (posterior) part of the cylinders. The pump mechanism transfers fluid from the proximal portion of the corporal cylinders to the distal (anterior) part of the device. Inflation is accomplished by squeezing the pump, whereas deflation is accomplished by bending the device cylinders in the midshaft to 90°, which facilitates transfer of the fluid back to the proximal cylinder reservoir. This device offers an excellent rigidity profile. For patients with a hostile pelvis, the 2-piece device is an excellent option. This device comes in standard sizes (2-cm increments, 14–22 cm), which may be customized by addition of extenders to the proximal tips (1–3 cm).

Three-Piece Inflatable Implant

Three-piece penile implant devices include American Medical Systems 700-CX, 700-CXR, and LGX implants, and the Coloplast Titan implant. These devices allow for both a flaccid and erect state. The 3-piece inflatable implant cycles fluid from a reservoir into the penile cylinders. Like the 2-piece device, the pump resides in the scrotum. Devices come in standard sizes (14–24 cm), which may be customized by addition of extenders to the proximal tips. The reservoir is classically placed in the space of Retzius but, for a variety of reasons, may be placed in an ectopic location.

Alternative, or ectopic, locations include subcutaneous and submuscular locations.

Complications of penile prosthesis use

The most serious complication of inflatable penile prostheses (IPPs) is infection. Infection may occur in the perioperative period or as a late complication. Additional surgical complications include bleeding, bruising, hematoma formation (genital or abdominal), wound separation, and severe pain. Long-term complications that may occur are mechanical malfunction, urethral perforation, visceral perforation, and device erosion, which typically necessitates device removal. Historical rates of infection have been as high as 5% in first-time implants.[53] Recent innovations, such as antibiotic impregnation and adaptations in technique, have reduced the rate of infection in modern series to 1% to 2% in the hands of experienced implanters.[54]

Device infections typically present within the first 8 weeks postoperatively with fever, pain, erythema, fixation of the scrotal pump to scrotal skin, pus drainage, or crepitus around the device pump or cylinders. Risk factors for infection include diabetes, immunosuppressed state, obesity, prior pelvic radiation, prolonged operative time, and an inexperienced surgeon.[55,56] Treatment is surgical with complete removal of all components of the infected device and extensive washout with a staged replacement of the implant 3 months later.[57] Broad-spectrum antibiotics should be administered and surgical drains are advocated by some authorities.

The chance of having a mechanical breakage of an IPP is approximately 5% to 10% after 10 years.[23] Patients with a malfunctioning implant report that the pump no longer compresses or that compression does not produce tumescence. A sound of air movement may be present. Although the most common approach is to remove and replace the entire device (especially >2 years after placement), some authorities repair or replace only the malfunctioning component.[58] Common defects include shearing or fracture of one of the tubes coming off the pump (to the reservoir or cylinders) or a blowout in the tubing from the pump to the reservoir. It is unusual to have a reservoir defect. Cylinder defects are rare.

REFERENCES

1. Esposito K, Ciotola M, Giugliano F, et al. Effects of intensive lifestyle changes on erectile dysfunction in men. J Sex Med 2009;6(1):243–50.
2. Derby CA, Mohr BA, Goldstein I, et al. Modifiable risk factors and erectile dysfunction: can lifestyle changes modify risk? Urology 2000;56(2):302–6.
3. Corona G, Mannucci E, Schulman C, et al. Psychobiologic correlates of the metabolic syndrome and associated sexual dysfunction. Eur Urol 2006;50(3):595–604 [discussion: 604].
4. Esposito K, Ciotola M, Giugliano F, et al. Mediterranean diet improves erectile function in subjects with the metabolic syndrome. Int J Impot Res 2006;18(4): 405–10.
5. Janiszewski PM, Janssen I, Ross R. Abdominal obesity and physical inactivity are associated with erectile dysfunction independent of body mass index. J Sex Med 2009;6(7):1990–8.
6. Hannan JL, Maio MT, Komolova M, et al. Beneficial impact of exercise and obesity interventions on erectile function and its risk factors. J Sex Med 2009; 6(Suppl 3):254–61.
7. Grimm RH Jr, Grandits GA, Prineas RJ, et al. Long-term effects on sexual function of five antihypertensive drugs and nutritional hygienic treatment in hypertensive men and women. Treatment of Mild Hypertension Study (TOMHS). Hypertension 1997;29(1 Pt 1):8–14.
8. Wassertheil-Smoller S, Blaufox MD, Oberman A, et al. Effect of antihypertensives on sexual function and quality of life: the TAIM Study. Ann Intern Med 1991; 114(8):613–20.
9. Polsky JY, Aronson KJ, Heaton JP, et al. Smoking and other lifestyle factors in relation to erectile dysfunction. BJU Int 2005;96(9):1355–9.
10. Kupelian V, Link CL, McKinlay JB. Association between smoking, passive smoking, and erectile dysfunction: results from the Boston Area Community Health (BACH) Survey. Eur Urol 2007;52(2):416–22.
11. Chew KK. Alcohol consumption and male erectile dysfunction: an unfounded reputation for risk? J Sex Med 2009;6(8):2340.
12. Smith AM, Ferris JA, Simpson JM, et al. Cannabis use and sexual health. J Sex Med 2010;7(2 Pt 1):787–93.
13. Andrew PJ, Mayer B. Enzymatic function of nitric oxide synthases. Cardiovasc Res 1999;43(3):521–31.
14. Chen J, Wollman Y, Chernichovsky T, et al. Effect of oral administration of high-dose nitric oxide donor L-arginine in men with organic erectile dysfunction: results of a double-blind, randomized, placebo-controlled study. BJU Int 1999; 83(3):269–73.
15. Choi HK, Seong DH, Rha KH. Clinical efficacy of Korean red ginseng for erectile dysfunction. Int J Impot Res 1995;7(3):181–6.

16. Hong B, Ji YH, Hong JH, et al. A double-blind crossover study evaluating the efficacy of Korean red ginseng in patients with erectile dysfunction: a preliminary report. J Urol 2002;168(5):2070–3.

17. Jiang Z, Hu B, Wang J, et al. Effect of icariin on cyclic GMP levels and on the mRNA expression of cGMP-binding cGMP-specific phosphodiesterase (PDE5) in penile cavernosum. J Huazhong Univ Sci Technolog Med Sci 2006;26(4): 460–2.

18. Dell'Agli M, Galli GV, Dal Cero E, et al. Potent inhibition of human phosphodiesterase-5 by icariin derivatives. J Nat Prod 2008;71(9):1513–7.

19. Zhang ZB, Yang QT. The testosterone mimetic properties of icariin. Asian J Androl 2006;8(5):601–5.

20. Laws KR, Sweetnam H, Kondel TK. Is Ginkgo biloba a cognitive enhancer in healthy individuals? A meta-analysis. Hum Psychopharmacol 2012;27(6):527–33.

21. Birks J, Grimley Evans J. Ginkgo biloba for cognitive impairment and dementia. Cochrane Database Syst Rev 2009;(1):CD003120.

22. Cohen AJ, Bartlik B. Ginkgo biloba for antidepressant-induced sexual dysfunction. J Sex Marital Ther 1998;24(2):139–43.

23. Corazza O, Martinotti G, Santacroce R, et al. Sexual enhancement products for sale online: raising awareness of the psychoactive effects of yohimbine, maca, horny goat weed, and Ginkgo biloba. Biomed Res Int 2014;2014:841798.

24. Sikora RSM, Engelke B, et al. Randomized placebo-controlled study on the effects of oral treatment with gingko biloba extract in patients with erectile dysfunction. J Urol 1998;159(5 (Suppl. 240)).

25. Kang BJ, Lee SJ, Kim MD, et al. A placebo-controlled, double-blind trial of Ginkgo biloba for antidepressant-induced sexual dysfunction. Hum Psychopharmacol 2002;17(6):279–84.

26. Wheatley D. Triple-blind, placebo-controlled trial of Ginkgo biloba in sexual dysfunction due to antidepressant drugs. Hum Psychopharmacol 2004;19(8): 545–8.

27. Corbin JD, Francis SH. Pharmacology of phosphodiesterase-5 inhibitors. Int J Clin Pract 2002;56(6):453–9.

28. Boolell M, Allen MJ, Ballard SA, et al. Sildenafil: an orally active type 5 cyclic GMP-specific phosphodiesterase inhibitor for the treatment of penile erectile dysfunction. Int J Impot Res 1996;8(2):47–52.

29. Rosen RC. Sexual pharmacology in the 21st century. J Gend Specif Med 2000; 3(5):45–52.

30. Umrani DN, Goyal RK. Pharmacology of sildenafil citrate. Indian J Physiol Pharmacol 1999;43(2):160–4.

31. Wallis RM. The pharmacology of sildenafil, a novel and selective inhibitor of phosphodiesterase (PDE) type 5. Nihon Yakurigaku Zasshi 1999;114(Suppl 1):22P–6P.

32. Bischoff E. Vardenafil preclinical trial data: potency, pharmacodynamics, pharmacokinetics, and adverse events. Int J Impot Res 2004;16(Suppl 1):S34–7.

33. Hatzichristou D, Cuzin B, Martin-Morales A, et al. Vardenafil improves satisfaction rates, depressive symptomatology, and self-confidence in a broad population of men with erectile dysfunction. J Sex Med 2005;2(1):109–16.

34. Hellstrom WJ, Gittelman M, Karlin G, et al. Vardenafil for treatment of men with erectile dysfunction: efficacy and safety in a randomized, double-blind, placebo-controlled trial. J Androl 2002;23(6):763–71.

35. Coward RM, Carson CC. Tadalafil in the treatment of erectile dysfunction. Ther Clin Risk Manag 2008;4(6):1315–30.

36. Brock GB, McMahon CG, Chen KK, et al. Efficacy and safety of tadalafil for the treatment of erectile dysfunction: results of integrated analyses. J Urol 2002; 168(4 Pt 1):1332–6.

37. Kim E, Seftel A, Goldfischer E, et al. Comparative efficacy of tadalafil once daily in men with erectile dysfunction who demonstrated previous partial responses to as-needed sildenafil, tadalafil, or vardenafil. Curr Med Res Opin 2015;31(2): 379–89.

38. Kyle JA, Brown DA, Hill JK. Avanafil for erectile dysfunction. Ann Pharmacother 2013;47(10):1312–20.

39. Wang H, Yuan J, Hu X, et al. The effectiveness and safety of avanafil for erectile dysfunction: a systematic review and meta-analysis. Curr Med Res Opin 2014; 30(8):1565–71.

40. Katz EG, Tan RB, Rittenberg D, et al. Avanafil for erectile dysfunction in elderly and younger adults: differential pharmacology and clinical utility. Ther Clin Risk Manag 2014;10:701–11.

41. Porst H, Rosen R, Padma-Nathan H, et al. The efficacy and tolerability of vardenafil, a new, oral, selective phosphodiesterase type 5 inhibitor, in patients with erectile dysfunction: the first at-home clinical trial. Int J Impot Res 2001;13(4): 192–9.

42. Yuan J, Zhang R, Yang Z, et al. Comparative effectiveness and safety of oral phosphodiesterase type 5 inhibitors for erectile dysfunction: a systematic review and network meta-analysis. Eur Urol 2013;63(5):902–12.

43. Fink HA, Mac Donald R, Rutks IR, et al. Sildenafil for male erectile dysfunction: a systematic review and meta-analysis. Arch Intern Med 2002;162(12):1349–60.

44. Porst H, Burnett A, Brock G, et al. SOP conservative (medical and mechanical) treatment of erectile dysfunction. J Sex Med 2013;10(1):130–71.

45. Atiemo HO, Szostak MJ, Sklar GN. Salvage of sildenafil failures referred from primary care physicians. J Urol 2003;170(6 Pt 1):2356–8.

46. Corona G, Razzoli E, Forti G, et al. The use of phosphodiesterase 5 inhibitors with concomitant medications. J Endocrinol Invest 2008;31(9):799–808.

47. Sur RL, Kane CJ. Sildenafil citrate-associated priapism. Urology 2000;55(6):950.

48. Giuliano F, Jackson G, Montorsi F, et al. Safety of sildenafil citrate: review of 67 double-blind placebo-controlled trials and the postmarketing safety database. Int J Clin Pract 2010;64(2):240–55.

49. Bosshardt RJ, Farwerk R, Sikora R, et al. Objective measurement of the effectiveness, therapeutic success and dynamic mechanisms of the vacuum device. Br J Urol 1995;75(6):786–91.

50. Ganem JP, Lucey DT, Janosko EO, et al. Unusual complications of the vacuum erection device. Urology 1998;51(4):627–31.

51. Baltaci S, Aydos K, Kosar A, et al. Treating erectile dysfunction with a vacuum tumescence device: a retrospective analysis of acceptance and satisfaction. Br J Urol 1995;76(6):757–60.

52. Linet OI, Ogrinc FG. Efficacy and safety of intracavernosal alprostadil in men with erectile dysfunction. The Alprostadil Study Group. N Engl J Med 1996;334(14): 873–7.

53. Carson CC 3rd. Efficacy of antibiotic impregnation of inflatable penile prostheses in decreasing infection in original implants. J Urol 2004;171(4):1611–4.

54. Mulcahy JJ. Long-term experience with salvage of infected penile implants. J Urol 2000;163(2):481–2.

55. Wilson SK, Delk JR, Salem EA, et al. Long-term survival of inflatable penile prostheses: single surgical group experience with 2,384 first-time implants spanning two decades. J Sex Med 2007;4(4 Pt 1):1074–9.

56. Henry GD, Kansal NS, Callaway M, et al. Centers of excellence concept and penile prostheses: an outcome analysis. J Urol 2009;181(3):1264–8.

57. Henry GD, Donatucci CF, Conners W, et al. An outcomes analysis of over 200 revision surgeries for penile prosthesis implantation: a multicenter study. J Sex Med 2012;9(1):309–15.

58. Garber BB. Mentor Alpha 1 inflatable penile prosthesis: patient satisfaction and device reliability. Urology 1994;43(2):214–7.

Hypogonadism
Therapeutic Risks, Benefits, and Outcomes

John T. Sigalos, BA[a], Alexander W. Pastuszak, MD, PhD[b,c],
Mohit Khera, MD, MBA, MPH[c,*]

KEYWORDS

- Hypogonadism • Cardiovascular risk • Testosterone therapy • Outcomes

KEY POINTS

- Hypogonadism is a common condition defined by the presence of low serum testosterone levels and hypogonadal symptoms, and most commonly treated using testosterone therapy (TTh).
- The accuracy of diagnosis and appropriateness of treatment, along with proper follow-up, are increasingly important given the large increase in testosterone prescriptions and the recent concern for cardiovascular (CV) risk associated with TTh.
- Only a few recent studies with significant methodological flaws have supported an increased CV risk in men on testosterone. In contrast, the body of literature evaluating TTh over the past 75 years, as well as more recent work, has shown that TTh may improve CV outcomes rather than increase risks.
- Given the association between low serum testosterone levels and CV events and morbidity, it is prudent to treat hypogonadal men until studies that more definitively elucidate the risk of TTh on CV outcomes become available.

INTRODUCTION

According to the Endocrine Society practice guidelines, hypogonadism is defined as "a clinical syndrome that results from failure of the testis to produce physiological

A.W. Pastuszak is a K12 scholar supported by a Male Reproductive Health Research (MRHR) Career Development Physician-Scientist Award (grant # HD073917-01) from the Eunice Kennedy Shriver National Institute of Child Health and Human Development (NICHD) Program.
Conflicts of Interest: Endo Pharmaceuticals, speaker and advisor; Boston Scientific/AMS, research support (Dr A.W. Pastuszak). Consultant for Endo, ATYU, Coloplast, Boston Scientific, Abbvie (Dr M. Khera). None (J.T. Sigalos).
[a] Baylor College of Medicine, 1 Baylor Plaza, Houston, TX 77030, USA; [b] Center for Reproductive Medicine, Baylor College of Medicine, 1 Baylor Plaza, Room N730 Houston, TX 77030, USA; [c] Scott Department of Urology, Baylor College of Medicine, 7200 Cambridge Street, Houston, TX 77030, USA
* Corresponding author. Scott Department of Urology, Baylor College of Medicine, 7200 Cambridge Street, Houston, TX 77030.
E-mail address: mkhera@bcm.edu

levels of testosterone (T) (androgen deficiency) and a normal number of spermatozoa due to disruption of one or more levels of the hypothalamic-pituitary-testicular axis."[1] In contrast, the US Food and Drug Administration (FDA) defines hypogonadism as a serum T level less than or equal to 300 ng/dL. The production of T in the testis is stimulated by secretion of gonadotropin-releasing hormone (GnRH) from the hypothalamus, resulting in secretion of follicle-stimulating hormone (FSH) and luteinizing hormone (LH) from the anterior pituitary gland.[2] LH and FSH stimulate production of T and spermatogenesis, respectively. Over the lifetime, T is essential for maintaining the male phenotype. Specifically, T facilitates the development and maintenance of secondary sex characteristics, muscle mass, bone density, stimulation of erythropoiesis, and libido. T also has central nervous effects on mood and cognition.[3]

Given these benefits, it is imperative to assess men for gonadal function. The reported prevalence of hypogonadism in men 30 to 79 years old from the Boston Area Community Health survey using a combination of hypogonadal symptoms and T level of less than 300 ng/dL is ~6%.[4] This rate increases with increasing age.[4,5] Increased awareness of hypogonadism by the lay public, as well as direct-to-consumer marketing of T products, has led to dramatic increases in T use around the world.[6] Between 2000 and 2011 the prevalence of T use increased 10-fold in the United States, and 40-fold in Canada.[6] In economic terms, US sales of T products increased from $324 million in 2002 to $2 billion in 2012, and the number of T doses prescribed increased from 100 million in 2007 to 500 million in 2012, not including prescriptions filled by compounding pharmacies, the Internet, and direct-to-patient clinic sales.[7] Up to 25% of men who were prescribed T did not have baseline serum T levels checked before obtaining a prescription.[8,9] Potential misuse of T therapy (TTh) and conflicting data regarding the therapeutic risks of TTh have led to increased scrutiny by the FDA, which in March 2015 mandated a change to T labels warning of potential cardiovascular (CV) risks related to TTh.[10] However, the FDA's stance is based on several recent studies that supported a weak, but significant, association between increased CV risk and TTh that the FDA decided could not be ignored. Given this controversy, as well as the clear missteps in the diagnosis and treatment of hypogonadism that have come to light in recent years, this article discusses the diagnosis and treatment of hypogonadism and reviews the literature regarding the association between TTh and CV risk.

DIAGNOSIS OF HYPOGONADISM

The causes of hypogonadism can be divided into 2 categories: primary hypogonadism, which represents a failure of the testes to produce T, and secondary (hypogonadotropic) hypogonadism, which is failure of the pituitary gland to secrete sufficient LH to stimulate testicular T production. Primary hypogonadism is associated with increased LH levels, whereas secondary hypogonadism is reflected by low or inappropriately normal LH levels.[1] The common causes of primary and secondary hypogonadism are summarized in **Table 1**.[11]

The diagnosis of hypogonadism relies on the presence of low serum T levels, considered to be less than 300 ng/dL by most practice recommendations,[1,12] as well as the presence of clinical symptoms associated with low T levels.[1,13] However, a standardized definition of hypogonadism is lacking. Clinical signs and symptoms suggestive of T deficiency that warrant further laboratory work-up include delayed puberty, decreased libido, decreased spontaneous erections, erectile dysfunction, gynecomastia and breast tenderness, loss of body hair, testicular atrophy, low sperm count, low bone mineral density, and hot flashes. Other symptoms that are less

Table 1
Causes of primary and secondary hypogonadism

Primary Hypogonadism	Secondary Hypogonadism
Klinefelter syndrome	Pituitary neoplasms
Uncorrected	Hyperprolactinemia
cryptorchidism	Hemochromatosis
Chemotherapy	Infiltrative disorders
Radiation therapy	Genetic disorders of GnRH secretion including idiopathic
Trauma	hypogonadotropic hypogonadism with and without anosmia
Mumps	Genetic disorders of gonadotropin secretion or action
Orchitis	Genetic disorders of pituitary development
Orchiectomy	Eating disorders
	Anabolic steroid abuse

specific for hypogonadism include decreased energy, depressed mood, poor concentration, anemia, and body composition changes, including reduced muscle mass/strength in conjunction with increased body fat.[1] Questionnaires such as the Aging Male Symptom Score (AMS) and Androgen Deficiency in Aging Men (ADAM) have been used in clinical practice to help identify and quantify the severity of hypogonadism but lack specificity in preferentially identifying men with the condition.[14]

All men with suspected hypogonadism should undergo a physical examination, with emphasis on the genitalia. Testicular volume less than 10 cm^3 is a strong predictor of hypogonadism, and should prompt more questioning for evaluation of sources of testicular injury, such as prior trauma, radiation/chemotherapy, and surgery.[14,15] A testicular volume less than 5 cm^3 is suggestive of Klinefelter syndrome and warrants evaluation with a karyotype.[16] In addition to low testicular volume, the presence of gynecomastia or a small prostate for age may indicate a history of chronic low T levels.[16]

In men with clinical symptoms of hypogonadism, most practice guidelines recommend 2 morning serum total T measurements to confirm a diagnosis of hypogonadism. Transient decreases in serum T may be caused by acute illness; therefore, clinicians should inquire about acute illness and a subsequent second measurement of T should be performed to rule out a transient decrease in total T.[17] Blood samples should be drawn between 7 AM and 11 AM, because during this window serum T levels are likely to be at their peak.[18] In general, the guidelines for laboratory assessment of low T level consider T level low if less than 350 ng/dL (12.1 nmol/L) or lower than the reference range for the laboratory performing the assessment.[1,13,14,17,19] Given the lack of age-specific normal T ranges, younger men with T levels less than 400 ng/dL with clinical symptoms may be likely to benefit from therapy.[20] Men with normal T levels with clinical symptoms may also benefit from treatment.[16] In symptomatic men with normal T levels, increases in sex hormone–binding globulin (SHBG), which binds T, may result in lower free T levels.[16] Thus, determining free T levels may be helpful in men with normal total T levels and hypogonadal symptoms, particularly older or overweight men with increased SHBG levels.

If low T levels are confirmed, determination of LH and FSH levels is recommended to determine whether hypogonadism is primary or secondary. If primary hypogonadism is suspected, karyotype to rule out Klinefelter syndrome can be performed. If findings are consistent with secondary hypogonadism, prolactin, estrogen (E), and iron saturation are recommended to rule out hyperprolactinemia, determine the T/E ratio, and evaluate for hemochromatosis, respectively. MRI examination of the pituitary can be considered in the presence of increased prolactin levels to assess for the presence of tumors.[1,14]

TREATMENT OF HYPOGONADISM

First-line treatment of hypogonadism is TTh, and common T formulations are summarized in **Table 2**. The Endocrine Society practice guidelines recommend against TTh in the presence of prostate or breast cancer, hematocrit greater than 50%, untreated sleep apnea, severe lower urinary tract symptoms (LUTS) (International Prostate Symptom Score >19), poorly controlled heart failure, and in patients desiring fertility.[1] Although some of these recommendations, including breast cancer, fertility desire, increased hematocrit, and poorly controlled heart failure, remain contraindications to TTh, recent work has shown that some men with prostate cancer or LUTS can be safely treated with TTh.[14] Current Endocrine Society and International Society for Sexual Medicine (ICSM) guidelines state that TTh is not contraindicated in men with a history of organ-defined prostate cancer if followed by a urologist and if appropriate surveillance and follow-up occur.[1,19] Furthermore, there is no evidence supporting an increased risk of prostate cancer in men with normal serum T levels, and men with prostate cancer on active surveillance or at risk for developing prostate cancer have not shown increased risk of progression while on TTh.[12,21–24] However, prospective, randomized, placebo-controlled studies are needed to more definitively assess the safety of TTh in this population. The recommendation against TTh in men with severe LUTS has also been relaxed with recent evidence,[14,19] because no increase in LUTS in men on TTh has been observed in several randomized, placebo-controlled trials.[19] Thus, there are no convincing data to support that hypogonadal men with LUTS cannot be treated with TTh.[17,19]

Given the variety of T formulations, each with different pharmacokinetics and adverse effect profiles, it is important to use shared decision making to identify the best therapy for each patient (see **Table 2**). Intramuscular (IM) injections reliably increase T levels and represent a cost-effective option for patients. Fluctuations in libido and mood may occur with IM injections because of large variations in serum T level during the dosing interval. More controlled serum T ranges can be achieved with more frequent (weekly or twice weekly) dosing given the resulting decreased variability in T levels. Transdermal patches result in physiologic T levels with the common side effect of skin irritation. However, pretreatment of the application site with 0.1% triamcinolone cream reduces the risk of irritation without reducing T absorption.[2] Transdermal formulations have a lower incidence of skin irritation than patches but result in variable increases in T levels. Patients on transdermal T formulations should be counseled regarding possible transfer of drug to partners or children via direct skin contact; the US FDA issued a black box warning after cases of precocious pseudopuberty were reported in children. Subcutaneous T pellets offer a longer term therapy lasting 3 to 6 months, although dosing requires a minor procedure.[2] In addition, buccal, nasal, and oral formulations can be considered because of their ease of administration, although these formulations require daily or twice-daily dosing, and oral T undecanoate is not currently available in the United States.[2]

Monitoring men on TTh is essential both to determine treatment response and to monitor for adverse effects. A baseline prostate serum antigen test and digital rectal examination are recommended in men 40 years and older.[1,13,17,19] Follow-up visits should occur at 3, 6, and 12 months in the first year of treatment, followed by annual visits, with regular determination of hormone levels and hematocrit, and screening for prostate cancer.[1,17,19] Therapeutic phlebotomy is a useful adjunct in men with increased hematocrit on TTh; the precise threshold to initiate this treatment remains to be determined but is generally accepted at a hematocrit of 50% or higher.[19]

Table 2
Common testosterone formulations

Name	Dose	Route	Pharmacokinetics	Advantages	Disadvantages
T enanthate[1,60]	150–200 mg Q2 wk or 75–100 mg Q1 wk	IM	Half-life 5–7 d, supraphysiologic T at first, then hypogonadal at end of dosing period	Inexpensive, flexible dosing	Fluctuation of T levels over dosing interval
T cypionate[1,60]	150–200 mg Q2 wk or 75–100 mg Q1 wk	IM	Half-life 5–7 d, supraphysiologic T at first, then hypogonadal at end of dosing period	Inexpensive, flexible dosing	Fluctuation of T levels over dosing interval
T propionate[14,60]	100 mg Q2 d	IM	Shorter half-life than other IM formulations	Inexpensive	Fluctuation of T levels over dosing interval, multiple injections per week
T undecanoate[1,13,60] (injection)	1000 mg Q10–14 wk	IM	T maintained in normal range	Long lasting	Pain at injection site, large-volume injection
T patch[1,14,60]	5–10 mg QD	Transdermal	T maintained in normal range	Mimics circadian rhythm	Skin irritation, daily administration
T gel[1,2,60]	40–80 mg QD	Transdermal	T maintained in normal range	Flexible dose modification	Possible transfer with contact, daily administration
T axillary[14,60]	60–120 mg QD	Transdermal	T maintained in normal range	Mimics circadian rhythm	Skin irritation, daily administration, possible transfer with contact
T pellets[1,13,14,60]	4–6 implants: dose varies with formulation	Subcutaneous	Serum T peaks at 1 mo and then is sustained in normal range for 3–6 mo	Long lasting	Invasive, implant site infection
T buccal[1,13,60]	30 mg BID	Buccal	T maintained in normal range	Oral administration	Twice daily dosing, unpleasant taste
T undecanoate[1,13,60,a] (oral)	120–240 mg BID or TID	Oral	Absorbed via lymphatics, by passes portal system	Oral administration, flexible dose modification	T variability in individual on different days and among individuals, multiple administrations daily

Abbreviations: BID, twice a day; IM, intramuscular; Q, every; QD, every day; TID, 3 times a day.
[a] Not available in the United States.

Adjunct medications that can be considered in men on TTh therapy include aromatase inhibitors (ie, anastrozole, letrozole), because these can increase the T/E ratio in men with increased estradiol levels and symptoms such as leg swelling or breast swelling and tenderness.[25–27] Tamoxifen, given its role as an E receptor antagonist, can be considered as well, especially in men with symptoms of increased estradiol level.[28] Concomitant use of human chorionic gonadotropin (HCG) should be considered in men interested in starting on TTh with plans for fertility in the near future, although cessation of TTh in such patients and/or initiation of therapies that do not increase risk of infertility are preferred.[29] In younger men in whom fertility preservation is paramount and TTh is not advisable, clomiphene citrate can be considered.[30,31] Clomiphene citrate is not FDA approved for treatment of hypogonadism, although current literature supports a beneficial effect on T levels and symptoms, particularly in younger men, without a negative impact on fertility.[14,32] These adjunct medications generally have few side effects, are well tolerated, and are considered safe.[14,33–35] HCG may cause or exacerbate gynecomastia and aromatase inhibitors may cause sexual side effects that require monitoring on follow-up.[35]

TESTOSTERONE THERAPY AND CARDIOVASCULAR RISK

Recent controversy implicating TTh in increased CV risk arises primarily from a few flawed studies supporting an increased CV risk in men treated with TTh. In its 2014 review, the FDA cited 3 studies that observed an increased CV risk in men on TTh, which led to the 2015 T label change to include a warning for potential CV risk.[36] Basaria and colleagues[37] performed a randomized controlled trial of 209 older (mean age, 74 years) community-dwelling men with T levels of 100 to 350 ng/dL who were randomized to placebo or T gel. However, the trial was stopped early given a significantly higher rate of cardiac events in 23 men in the treatment arm versus 5 men in the placebo arm. Limitations of this trial included a small sample size and that it was not powered to assess CV risk but to determine the effects of TTh on men with limited mobility and their ability to recover mobility on TTh.

Vigen and colleagues[38] retrospectively examined all-cause mortality and CV risk in 8709 veterans after coronary angiography with a T level less than 300 ng/dL who had or had not been treated with TTh, finding a significantly higher risk of death, myocardial infarction (MI), or stroke in men on TTh (hazard ratio [HR], 1.29; 95% confidence interval [CI], 1.04–1.58). Major limitations of this study included evaluation of a cohort of men who had undergone coronary angiography and were therefore likely at increased risk for a CV event. In addition, there was no clear evidence that men were taking T, which was determined by a single T prescription being filled during the observation period. Further, the initial publication observed an absolute rate of CV events of 19.9% in the non-TTh group, and 25.7% in the TTh group, at 3 years after angiography. However, the fraction of individuals having a CV event was 10.1% in the TTh group and 21.2% in the non-TTh group, suggesting a beneficial effect of TTh. Perhaps even more concerning was the inclusion of 100 women in the TTh group.[39] For these reasons, 29 international medical societies and 160 physician scientists petitioned *JAMA* to retract the article, which has not occurred.[40]

A 2014 study by Finkle and colleagues[41] also contributed to the FDA's recent recommendation. The article examined the incidence of nonfatal MI in the 90 days following initiation of TTh compared with the year before TTh. A separate before/after treatment design was used for men on phosphodiesterase 5 (PDE5) inhibitors, who were used as a comparison group. For all ages combined (n = 55,593), an increased risk of nonfatal MI was observed during the post-TTh period (relative risk [RR], 1.36;

95% CI, 1.03–1.81). An increased risk was observed for men greater than or equal to 65 years of age (RR, 2.19; 95% CI, 1.27–3.77) and men less than 65 years of age with a history of heart disease (RR, 2.9; 95% CI, 1.49–5.62). In the PDE5 inhibitor comparison group (n = 167,279), no increased risk of nonfatal MI was observed (RR, 1.08; 95% CI, 0.93–1.24). This study was limited by the absence of clinical data for the included subjects; the cohort was tracked using only insurance claims data, diagnosis codes, and prescription information. Men on TTh were not evaluated and formally diagnosed with hypogonadism before TTh initiation. Further, no formal control group was used, and PDE5 inhibitors are vasodilators, which could have introduced bias into the study and should not have been used as a control group. In the postprescription interval, the CV end point was assessed at diagnosis of acute nonfatal MI, at first prescription refill, or at 90 days following initial prescription passed, whichever occurred first. A 90-day evaluation period is also fairly short, and would not typically be expected to adequately evaluate CV risk in men on TTh risk, and the observed CV events could have been a result of previously existing conditions, including hypogonadism.[39]

In addition, a systematic meta-analysis by Xu and colleagues[42] also supports an increased CV risk in men on TTh. The study included 27 trials encompassing 2994 men on TTh, observing an increased the risk of CV-related events (odds ratio, 1.54; 95% CI, 1.09–2.18). When examined more closely, 35% of the 180 CV events were observed in only 2 studies included in the meta-analysis, including the Basaria and colleagues[37] study, and others have criticized the inclusion criteria and study selection bias for the Xu and colleagues[42] meta-analysis.[40]

The observations discussed earlier are in direct contrast with previously published studies that support an increased risk of CV events in hypogonadal men. In a recent systematic review, Zarotsky and colleagues[43] observed that low T levels are associated with increased CV risk in 6 of the 8 population studies discussed, with hazard ratios for CV disease mortality ranging from 1.38 to 2.56 in these studies.[44–49] In addition, CV risk factors including obesity, fat mass, blood pressure, and glycemic control are known to be improved by TTh.[50]

In response to the controversy regarding the CV safety of TTh, a systematic review of the literature was published by Morgentaler and colleagues[50] in 2015. The systematic review examined decades of research and provided summary assessments based on levels of evidence. The investigators concluded that coronary artery disease severity is inversely proportional to T; that TTh helps with CV risk factors, including obesity; facilitates reductions in inflammatory markers; may be useful in some classes of congestive heart failure and patients with angina; and that the available evidence is insufficient to conclude whether a relationship exists between ischemic stroke and serum androgens. A recent overview of systematic reviews on this topic included 7 systematic reviews, with 6 that each included a meta-analysis showing no significant association between exogenous T and CV events, with summary HR estimates from 1.07 to 1.82 and insignificant confidence intervals.[51]

Since the publication of the studies and reviews discussed earlier, more recent publications have added to the literature on the CV safety of TTh. A recent retrospective review compared 8808 men who had ever been on TTh with a mean age of 58.4 years and with 1.4% having had prior CV events, with 35,527 men who had not previously been on TTh with a mean age of 59.8 years and with 2.0% having had prior CV events. Median follow-up was 4.2 years in both groups. The adjusted HR for the composite CV end point in the TTh group was 0.67 (95% CI, 0.62–0.73).[52] A recent European prospective multinational registry study (n = 999) also observed over 2 to 3 years of follow-up that CV event rates for men on TTh were not statistically different from those of untreated men (*P* = .70). Methodologically, this study benefits from clinical information because data collection included a complete medical history, physical examination, blood sampling, and patient questionnaires at multiple study visits over the follow-up period.[53] Although not powered to assess safety, 2 recent clinical trials have also shown no increased CV risk in the setting of TTh.[54,55]

Three more studies evaluating TTh over 5 to 10 years showing decreased CV event rates and mortality have been published during the past year as well.[56–58] Traish and colleagues[56] prospectively examined 656 hypogonadal men on TTh and 296 men not on TTh over a 10-year period (median follow-up, 7 years), observing a 10-year death rate of 0.1145 in the control group (95% CI, 0.0746–0.1756; $P<.000$) and 0.0092 in the TTh group (95% CI, 0.0023–0.0368; $P<.000$). The estimated reduction in mortality for the TTh group was 66% to 92%. Sharma and colleagues[59] retrospectively examined the risk of deep vein thrombosis (DVT) and pulmonary embolism (PE) in 71,407 male veterans with low T levels. The men treated with TTh were split into 3 groups: adequately treated, undertreated, and untreated. The incidence of DVT/PE was not significantly different because DVT/PE was observed in 0.5%, 0.4%, and 0.4% of men in those groups respectively.[59]

The true relationship between CV risk and TTh is challenging to assess given the large sample size needed for a randomized controlled trial. One trial currently in the recruitment phase, called the Cardiovascular Outcomes of Low Testosterone (CardioVOLT) trial, is set to perform a randomized controlled, double-blind trial in order to assess the cardiovascular outcomes of men with T levels less than 250 ng/dL compared with those treated with TTh. The estimated enrollment for this study is 379 participants. The CardioVOLT trial will be important in rigorously assessing cardiac end points in men with low serum T levels but the study size is still smaller than current estimates state would be needed for definitive assessment of safety. Current sample size estimates to determine CV risk in men on TTh using a 2-sided P-value of 0.05 and a power of 80% require at least 17,664 participants in each group.[51] However, available studies performed over the past several decades, although not definitive, largely support an increased CV risk in hypogonadal men, with no apparent negative effects on CV risk in men on TTh.

SUMMARY

Hypogonadism is a common condition that can manifest with nonspecific symptoms. Diagnosis of hypogonadism relies on assessment of symptoms and determination of serum T levels. Treatment is most commonly in the form of exogenous T, which is available in numerous formulations; including IM injections; subcutaneous pellets; and topical, intranasal, and oral formulations, all of which can increase serum T levels. Recent studies have supported an increased CV risk in men on TTh, leading the FDA to include a warning on T labels indicating a potential increased CV risk. However, these studies have had significant flaws that undermine their validity, and more recent studies have not supported an increased CV risk in men on TTh. Given the existing evidence that low T levels may increase CV risk and morbidity, and in the absence of rigorous studies to suggest otherwise, it is prudent to treat hypogonadal men until further definitive study elucidates the risk of TTh on CV outcomes.

REFERENCES

1. Bhasin S, Cunningham GR, Hayes FJ, et al. Testosterone therapy in men with androgen deficiency syndromes: an Endocrine Society clinical practice guideline. J Clin Endocrinol Metab 2010;95(6):2536–59.
2. Basaria S. Male hypogonadism. Lancet 2014;383(9924):1250–63.

3. Snyder PJ, Matsumoto AM, Martin KA. Testosterone treatment of male hypogonadism. Waltham (MA): UpToDate; 2012.

4. Araujo AB, Esche GR, Kupelian V, et al. Prevalence of symptomatic androgen deficiency in men. J Clin Endocrinol Metab 2007;92(11):4241–7.

5. Hall SA, Esche GR, Araujo AB, et al. Correlates of low testosterone and symptomatic androgen deficiency in a population-based sample. J Clin Endocrinol Metab 2008;93(10):3870–7.

6. Handelsman DJ. Global trends in testosterone prescribing, 2000-2011: expanding the spectrum of prescription drug misuse. Med J Aust 2013;199(8):548–51.

7. Perls T, Handelsman DJ. Disease mongering of age-associated declines in testosterone and growth hormone levels. J Am Geriatr Soc 2015;63(4):809–11.

8. Katz A, Katz A, Burchill C. Androgen therapy: testing before prescribing and monitoring during therapy. Can Fam Physician 2007;53(11):1936–42.

9. Baillargeon J, Urban RJ, Ottenbacher KJ, et al. Trends in androgen prescribing in the United States, 2001 to 2011. JAMA Intern Med 2013;173(15):1465–6.

10. US Food and Drug Administration. FDA drug safety communication: FDA cautions about using testosterone products for low testosterone due to aging; requires labeling change to inform of possible increased risk of heart attack and stroke with use. Available at: https://www.fda.gov/Drugs/DrugSafety/ucm436259.htm. Accessed June 4, 2015.

11. Bhasin S, Basaria S. Diagnosis and treatment of hypogonadism in men. Best Pract Res Clin Endocrinol Metab 2011;25(2):251–70.

12. Pastuszak AW, Rodriguez KM, Nguyen TM, et al. Testosterone therapy and prostate cancer. Transl Androl Urol 2016;5(6):909–20.

13. Dohle G, Arver S, Bettochi S. Guidelines on male hypogonadism. Arnhem (The Netherlands): European Association of Urology; 2015.

14. McBride JA, Carson CC, Coward RM. Diagnosis and management of testosterone deficiency. Asian J Androl 2015;17(2):177–86.

15. Corona G, Mannucci E, Ricca V, et al. The age-related decline of testosterone is associated with different specific symptoms and signs in patients with sexual dysfunction. Int J Androl 2009;32(6):720–8.

16. Morgentaler A, Khera M, Maggi M, et al. Commentary: who is a candidate for testosterone therapy? A synthesis of international expert opinions. J Sex Med 2014;11(7):1636–45.

17. Wang C, Nieschlag E, Swerdloff R, et al. Investigation, treatment, and monitoring of late-onset hypogonadism in males: ISA, ISSAM, EAU, EAA, and ASA recommendations. Eur Urol 2009;55(1):121–30.

18. Diver MJ, Imtiaz KE, Ahmad AM, et al. Diurnal rhythms of serum total, free and bioavailable testosterone and of SHBG in middle-aged men compared with those in young men. Clin EndoCrinol (Oxf) 2003;58(6):710–7.

19. Buvat J, Maggi M, Gooren L, et al. Endocrine aspects of male sexual dysfunctions. J Sex Med 2010;7(4 Pt 2):1627–56.

20. Scovell JM, Ramasamy R, Wilken N, et al. Hypogonadal symptoms in young men are associated with a serum total testosterone threshold of 400 ng/dL. BJU Int 2015;116(1):142–6.

21. Ory J, Flannigan R, Lundeen C, et al. Testosterone therapy in patients with treated and untreated prostate cancer: impact on oncologic outcomes. J Urol 2016; 196(4):1082–9.

22. Kacker R, Hult M, San Francisco IF, et al. Can testosterone therapy be offered to men on active surveillance for prostate cancer? Preliminary results. Asian J Androl 2016;18(1):16–20.

23. Ferreira U, Leitao VA, Denardi F, et al. Intermittent androgen replacement for intense hypogonadism symptoms in castrated patients. Prostate Cancer Prostatic Dis 2006;9(1):39–41.

24. Rhoden EL, Morgentaler A. Testosterone replacement therapy in hypogonadal men at high risk for prostate cancer: results of 1 year of treatment in men with prostatic intraepithelial neoplasia. J Urol 2003;170(6 Pt 1):2348–51.

25. Burnett-Bowie SA, Roupenian KC, Dere ME, et al. Effects of aromatase inhibition in hypogonadal older men: a randomized, double-blind, placebo-controlled trial. Clin Endocrinol 2009;70(1):116–23.

26. Leder BZ, Rohrer JL, Rubin SD, et al. Effects of aromatase inhibition in elderly men with low or borderline-low serum testosterone levels. J Clin Endocrinol Metab 2004;89(3):1174–80.

27. Dias JP, Melvin D, Simonsick EM, et al. Effects of aromatase inhibition vs. testosterone in older men with low testosterone: randomized-controlled trial. Andrology 2016;4(1):33–40.

28. Barros AC, Sampaio Mde C. Gynecomastia: physiopathology, evaluation and treatment. Sao Paulo Med J 2012;130(3):187–97.

29. Hsieh TC, Pastuszak AW, Hwang K, et al. Concomitant intramuscular human chorionic gonadotropin preserves spermatogenesis in men undergoing testosterone replacement therapy. J Urol 2013;189(2):647–50.

30. Ramasamy R, Scovell JM, Kovac JR, et al. Testosterone supplementation versus clomiphene citrate for hypogonadism: an age matched comparison of satisfaction and efficacy. J Urol 2014;192(3):875–9.

31. Katz DJ, Nabulsi O, Tal R, et al. Outcomes of clomiphene citrate treatment in young hypogonadal men. BJU Int 2012;110(4):573–8.

32. Moskovic DJ, Katz DJ, Akhavan A, et al. Clomiphene citrate is safe and effective for long-term management of hypogonadism. BJU Int 2012;110(10):1524–8.

33. Helo S, Wynia B, McCullough A. "Cherchez la femme": modulation of estrogen receptor function with selective modulators: clinical implications in the field of urology. Sex Med Rev 2017;5(3):365–86.

34. Rambhatla A, Mills JN, Rajfer J. The role of estrogen modulators in male hypogonadism and infertility. Rev Urol 2016;18(2):66–72.

35. Rahnema CD, Lipshultz LI, Crosnoe LE, et al. Anabolic steroid-induced hypogonadism: diagnosis and treatment. Fertil Steril 2014;101(5):1271–9.

36. Desroches B, Kohn TP, Welliver C, et al. Testosterone therapy in the new era of Food and Drug Administration oversight. Transl Androl Urol 2016;5(2):207–12.

37. Basaria S, Coviello AD, Travison TG, et al. Adverse events associated with testosterone administration. N Engl J Med 2010;363(2):109–22.

38. Vigen R, O'Donnell CI, Baron AE, et al. Association of testosterone therapy with mortality, myocardial infarction, and stroke in men with low testosterone levels. JAMA 2013;310(17):1829–36.

39. Morgentaler A, Lunenfeld B. Testosterone and cardiovascular risk: world's experts take unprecedented action to correct misinformation. Aging Male 2014; 17(2):63–5.

40. Elsherbiny A, Tricomi M, Bhatt D, et al. State-of-the-art: a review of cardiovascular effects of testosterone replacement therapy in adult males. Curr Cardiol Rep 2017;19(4):35.

41. Finkle WD, Greenland S, Ridgeway GK, et al. Increased risk of non-fatal myocardial infarction following testosterone therapy prescription in men. PLoS One 2014; 9(1):e85805.

42. Xu L, Freeman G, Cowling BJ, et al. Testosterone therapy and cardiovascular events among men: a systematic review and meta-analysis of placebo-controlled randomized trials. BMC Med 2013;11:108.

43. Zarotsky V, Huang MY, Carman W, et al. Systematic literature review of the risk factors, comorbidities, and consequences of hypogonadism in men. Andrology 2014;2(6):819–34.

44. Khaw KT, Dowsett M, Folkerd E, et al. Endogenous testosterone and mortality due to all causes, cardiovascular disease, and cancer in men: European Prospective Investigation into Cancer in Norfolk (EPIC-Norfolk) prospective population study. Circulation 2007;116(23):2694–701.

45. Hyde Z, Norman PE, Flicker L, et al. Low free testosterone predicts mortality from cardiovascular disease but not other causes: the Health in Men Study. J Clin Endocrinol Metab 2012;97(1):179–89.

46. Yeap BB, Hyde Z, Almeida OP, et al. Lower testosterone levels predict incident stroke and transient ischemic attack in older men. J Clin Endocrinol Metab 2009;94(7):2353–9.

47. Menke A, Guallar E, Rohrmann S, et al. Sex steroid hormone concentrations and risk of death in US men. Am J Epidemiol 2010;171(5):583–92.

48. Laughlin GA, Barrett-Connor E, Bergstrom J. Low serum testosterone and mortality in older men. J Clin Endocrinol Metab 2008;93(1):68–75.

49. Haring R, Volzke H, Steveling A, et al. Low serum testosterone levels are associated with increased risk of mortality in a population-based cohort of men aged 20-79. Eur Heart J 2010;31(12):1494–501.

50. Morgentaler A, Miner MM, Caliber M, et al. Testosterone therapy and cardiovascular risk: advances and controversies. Mayo Clin Proc 2015;90(2):224–51.

51. Onasanya O, Iyer G, Lucas E, et al. Association between exogenous testosterone and cardiovascular events: an overview of systematic reviews. Lancet Diabetes Endocrinol 2016;4(11):943–56.

52. Cheetham TC, An J, Jacobsen SJ, et al. Association of testosterone replacement with cardiovascular outcomes among men with androgen deficiency. JAMA Intern Med 2017;177(4):491–9.

53. Maggi M, Wu FC, Jones TH, et al. Testosterone treatment is not associated with increased risk of adverse cardiovascular events: results from the Registry of Hypogonadism in Men (RHYME). Int J Clin Pract 2016;70(10):843–52.

54. Brock G, Heiselman D, Maggi M, et al. Effect of testosterone solution 2% on testosterone concentration, sex drive and energy in hypogonadal men: results of a placebo controlled study. J Urol 2016;195(3):699–705.

55. Budoff MJ, Ellenberg SS, Lewis CE, et al. Testosterone treatment and coronary artery plaque volume in older men with low testosterone. JAMA 2017;317(7):708–16.

56. Traish AM, Haider A, Haider KS, et al. Long-term testosterone therapy improves cardiometabolic function and reduces risk of cardiovascular disease in men with hypogonadism: a real-life observational registry study setting comparing treated and untreated (control) groups. J Cardiovasc Pharmacol Ther 2017;22(5):414–33.

57. Haider A, Yassin A, Haider KS, et al. Men with testosterone deficiency and a history of cardiovascular diseases benefit from long-term testosterone therapy: observational, real-life data from a registry study. Vasc Health Risk Manag 2016;12:251–61.

58. Wallis CJ, Lo K, Lee Y, et al. Survival and cardiovascular events in men treated with testosterone replacement therapy: an intention-to-treat observational cohort study. Lancet Diabetes Endocrinol 2016;4(6):498–506.
59. Sharma R, Oni OA, Chen G, et al. Association between testosterone replacement therapy and the incidence of DVT and pulmonary embolism: a retrospective cohort study of the Veterans Administration database. Chest 2016;150(3): 563–71.
60. Corona G, Rastrelli G, Maggi M. Diagnosis and treatment of late-onset hypogonadism: systematic review and meta-analysis of TRT outcomes. Best Pract Res Clin Endocrinol Metab 2013;27(4):557–79.

Urologic Emergencies

Adarsh S. Manjunath, MD, Matthias D. Hofer, MD, PhD*

KEYWORDS

- Urologic emergencies • Acute urinary retention • Infected nephrolithiasis
- Paraphimosis • Penile fracture • Priapism • Fournier gangrene • Testicular torsion

KEY POINTS

- When evaluating a potential urologic emergency, the internist should have a high level of suspicion for a serious underlying illness or injury.
- Diagnosis often relies heavily on clinical history and physical examination, with imaging playing an increasingly vital role.
- Urologic consultation should be requested early if surgical intervention is thought to be necessary.

ACUTE URINARY RETENTION

Acute urinary retention (AUR) will be encountered by most health care professionals, and it should be distinguished from chronic urinary retention, which is usually due to the same cause but is less emergent because it develops over time.

Clinical Presentation

AUR can be secondary to obstructive causes or a dysfunctional (atonic) bladder. When obstructive, it presents an overwhelming majority of the time in men rather than in women. Most commonly, this is due to the presence of a large, obstructing prostate secondary to benign prostatic hyperplasia (BPH). Less common obstructive causes include narrowing of the urethra due to urethral strictures or bladder neck contractures, which are usually consequences of prior urologic surgery, prior Foley catheterization, straddle injuries or other trauma, sexually transmitted infections, or congenital causes such as hypospadias.

When AUR is due to a dysfunctional bladder, an inciting factor is usually present. This factor tends to be a side effect of a medication, especially an anticholinergic or opioid, or a side effect of general/locoregional anesthesia.[1] Although this cause is most common in women presenting with AUR, such medications in men can

Disclosure Statement: No disclosures for either author.
Department of Urology, Northwestern University Feinberg School of Medicine, 303 East Chicago Avenue 16-703, Chicago, IL 60611, USA
* Corresponding author. 675 North St. Clair Street, Suite 20-150, Chicago, IL 60611.
E-mail address: m-hofer@northwestern.edu

Med Clin N Am 102 (2018) 373–385
https://doi.org/10.1016/j.mcna.2017.10.013

exacerbate an already existing obstructive condition such as BPH. A typical example would be postoperative urinary retention after surgery.

Therefore, typical presenting symptoms of AUR include a history of difficulty with urination or prior urinary retention episodes, a lack of urination for several hours or longer, frequent urination of small amounts, overflow incontinence, abdominal or suprapubic pain, and a suprapubic mass on palpation caused by the distended bladder.

It is important to separate this from patients experiencing gross hematuria who can develop clots, which may be passed painfully in the urine. Clots accumulating in the bladder can obstruct the outlet and prevent passage of any urine leading to retention as well.

Last, neurologic illnesses can be responsible for retention via inability of the bladder to sufficiently contract. A thorough history and physical examination should always be performed to rule out spinal cord injury, compression, multiple sclerosis, Parkinson disease, or cauda equina syndrome as the cause of AUR.

Diagnosis

The diagnosis of AUR relies heavily on history-taking and the physical examination. Additional diagnostic tools, such as ultrasonic bladder scan, to determine urine volume can be used. It should be noted that the presence of ascites would lead to a false-positive reading by the bladder scanner because it will simply detect this intra-abdominal fluid. A bedside bladder ultrasound can also be performed to visualize the distended bladder and, if present, blood clots.

Treatment

Primary management of AUR involves emergent bladder drainage with insertion of a Foley catheter. The type of Foley used should be based on the clinical situation as detailed in later discussion (**Fig. 1**). In all cases, an α1-blocker such as tamsulosin should be started and continued for a minimum of 3 days before Foley removal because this has been demonstrated to increase the chances of a successful voiding trial.[2–4] In practice, however, a period of 1 to 2 weeks appears to be associated with a higher rate of successful decatheterizations.

In an uncomplicated case of AUR, a standard 16-French Foley catheter should be inserted under sterile technique. If resistance is met and the patient is an older man with BPH, increasing the Foley size to 18 or 20 French may be more successful because increased rigidity allows better passage of the enlarged prostate. A Coudé catheter with its curved tip also facilitates placement because the tip is designed to align itself with the curve in the bulbar urethra, making it more likely to pass between obstructing prostatic lobes. If resistance is consistently encountered, further attempts should be abandoned because a false urethral passage may form. Urology consultation should follow, because a flexible bedside cystoscopy may be necessary to place a guidewire into the bladder over which a Foley catheter can be advanced.

In a younger patient in whom BPH is unlikely and a urethral stricture is suspected (typically a history of congenital hypospadias, pelvic trauma, or radiation), decreasing the Foley size to 12- or 14 French often allows placement. Again, if resistance is consistently encountered, flexible cystoscopy by urology should be performed at the bedside to allow for immediate dilation of the stricture.

If gross hematuria or clots are present, placement of a larger 22- or 24-French 3-way Foley catheter for continuous bladder irrigation is recommended. Initially, irrigation by hand should be attempted with a 60-mL syringe to remove clots. If the irrigation fluid

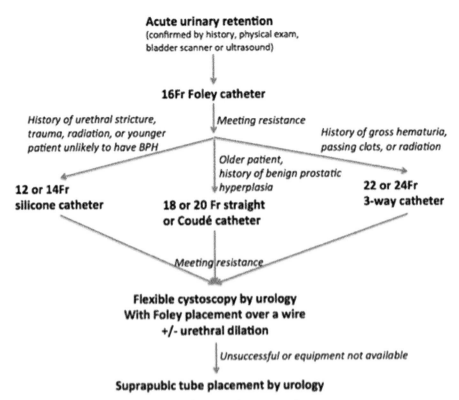

Fig. 1. Flowchart for management of acute urinary retention.

remains bloody and fails to clear up, continuous bladder irrigation through the third port of the catheter should be initiated.

NEPHROLITHIASIS

Kidney stone disease has been increasing in prevalence in US adults over the last several decades,[5] and evidence from the National Health and Nutrition Examination Survey suggests that the prevalence has doubled between 1994 and 2010.[6] Although asymptomatic kidney stones can be found in nearly 10% of patients,[7] it is those with refractory pain or a high stone burden that are treated surgically. Furthermore, concerns of concomitant urinary tract infections should trigger emergent urologic intervention to prevent bacteremia or sepsis. Bilateral obstructing stones or an obstructing stone in a solitary kidney is also an indication for intervention to avoid acute renal failure caused by total obstruction.

Clinical Presentation

Most patients presenting to the emergency room or outpatient office with kidney stones will complain of colicky flank or abdominal pain on the side of the stone, pain that radiates to the groin and specifically the scrotum in men or labia in women, nausea, and vomiting. In terms of urinary symptoms, patients may have frequency, dysuria, and gross hematuria. A history of hyperparathyroidism, type 1 renal tubular acidosis, inflammatory bowel disease, sarcoidosis, cystinuria, gout, metabolic syndrome, diabetes, and recurrent urinary tract infections is associated with stone formation.[7]

In a patient with an infected kidney stone, presentation with systemic symptoms such as fever and chills in addition to the aforementioned ones is common. Beware of immunocompromised patients who may not mount a sufficient immune reaction for these symptoms to be present. In these cases, most commonly in diabetic patients or those on chemotherapy, emergent stent placement may be indicated in the absence of systemic symptoms.

Diagnosis

The most useful diagnostic test when a stone is suspected is a computed tomographic (CT) scan, which allows determination of the location, size, and quantity of stones as well as the degree of hydronephrosis. Although ultrasound has become a more widely used modality in the initial evaluation of stones,[8,9] CT imaging remains the gold standard because it visualizes almost all stone types and has sensitivities and specificities of greater than 95%.[10,11]

Typically, a patient with an infected kidney stone will have leukocytosis, a positive urinalysis with nitrites, leukocyte esterase, bacteria, or white blood cells, and ultimately a positive urine culture. Bilateral obstructing stones or an obstructing stone in a solitary kidney will be visualized anywhere between the ureteropelvic junction and the ureterovesical junction. Hydronephrosis will be present proximal to the stone or stones, and the obstruction may lead to an acute kidney injury (AKI). It should be noted that these patients may have a mild AKI because of renal colic causing nausea, vomiting, and decreased fluid intake or appetite. Infected stones, bilateral obstructing kidney stones, or an obstructing stone in a solitary kidney warrants emergent treatment and urology consultation. In the case of an infected stone, broad-spectrum antibiotics should be started immediately as well.

Treatment

Emergent urologic treatment of these conditions consists of placement of a ureteral stent, which diverts the urine around the stone obstructing the kidney. Definitive stone treatment can occur via ureteroscopy with laser lithotripsy and stone extraction once the patient has stabilized and recovered. For intractable pain that is not manageable with oral medications, stent placement is also indicated because it will mitigate the pain.

PENILE EMERGENCIES: PARAPHIMOSIS

Paraphimosis refers to the entrapment of the foreskin behind the glans penis for a prolonged amount of time (**Fig. 2**). Because venous and lymphatic return from the glans and foreskin is reduced, painful edema of the trapped foreskin occurs and further impedes reduction of the foreskin. If not reduced in a timely fashion, paraphimosis can eventually result in tissue ischemia and necrosis.

Clinical Presentation

In the clinical presentation, patients present with severe pain for several hours. In an adult, the typical presentation is in the hospital setting in which a Foley catheter is placed in an uncircumcised male patient, and the foreskin is retracted during the procedure but not reduced thereafter. In a young child, it can be seen after a physical examination in which the foreskin was traumatically reduced or by aggressive parental attempts at hygiene.[12]

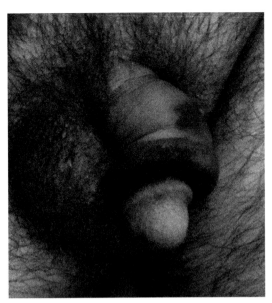

Fig. 2. Swollen and edematous foreskin trapped behind the glans penis, resulting in paraphimosis. Note the dystrophy of the foreskin, which may lead to ulceration or gangrene if untreated.

Diagnosis

Diagnosis relies on physical examination, and there is no role for imaging studies.

Treatment

Treatment involves pain control and reduction of the edematous foreskin, which is successful in the vast majority of cases. In addition to pain medication, an icepack on the area can minimize swelling and also be helpful as a local analgesic. To perform the reduction, gentle steady pressure should be applied to the foreskin for 5 to 10 minutes to compress the edema and decrease swelling.[13] Then, 2 thumbs should be placed on the glans and pushed against it while the fingers pull outwards on the foreskin. If this maneuver fails, it can be repeated with longer compression time. However, if this also remains unsuccessful, then urology should be consulted because an emergent dorsal slit procedure at the bedside may be necessary. This procedure consists of incising the foreskin at the dorsal aspect to facilitate foreskin reduction, and the dorsal slit can be extended to a full circumcision later.

PENILE EMERGENCIES: PENILE FRACTURE

Fracture of an erect penis should be promptly explored and surgically repaired to prevent long-term complications, specifically erectile dysfunction and Peyronie disease.

Clinical Presentation

Nearly all penile fractures occur during sexual intercourse,[14] because the penis must be erect for this to happen. The otherwise relatively thick tunica albuginea that encases the corpora cavernosa is thinned out due to the stretch during an erection. Patients often provide a history of having vigorous sexual intercourse when the erect penis slipped out and struck the perineum or pubic bone of their partner. This buckling injury causes the erect penis to bend abnormally and results in a laceration of the tunica albuginea[15] and is typically associated with a "popping" or "cracking" sound and rapid detumescence.

Diagnosis

Diagnosis relies on the history provided by the patient in conjunction with the physical examination. It is important to note that patients often provide incomplete details likely because of embarrassment or fear. On examination, the penis may be discolored and swollen. A penile hematoma will result in a typical "eggplant deformity" as the fascial organization of the penis typically limits the hematoma formation to this organ (**Fig. 3**). The hematoma can, in some cases, also extend to the scrotum, perineum, and suprapubic regions. Because the urethra may often be injured simultaneously, gross hematuria, blood at the meatus, or inability to void may be present.

In men in whom the clinical suspicious of penile fracture is high, imaging studies are unnecessary. When the suspicion is low, ultrasound is rapid, noninvasive, inexpensive, and accurate at determining whether a tear in the tunica albuginea layer is present and warrants surgical repair.[16,17] Although MRI has been described as a diagnostic tool in equivocal cases,[18] it is not recommended because of the time required, limited availability, and expense.[19]

Treatment

Treatment of penile fracture involves prompt surgical exploration and repair. Flexible cystoscopy is done in the operating room to visualize urethral injury. Through a vertical penoscrotal incision[20] or a distal circumcising incision, the penis is explored for lacerations of the tunica albuginea layer as demonstrated in **Fig. 4**. The lacerations are sutured closed, and urethral injuries are repaired primarily as well. The Foley catheter may be maintained postoperatively depending on the degree of urethral injury, and

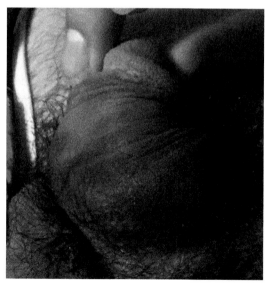

Fig. 3. Patient who presented with a history consistent with penile fracture and the physical examination findings above. Note the discolored and swollen penis resulting in a typical "eggplant deformity."

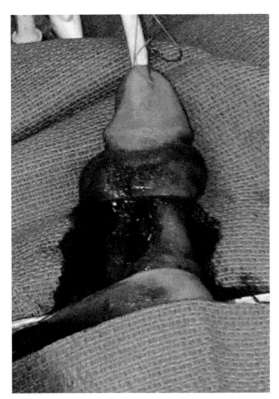

Fig. 4. Exploration of a penile fracture in the operating room. A tear in the midline in the corpora cavernosa is visualized that requires repair.

sexual abstinence is recommended for several weeks to give the tunica albuginea sufficient time to heal.

PENILE EMERGENCIES: PRIAPISM

Priapism is defined as having an erection without sexual stimulation lasting for more than 4 hours. It can be subdivided into ischemic, stuttering, and nonischemic types. This section focuses on ischemic priapism because it requires emergent treatment, as minimal or no arterial inflow into the corpora cavernosa is present, and if untreated, often results in permanent erectile dysfunction (ED). In fact, erectile function was preserved in 92% of patients in one study if ischemic priapism was reversed in less than 24 hours compared with 22% preservation with priapism lasting longer than 7 days.[21]

Clinical Presentation

A thorough history is essential to determine predisposing factors and the time course of the persistent erection. Patients at risk include those with hematologic dyscrasias, such as sickle cell disease (SCD), those with elevated white blood cell counts as in leukemia, and patients with neurologic conditions affecting the spinal cord. Although the overall incidence of priapism is low, the lifetime probability of developing ischemic priapism in a man with SCD is 29% to 42%.[22] Medications associated with priapism are trazodone and intracavernous injections for men with ED. Prolonged erection and priapism have been reported to be as high as 35% in this population.[12] Notably, priapism is rare with PDE5 inhibitor therapy, and case reports describe other concomitant risk factors, such as SCD, recreational use of the medication, and use in combination with intracavernous injections.[23–25] In addition to a history of these predisposing conditions or medication use, patients will have progressive penile pain associated with the duration of the erection.

On physical examination, patients with ischemic priapism will have a rigid, erect penis. If signs of trauma or bruising are present in the perineum to suggest straddle injury, it is more likely to be nonischemic priapism, in which case the penis will be erect but not completely rigid.

Diagnosis

After a history, physical examination, and basic laboratory analysis, a corporal blood gas analysis should be obtained to differentiate between ischemic and nonischemic priapism. Although this distinction can often be made on the basis of history and physical examination alone, corporal aspiration serves both diagnostic and therapeutic purposes. To obtain this aspirate, 1% lidocaine without epinephrine should first be injected to provide anesthetic, either circumferentially around the penile base in a ring block fashion or dorsally at the penile base. A single, large-bore 14-gauge to 18-gauge butterfly needle should be inserted into the proximal penile shaft at the 3 or 9 o'clock position. The penile shaft should be compressed with one hand and blood be aspirated from the corpora. Initially, the blood will be dark and deoxygenated. Diagnostically, sending this off for venous blood gas analysis will reveal hypoxia ($Po_2<30$), hypercarbia ($Pco_2>60$), and acidosis (pH<7.25) to suggest ischemic priapism. This needle should be left in place for therapeutic purposes as detailed in the next section.

Treatment

Oral agents such as pseudoephedrine and terbutaline have been used for prolonged erection with variable success rates,[26] but are not recommended for acute ischemic priapism.

Treatment centers on continued corporal aspiration of blood, saline irrigation, and use of phenylephrine. The goal is to empty the cavernosal spaces sufficiently and free them of partially clotted blood so that new arterial blood can flow into the cavernosal spaces to preserve the smooth muscle fibers needed for erection. Using the already placed needle at the 3 or 9 o'clock position, aspiration with empty syringes should be continued until the blood coming out from the corpora becomes brighter in color, suggesting that the hypoxic, hypercarbic, and acidotic blood is being removed and fresh, oxygenated blood is now supplying the penis. Aspiration can be successful in softening the erection, relieving pain, and relieving priapism in 36% of cases.[27] Irrigation of the corpora with saline will facilitate the aspiration of blood clots.

If corporal aspiration and irrigation is unsuccessful, phenylephrine should be injected.[27,28] As an α-adrenergic agent, phenylephrine causes cavernous smooth muscle contraction. The pharmacy should be asked to prepare phenylephrine diluted in normal saline to a concentration of between 100 and 200 µg/mL in 1-mL syringes. These injections can be repeated every 3 to 5 minutes, up to a maximum dose of 1 mg. Corporal aspiration should continue between successive phenylephrine injections. As a sympathomimetic, phenylephrine can cause hypertension, reflex bradycardia, tachycardia, and arrhythmias, especially in the elderly and those with preexisting cardiac conditions. Close monitoring of vitals should be performed on a cardiac or electrocardiogram monitor during and after injections. If aspiration, irrigation, and phenylephrine injections fail, then surgical therapy will be necessary with distal or proximal shunting procedures in the operating room.

SCROTAL EMERGENCIES: FOURNIER GANGRENE

A necrotizing fasciitis of the male genital skin, urethra, or rectum, Fournier gangrene is a severe complication of an initially localized bacterial infection that can rapidly progress to sepsis and death. It requires aggressive treatment and emergent surgical debridement because the mortality rate averages 20%.[29]

Clinical Presentation

Patients often have a history of diabetes mellitus, local trauma, instrumentation, and perirectal or perianal infections. They present initially with systemic symptoms, such as fever and chills, as well as local symptoms, such as cellulitis and a swollen, erythematous, and tender penis, scrotum, inguinal area, or perineum.[30] Genitourinary symptoms include dysuria and obstructed voiding. These symptoms rapidly progress to include crepitus and a dark purple or black discoloration of the skin (**Fig. 5**). When septic, patients commonly have altered mental status and abnormal vitals.

Diagnosis

The diagnosis of Fournier gangrene relies heavily on clinical history and physical examination. Differentiating cellulitis from Fournier gangrene is important and can be distinguished by the presence of marked systemic toxicity out of proportion to the local findings. The hallmark is palpable crepitus underneath the skin, which is sufficient to make the diagnosis.

Laboratory analyses are only an adjunct and may reveal a leukocytosis, hyponatremia, hypocalcemia, elevated serum creatinine levels, and elevated lactate. Cultures

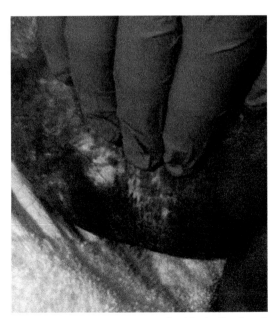

Fig. 5. Presentation of Fournier gangrene. Note the black discoloration of the scrotum. Crepitus will be present underneath.

should be obtained from the blood, urine, and any wound, which often show multiple organisms including *Klebsiella*, *Proteus*, *Staphylococcus*, and *Streptococcus*. Ultrasound can show scrotal wall thickening containing gas, and CT can often diagnose Fournier gangrene radiographically. However, it is not recommended to delay treatment to obtain imaging.

A severity index was created and validated to determine prognostic factors for a patient with Fournier gangrene. Elevated heart rate, respiratory rate, creatinine, bicarbonate, lactate, and calcium levels were found to be associated with increased mortality. Of patients with a severity index score of less than 9, there was a 96% survival rate. On the other hand, patients with a severity index score of 9 or more had mortality of 46%.[31]

Treatment

Sepsis management principles are essential, including adequate intravenous hydration and antimicrobial therapy with broad-spectrum antibiotics. Immediate surgical debridement is required to extensively resect all infected tissue. The wound is left open, and a second debridement in the operating room may be performed 24 to 48 hours later if additional necrotic tissue is detected or if the patient remains unstable. Vacuum-assisted closure devices are effective at helping these wounds heal. Once the patient has stabilized and the wound healed, it can be closed primarily or, if more extensive, with skin grafts or skin flaps.

SCROTAL EMERGENCIES: TESTICULAR TORSION

Testicular torsion refers to a twisting of the spermatic cord causing lack of blood flow through the testicular artery to the testicle. It is commonly attributed to excess mobility of the testis within a bell-clapper deformity, where the tunica vaginalis is abnormally fixed proximally on the cord.

Although the list of differential diagnoses is long, including torsion of an appendix testis, epididymitis, orchitis, strangulated hernia, hydrocele, varicocele, intrascrotal mass, and referred pain, suspicion of testicular torsion requires urgent evaluation and management. The viability of the testis is inversely related to the duration of the torsion. In more than 1100 patients, the risk of orchiectomy was 5% at 0 to 6 hours after onset of pain, 20% at 7 to 12 hours, and 80% at more than 24 hours.[32] Although the impact on fertility is poorly understood, subtle abnormalities of semen quality are common in patients after treatment of testicular torsion.[33]

Clinical Presentation

Torsion is most common after 10 years of age but can occur at any age.[34] Boys present with acute onset, one-sided testicular pain that lasts several hours in duration. On examination, the testicle can be exquisitely tender, can be high riding, and might even be oriented horizontally because of twisting of the spermatic cord. The testicle can be indurated, the cord thickened, and the scrotum edematous. The cremasteric reflex (elevation of the testis when scratching the inner thigh) can be reduced or absent.[35] Preservation of this reflex is associated with sufficient testicular blood flow but can still be seen in patients in whom torsion was subsequently confirmed.[36]

In contrast to testicular torsion, patients with epididymitis will present with gradual onset pain over days to weeks, and their cremasteric reflex will be intact. A history of urinary tract infections, sexual activity, intermittent catheterization, or recent Foley catheter use may be present.

Diagnosis

Diagnosis hinges on the clinical presentation as noted above. With the advent of rapid and reliable scrotal imaging, color Doppler ultrasound is often performed to confirm the diagnosis before taking a patient to the operating room. Lack of intratesticular flow on ultrasound is 86% sensitive and 100% specific in the diagnosis of torsion.[37] In practice, surgical exploration will often be performed if the ultrasound is equivocal and clinical signs and symptoms are suggestive of torsion.

Treatment

Once testicular torsion is suspected, manual detorsion should be attempted at the bedside in order to relieve symptoms after premedicating with narcotics. Manual detorsion is performed via the "open-the-book" maneuver. The testicle should be grasped and rotated away from the midline. Although the testicle may be partially or completely unwound in this manner, the patient should still be taken for surgical exploration or at least for a repeat ultrasound because manual detorsion can fail to completely relieve torsion in up to 32% of cases.[38]

In the operating room, the affected testicle is untwisted and examined for a healthy color and overall viability. The testis is then sutured to the inner lining of the scrotum (orchiopexy) to prevent retorsion. The contralateral testis should also be sutured to the scrotum as well. If the testis is deemed nonviable intraoperatively, it is removed.

REFERENCES

1. McNeil SA. Spontaneous versus precipitated AUR: the same? World J Urol 2006; 24(4):354–9.
2. Fitzpatrick JM, Desgrandchamps F, Adjali K, et al. Management of acute urinary retention: a worldwide survey of 6074 men with benign prostatic hyperplasia. BJU Int 2012;109(1):88–95.
3. Zeif HJ, Subramonian K. Alpha blockers prior to removal of a catheter for acute urinary retention in adult men. Cochrane Database Syst Rev 2009;(4):CD006744.
4. McNeill SA, Hargreave TB, Members of the Alfaur Study Group. Alfuzosin once daily facilitates return to voiding in patients in acute urinary retention. J Urol 2004;171(6 Pt 1):2316–20.
5. Stamatelou KK, Francis ME, Jones CA, et al. Time trends in reported prevalence of kidney stones in the United States: 1976-1994. Kidney Int 2003;63(5):1817–23.
6. Scales CD Jr, Smith AC, Hanley JM, et al, Urologic Diseases in America Project. Prevalence of kidney stones in the United States. Eur Urol 2012;62(1):160–5.
7. Lorenz EC, Lieske JC, Vrtiska TJ, et al. Clinical characteristics of potential kidney donors with asymptomatic kidney stones. Nephrol Dial Transplant 2011;26(8):2695–700.
8. Dalziel PJ, Noble VE. Bedside ultrasound and the assessment of renal colic: a review. Emerg Med J 2013;30(1):3–8.
9. Smith-Bindman R, Aubin C, Bailitz J, et al. Ultrasonography versus computed tomography for suspected nephrolithiasis. N Engl J Med 2014;371(12):1100–10.
10. White WM, Zite NB, Gash J, et al. Low-dose computed tomography for the evaluation of flank pain in the pregnant population. J Endourol 2007;21(11):1255–60.
11. Heidenreich A, Desgrandschamps F, Terrier F. Modern approach of diagnosis and management of acute flank pain: review of all imaging modalities. Eur Urol 2002;41(4):351–62.
12. Wein AJ, Kavoussi LR, Campbell MF. Campbell-Walsh urology. In: Wein AJ, Kavoussi LR, Partin AW, et al, editors. 11th edition. Philadelphia: Elsevier Saunders; 2015.

13. Ludvigson AE, Beaule LT. Urologic emergencies. Surg Clin North Am 2016;96(3): 407–24.

14. Mydlo JH. Surgeon experience with penile fracture. J Urol 2001;166(2):526–8 [discussion: 528–9].

15. Bitsch M, Kromann-Andersen B, Schou J, et al. The elasticity and the tensile strength of tunica albuginea of the corpora cavernosa. J Urol 1990;143(3):642–5.

16. el-Assmy A, el-Tholoth HS, Mohsen T, et al. Does timing of presentation of penile fracture affect outcome of surgical intervention? Urology 2011;77(6):1388–91.

17. Koifman L, Barros R, Junior RA, et al. Penile fracture: diagnosis, treatment and outcomes of 150 patients. Urology 2010;76(6):1488–92.

18. Uder M, Gohl D, Takahashi M, et al. MRI of penile fracture: diagnosis and therapeutic follow-up. Eur Radiol 2002;12(1):113–20.

19. Morey AF, Metro MJ, Carney KJ, et al. Consensus on genitourinary trauma: external genitalia. BJU Int 2004;94(4):507–15.

20. Mazaris EM, Livadas K, Chalikopoulos D, et al. Penile fractures: immediate surgical approach with a midline ventral incision. BJU Int 2009;104(4):520–3.

21. Kulmala RV, Lehtonen TA, Tammela TL. Preservation of potency after treatment for priapism. Scand J Urol Nephrol 1996;30(4):313–6.

22. Emond AM, Holman R, Hayes RJ, et al. Priapism and impotence in homozygous sickle cell disease. Arch Intern Med 1980;140(11):1434–7.

23. Kassim AA, Fabry ME, Nagel RL. Acute priapism associated with the use of sildenafil in a patient with sickle cell trait. Blood 2000;95(5):1878–9.

24. Kumar R, Jindal L, Seth A. Priapism following oral sildenafil abuse. Natl Med J India 2005;18(1):49.

25. McMahon CG. Priapism associated with concurrent use of phosphodiesterase inhibitor drugs and intracavernous injection therapy. Int J Impot Res 2003;15(5): 383–4.

26. Priyadarshi S. Oral terbutaline in the management of pharmacologically induced prolonged erection. Int J Impot Res 2004;16(5):424–6.

27. Montague DK, Jarow J, Broderick GA, et al. American Urological Association guideline on the management of priapism. J Urol 2003;170(4 Pt 1):1318–24.

28. Salonia A, Eardley I, Giuliano F, et al. European Association of Urology guidelines on priapism. Eur Urol 2014;65(2):480–9.

29. Baskin LS, Carroll PR, Cattolica EV, et al. Necrotising soft tissue infections of the perineum and genitalia. Bacteriology, treatment and risk assessment. Br J Urol 1990;65(5):524–9.

30. Paty R, Smith AD. Gangrene and Fournier's gangrene. Urol Clin North Am 1992; 19(1):149–62.

31. Corcoran AT, Smaldone MC, Gibbons EP, et al. Validation of the Fournier's gangrene severity index in a large contemporary series. J Urol 2008;180(3): 944–8.

32. Visser AJ, Heyns CF. Testicular function after torsion of the spermatic cord. BJU Int 2003;92(3):200–3.

33. Arap MA, Vicentini FC, Cocuzza M, et al. Late hormonal levels, semen parameters, and presence of antisperm antibodies in patients treated for testicular torsion. J Androl 2007;28(4):528–32.

34. Makela E, Lahdes-Vasama T, Rajakorpi H, et al. 19-year review of paediatric patients with acute scrotum. Scand J Surg 2007;96(1):62–6.

35. Kadish HA, Bolte RG. A retrospective review of pediatric patients with epididymitis, testicular torsion, and torsion of testicular appendages. Pediatrics 1998; 102(1 Pt 1):73–6.

36. Murphy FL, Fletcher L, Pease P. Early scrotal exploration in all cases is the investigation and intervention of choice in the acute paediatric scrotum. Pediatr Surg Int 2006;22(5):413–6.
37. Burks DD, Markey BJ, Burkhard TK, et al. Suspected testicular torsion and ischemia: evaluation with color Doppler sonography. Radiology 1990;175(3):815–21.
38. Sessions AE, Rabinowitz R, Hulbert WC, et al. Testicular torsion: direction, degree, duration and disinformation. J Urol 2003;169(2):663–5.

The Current State of Telemedicine in Urology

Adam Miller, MD[a], Eugene Rhee, MD, MBA[b], Matthew Gettman, MD[a], Aaron Spitz, MD[c],*

KEYWORDS

- Telemedicine • Telehealth • Tele-mentoring • Tele-surgery • Tele-rounding
- Tele-imaging • Urology

KEY POINTS

- Telemedicine services can be implemented through a multitude of modalities, including videoconferencing software, mobile applications, and wearable devices and monitors.
- Telemedicine improves access to health care while maintaining physician and patient satisfaction.
- Many formats of telemedicine are readily reproducible and relevant to surgical and nonsurgical practices alike, including video visits, online services, electronic consults, and tele-rounding.
- Telemedicine is covered by Medicaid in almost all states.
- Barriers currently exist for Medicare reimbursement; however, this is an evolving process.

INTRODUCTION

In an era of medicine when there is pressure to do more with less, telemedicine becomes relevant to nearly all medical specialties. Urology has been innovative with this field. The authors review herein how this is relevant and applicable to internal medicine practices.

Both the increasing cost of health care and the shortage of physicians across multiple specialties have required the development of efficient, accessible, and cost-effective health care delivery models.[1] One initiative has been the implementation of remote medical care, known as telemedicine.

Disclosure Statement: A. Spitz is a speaker for Endo Pharmaceuticals and AbbVie Pharmaceuticals. The other authors have nothing to disclose.
[a] Department of Urology, Mayo Clinic, 200 First Street Southwest, Rochester, MN 55905, USA; [b] Department of Urology, Kaiser Permanente San Diego, Administration, 2nd Floor Finance, 4511 Orcutt Avenue, San Diego, CA 92120, USA; [c] Department of Urology, University of California–Irvine, Orange County Urology Associates, 25200 La Paz Road Suite 200, Laguna Hills, CA 92653, USA
* Corresponding author.
E-mail address: aaronspitz100@gmail.com

Telemedicine is the interactive exchange of health care information electronically between patients, providers, and consultants for the purpose of education, evaluation, decision-making, and treatment. These interactions can be implemented through a multitude of modalities, including videoconferencing software, mobile applications, and wearable devices and monitors; they can exist as synchronous or asynchronous encounters.

Preliminary data suggest that telemedicine has the potential to reduce costs and travel time for patients, improve patient satisfaction, and facilitate quality care for complex patients.[2] Innovative urologists have been adopting telemedicine successfully, with academic pilots leading to standard operating procedures in the Veterans Affairs (VA) system, for example.[3,4]

In this article, the authors discuss the current role of telemedicine in urology. Key topics, including logistics of telemedical implementation, different telemedical modalities, regulatory and reimbursement aspects of telemedicine, and limitations, are addressed.

CURRENT USE OF TELEMEDICINE

Telemedical applications are being applied to a host of acute and chronic conditions across a wide array of specialties. For example, psychiatrists have been using telemedicine in the emergency department,[5] intensivists are using telemedical platforms to manage complex intensive care unit patients from afar,[6] and pediatric surgeons are expanding their accessibility to rural hospitals[7] and institutions that lack pediatric surgical expertise. In the outpatient setting, the virtual consultation is being used more frequently by dermatologists,[8] orthopedists,[9] general surgeons,[10] and ophthalmologists.[11] Moreover, telemedical visits are being hosted in a wide range of settings, including satellite clinics,[12] retail minute clinics,[13] and elementary schools.[14]

In urology, pediatric urologists were among the pioneering groups to begin implementing telemedicine into daily practice.[15–17] Now, academic and private practice groups have found numerous roles for telemedicine and are now providing hospital consultation as well as postoperative follow-up care through telemedical interfaces. Routine urology office visits are being conducted from patients' homes or workplaces; hospital rounds are taking place via a robot or ipad, saving the physician time traveling between hospitals while maintaining high patient satisfaction and increasing the opportunity for a multidisciplinary team approach.

As telemedicine has evolved, systems and procedures have been established making it easier for practices of all types to incorporate this technology.

NECESSARY SYSTEMS AND PROCEDURES

In general, telemedicine involves live, real-time applications (ie, synchronous telemedicine) or store and forward applications (ie, asynchronous telemedicine). In urologic practice, an example of an asynchronous application would be a recorded cystoscopy video that is stored and viewed at a later date, whereas a synchronous application may involve a real-time interview with patients in a remote location. Asynchronous applications are often less difficult to implement, as technology requirements increase with real-time interactions. It is best to select the least cumbersome application that will fulfill the goals of practice.

In addition to considering the types of telemedical visits that will be offered, a practice must also consider the diagnoses and indications for which the technology will be used. For example, at the VA urology clinic in Los Angeles, California, any new diagnosis may be initially managed telemedically,[4] whereas other institutions, such as the University of California–Davis Department of Urology, will determine which conditions it will see telemedically and what records, laboratory tests, and imaging may be required before the initial tele-consultation. In other practices, telemedical visits may be limited to select follow-up patients.

Telemedicine must be delivered using a secure and robust Internet-based system, typically involving the use of a virtual private network combined with point-to-point encryption software that meets recognized standards. The goal should be to securely transmit and store data across a wide variety of settings, including patients' homes or other noninstitutional settings. A mobile device, computer, or remotely controlled robotic platform can be used as the interface for a live telemedical encounter. There are several Internet-based videoconferencing software programs that are commercially available for synchronous applications, but the electronic medical record may be all that is required for asynchronous applications.

Informed consent and privacy are two important considerations when using video encounters. Video encounters should be carried out in an environment that maximizes privacy for both the provider and patients. A consent should be obtained in real time and should include a discussion about the structure and timing of services, record keeping, scheduling, privacy, risks, confidentiality, mandatory reporting, and billing. Additionally, expectations regarding the video visit and any subsequent visits should be discussed. These items should be documented in the medical record. It is important that video visits also be completed in accordance with a given state's telemedicine laws.

Technology failure can lead to interruptions during the telemedical encounter. A plan should be in place in the event of equipment failure, and patients should have contact information for technical support in case troubleshooting is required. Rather than have patients manage the requirements of a video visit, another option is for patients to report to a telemedicine center where the hardware, software, and connectivity are provided and standardized for maximum reliability and staff are available to troubleshoot problems as they arise.

Documentation of a telemedical encounter is similar to an in-person encounter. It is important to note that patients were seen using telemedicine technologies. For example, an electronic consultation without video might include the following claim: *This patient was not personally interviewed or examined. The history and examination findings are based on the clinical documentation provided and/or discussion with a physician or provider who had personally interviewed and examined the patient*. Otherwise, the medical record entry should include an assessment and plan, patient information, contact information, history, informed consent, and information regarding fees and billing.

TECHNIQUES/TYPES OF SERVICES

Telemedicine can be implemented through a multitude of modalities, including videoconferencing software, mobile applications, and wearable devices and monitors. The authors describe an array of formats and examples next.

Video Visits

A video visit consists of a live face-to-face electronic audiovisual interaction between the provider and patients. Despite the limitations of tactile feedback, video visits have proven to be a reasonable alternative to traditional in-person visits across a variety of settings.

Chu and colleagues[4] have conducted face-to-face audiovisual encounters with more than 1000 new VA patients with urologic complaints at the Los Angeles VA. Many of these patients live at a great distance from the Los Angeles VA, and their travel to the clinic is burdensome. This barrier has been overcome by video visits with these patients at satellite clinics that are closer to their homes, saving time and money on patient travel. Andreassi and colleagues[18] at the University of California–Davis Department of Urology have a similar practice. In both practices, all conditions are initially evaluated telemedically and in-office visits and procedure are scheduled as needed. The top chief complaints seen by these two groups include bothersome lower urinary tract symptoms, elevated prostate-specific antigen, and prostate cancer. In patient surveys, 95% of patients score satisfaction as very good to excellent and 80% of urologists score the encounters as excellent.[4] In a similar group receiving telemedical care at the VA Medical Center in Omaha, Nebraska, patients traveled 277 fewer miles and saved $200 on travel when virtual consultations were used.[4]

Like many large academic institutions, patients traveling to the Mayo Clinic Department of Urology in Rochester, Minnesota travel great distances and often across state lines to seek care. Viers and colleagues[2] randomly assigned patients to video visits or traditional office visits and found that video visits resulted in a similar patient-to-provider face time (mean 14.5 minutes vs 14.3 minutes; $P = .96$), patient wait time (18.4 minutes vs 13.0 minutes; $P = .20$), and total time devoted to care (17.9 minutes vs 17.8 minutes; $P = .97$) while reducing the patients' time away from work and eliminating the costs associated with travel. In other words, this demonstrated a major convenience to patients; overall, the patients in the study were highly satisfied with video visits and provider satisfaction was nearly identical to in-person encounters.[2]

Dr Robert Nguyen[19] pioneered a postoperative telemedical program at Boston Children's Hospital where remote-controlled telemedical robots (VGo Communications, Cambridge, MA) were sent home with children who were discharged from the hospital after urologic surgery.[19] The robots were equipped with video cameras and a set of wheels for mobilizing around the home environment. The robots were also equipped with features for analyzing urine and blood, along with the ability to provide education to patients and family members related to the patient's diagnosis or procedure performed. These features allowed Dr. Nguyen and his team to easily monitor patients in the critical postoperative period without prolonging hospitalization or requiring frequent follow-up appointments.

Spitz and colleagues, in collaboration with OptumHealth, have also used a rounding robot to provide new patient consultations as well as follow-up care for residents of a local skilled nursing facility.[18] This practice has allowed for a great reduction in the burden associated with the transfer of these convalescing patients to and from the facility. Moreover, this has been met with high patient and family satisfaction and even instances of earlier discharge from the facility.[18]

Regular follow-up visits are being performed using a telemedicine interface (personal communication, 2016, Geisler, Austin, TX; Spitz, Orange County, CA). A focus of delivery has been to local preferred provider organizations or capitated patients in the form of follow-up visits for those who would otherwise not require a hands-on physical examination or procedure. These encounters are performed with the aid of mobile devices or personal computers equipped with cameras. The patients report great satisfaction with the convenience of conducting these visits from their home, place of employment, or even while traveling out of town. These visits have augmented the two practices in that physical office space is able to be reserved for more complex patients requiring in-person evaluations.

Finally, pediatric urology groups have noted good results with early use of telemedicine technology. Devries and colleagues at the University of Utah reach remote pediatric patients in their homes using telemedical technology.[18] Kennedy and colleagues at Lucile Packard Children's Hospital at Stanford care for numerous patients telemedically with the aid of practitioners at rural clinics as well as an inner-city satellite hospital.[18] Most families prefer the telemedical visit and enjoy a 50% reduction in wait times.[15] Moreover, Canon and associates[17] at Arkansas Children's Hospital are using telemedicine linked to local clinics to reduce the travel and expense for preoperative consultations and postoperative follow-up for patients in remote rural areas. Travel in this group was reduced from 335 km to 35 km, and there was no increase in complications.[15]

Online Services

Online health care interfaces allow patients to access portions of their electronic medical record and communicate with their care team. Value-added services include online appointment scheduling; form submission, such as history intake questionnaires; online bill payment; and access to clinical notes, reports, and imaging contained within patients' records. Additionally, this interface can incorporate education by providing articles related to certain diagnoses and definitions for medical jargon that patients may find in the chart. Alerts for preventative services can also be incorporated into the online portal, allowing reminders to be sent to patients. Although these services are typically not billable, they bring value to patients and they help satisfy the government's mandated meaningful use criteria for electronic health records.[20]

Electronic Consults

Electronic consults (eConsults) are virtual consultations that allow a particular provider to asynchronously answer another provider's focused questions about the diagnosis or management of a specific patient. The consulted provider reviews the supporting material from the electronic health record and provides a formal response to the focused question. Consultations are most likely to be solicited from large academic centers but can also be solicited from large private groups.

eConsults are performed using electronic software and hardware specifically for electronic consultations. There are several programs that are commercially available specifically for this use. The response is then documented in the medical record, similar to an in-person encounter.

eConsults are convenient for requesting providers (and indirectly to patients) because they provide timely access to specialty expertise without requiring patients to travel. The patient evaluation can be completed in a shorter timeframe, which streamlines the delivery of care.

Both synchronous and asynchronous eConsults exist. With the former, a real-time conversation is held with the referring provider and is generally scheduled during regular business hours. In the latter, the eConsult can be performed at any time because there is no real-time interaction with the referring provider, allowing for extremely flexible scheduling and the freedom of the consulted physician to decide when to perform the consult.

The Mayo Clinic in Rochester, Minnesota has been piloting an eConsult program whereby each provider sees, on average, 1 to 2 asynchronous eConsults per clinic day. Although this is still a relatively new program, empirical evidence would suggest this has been well received.

Tele-Rounding

During tele-rounding, the provider interacts with patients via a rounding robot or mobile device. For the provider covering many locations, tele-rounding is a mechanism to decrease the time burden associated with traveling to multiple hospitals for traditional rounding. The use of tele-rounding technology allows physicians to provide remote medical care across a wide range of settings. Moreover, tele-rounding instantly bridges distance, decreasing time in transit from one physical location to another, freeing up the urologist to be more available and less rushed on hospital rounds. Another distinct advantage of tele-rounding is the opportunity for multidisciplinary care, involving all members of the care team to come together simultaneously in an effort to enhance delivery of care to patients.

Kavoussi and colleagues[21] were the first to introduce the concept of tele-rounding in 2004. Tele-rounding was initially performed using a remote-controlled robot with a microcomputer, video monitor, and a microphone. Data transmission was accomplished with high-speed data lines using wireless connections. During tele-rounding, the urologist interacted with patients via the digital video camera, flat-screen monitor, microphone, and a joystick controller. Using a prospective randomized trial that enrolled 270 adult postoperative urology patients early after surgery, patient satisfaction between traditional rounding and robotic tele-rounding was not significantly different.[21] In the same study, tele-rounding was not associated with adverse events, such as increased or missed complications or increased lengths of stay. The investigators found that if their attending surgeon was out of town, two-thirds of patients preferred a tele-rounding encounter from their own surgeon rather than be seen in person by another attending surgeon.[21] Moreover, tele-rounding was shown to have a significant positive impact on patient-reported satisfaction during postsurgical hospitalization with improved perception of surgeon availability, quality of medical information delivered, thoroughness of the examination, and postoperative care coordination.[21]

Bretan and colleagues[22] pioneered the use of the rounding robot (RP-Vita, InTouch Health, Santa Barbara, CA). His team has provided remote urologic consults to 6 rural hospitals and a prison that average a distance of 100 miles from his office. Using the robot and the help of on-site nurse practitioners to assist in his evaluation, Dr Bretan is able to perform a range of emergency department and inpatient consultations.[22]

In Irvine, California, Spitz and colleagues similarly use a rounding robot to perform urologic consultations with a local emergency department. By using the remote consultation approach, disruption of the office practice is minimized and delivery of emergency department care is streamlined.

Laptop computers have also played a role in tele-rounding. Kau and colleagues[23] successfully used laptop computers equipped with built-in webcams and videoconferencing software for tele-rounding. Out of the 10 patients studied, 90% of the patients agreed or strongly agreed that the system permitted easy communication with the urologist; all patients agreed that tele-rounding should be a regular part of patient care.[23] All physicians and nurses involved in the study agreed that tele-rounding enhanced patient care and would be an improvement in health care delivery, perhaps because of the ease of incorporating a multidisciplinary approach to rounding. Moreover, the investigators also reported that the rounding system using laptop computers was simple to use and more cost-effective than tele-rounding robots.[23]

Tablet devices have also been used for tele-rounding. Kaczmarek and colleagues[24] enrolled 32 patients to compare tablet tele-rounding on postoperative day 1 with traditional rounding with direct patient contact on day 2. Tablet devices were equipped with videoconferencing software and a wireless internet connection. The authors found that tablet tele-rounding was favorable, with 91% of patients saying their care was better with tele-rounding and 97% saying that tele-rounding should be incorporated into routine care.

Tele-Monitoring

Tele-monitoring is the use of technology to remotely track health parameters using wearable devices, monitors, and various remote sensing software. With this, providers are able to follow details like vital signs outside of the hospital or office setting.

Holzbeirlein and colleagues (personal communication, 2017), at the University of Kansas Medical Center Department of Urology, have piloted a program whereby wearable activity-tracking devices (Garmin Ltd, Schaffhausen, Switzerland) are sent home with postoperative cystectomy patients in order to track activity levels following surgery. Activity goals are set by the health care team, and the patients and team are able to ensure these goals are met in an effort to optimize recovery. Moreover, these patients are sent home with ipads preloaded with software capable of tracking weight, urine output, medication administration, and vital signs, enabling the surgical team to closely track these patients in the critical postoperative period. Early unpublished data have demonstrated good compliance and positive feedback from patients.

Similarly, wearable activity-tracking devices are also being piloted at the Mayo Clinic to track activity levels of postoperative prostatectomy patients. To date, a total of 46 patients have been included in the study with a median age of 63 years and a body mass index of 29. Initial data have shown the obese and those older than 65 years took significantly fever steps after surgery, but there was no difference in nonobese or those less than 65 years old. Most of the patients felt a medical benefit using the fitness trackers, and patient satisfaction was high (unpublished data). These data regarding postoperative activity levels are not only important for postoperative monitoring but also for patient counseling in the perioperative setting.

Tele-Mentoring, Tele-Proctoring, and Education

Tele-mentoring involves remote guidance or teaching, whereas tele-proctoring refers to the remote evaluation of performance. Both have significant implications on medical education. Urologists have used these strategies to overcome the burdensome process of mentoring and proctoring that often leads to logistical roadblocks to training by using a tele-mentoring and tele-proctoring system associated with robotic-assisted radical prostatectomies.[25] These modalities can be applied to almost all areas of medicine, however.

Patient education is another way that telemedical technology can be used. Patients presenting to the Mayo Clinic for a men's health consult are provided with numerous online educational videos and resources regarding various men's health topics and related treatments. In one study looking at video-based prostate cancer education, Wang and colleagues[26] found that video-based educational tools are an effective method for overcoming the severe lack of comprehension of prostate health terminology among patients and enhancing patient participation in shared and informed decision-making.

Tele-Simulation

Tele-simulation is a teaching process that uses simulators and an Internet connection to educate learners in remote locations. Surgical simulators are now being used as educational tools to teach minimally invasive techniques.[27] However, there is a wealth of medical and nonsurgical applications for this technology. Applied more broadly, this type of technology could be used to teach trainees a wealth of topics, including how to perform components of the physical examination.

REIMBURSEMENT

Health care reform, with its emphasis on value, is bringing more attention to the prospect of telemedicine. Twenty-nine states have telemedicine parity laws whereby private payers are required to cover telemedicine services at rates equal to those paid as if the service was provided as an in-person encounter. Telemedicine is covered by Medicaid in almost all states. Medicare, however, is a different matter.

Although fee-for-service Medicare reimbursement for telemedicine is still very restrictive and limits coverage to patients in remote locations or specific chronic conditions, the Centers for Medicare and Medicaid Services (CMS) are currently working to liberalize its implementation in alternative payment models, such as accountable care organizations and integrated health systems that take upside and downside risk with Medicare patients. In these models, if telemedicine does not increase the overall cost, then there is no compelling reason to restrict it. Moreover, group practices can be well positioned to participate in alternative payment models, which would compensate for telemedical services.

Regulations governing telemedicine vary by state. There are varying requirements for what constitutes a valid doctor-patient relationship via telemedical communication. There are varying criteria for the patients' consent to participate, and states differ on whether a provider must be in physical proximity to patients. Currently, telemedicine can only be practiced in the state in which a physician is licensed, as with traditional practice. Such restrictions may soon be circumvented by new Tricare telemedical legislation and pending VA and Medicare legislation.[28]

Retail providers of telemedicine use several strategies for reimbursement. They may privately contract patients or they may be contracted with insurance companies on a fee-for-service basis. Teledoc, one of the nation's largest retailers of telemedical services, engages in capitation arrangement directly with private insurance payers and large employers while also requiring a copay.

In highly integrated health care systems, fee-for-service considerations do not influence the adoption of telemedicine. Telemedicine is provided for efficiency, access, and patient and provider satisfaction, which explains the more robust adoption of telemedicine by the VA, the Department of Defense, prisons,[29] and other commercial-capitated entities, such as Kaiser Permanente.

For billing purposes, modifier –GT is appended to the service reported to indicate the use of telemedicine technology. A list of 89 covered services and specific requirements was included in the final rule for payment for Medicare in 2017. Telephone calls as part of an office visit or follow-up of an office visit often do not qualify for payment under current telemedical coverage rules. Moreover, services such as previsit history and demographics, follow-up for test results, and prescription refills fall into the bundled category of services and are not paid separately.[30]

TELEMEDICINE IN PRACTICE

The Physician Quality Reporting System (PQRS) is a well-known health care quality improvement incentive program initiated by the CMS in 2006. By reporting health care quality data to the CMS, providers are rewarded with reimbursement incentives. Next is an example of how telemedicine can be used in medical practice to achieve these incentives.

For this example, the authors use a 68-year-old otherwise healthy woman who presents to her primary care physician for routine health maintenance. Her provider systematically runs through a full systems review. The provider specifically asks the patient about urinary incontinence in reference to the PQRS measure (number 048 in the 2016 PQRS Measure List) addressing percentage of female patients aged 65 years and older who were assessed for presence or absence of urinary incontinence. The patient admits to occasional urinary urge with urge incontinence.

The standard workup for urinary urgency is performed; the patient is not in urinary retention, and urinalysis returns negative for evidence of infection. The physical examination is negative for pelvic abnormalities, including prolapse. She is subsequently referred to urology by way of an eConsult. The consulted urologist asks the primary care provider to obtain a bladder diary and reviews the patient record within 1 to 2 days of receiving the consult. The urologist sees that the patient has been consuming 100-oz liquid (primarily coffee) per day and voids supraphysiologic amounts every 5 hours on average. Recommendations for a 60-oz fluid restriction, time voiding schedule every 3 to 4 hours while awake, avoidance of coffee, and Kegel-strengthening exercises are provided.

These recommendations are then passed along to the patient, who makes the recommended lifestyle changes and has a significant improvement in her symptoms. The patient is satisfied because her problem has been addressed in a timely manner and did not require her to travel further than her primary care physician's office. Her primary care provider is satisfied because he or she can now report this quality measure for reimbursement incentives and was able to satisfactorily treat the patient. The urologist is pleased with an efficient consult and the flexibility to perform the consult during a convenient time.

CHALLENGES/LIMITATIONS

Telemedicine is not without limitations. Perhaps the most obvious limitation is the physical examination, as providers must rely primarily on sight and sound. One solution for augmenting the physical examination involves a medical assistant alongside patients who can act as a surrogate during the physical examination portion of the encounter. With the physical examination largely limited to sight and sound, another limitation of telemedical encounters becomes the quality of the audiovisual data transferred back to the provider. One could imagine that with poor audiovisual data comes a severely limited patient encounter.

Perhaps the most appropriate setting for the telemedical encounter is when the physical examination is not critical. For example, this would include encounters whereby the primary goal is to review a test result or to evaluate a response to therapy. However, it could be argued that providers can derive adequate information from the audiovisual encounter, when combined with imaging, laboratory tests, and surrogate examinations, ultimately leading to proper evaluation of a broad range of presenting complaints. Naturally, many patients will require in-person follow-up for physical examinations or procedures, but this can be arranged following an initial virtual consultation.

Another limitation of telemedicine is the disparity of access to technology. Lower income rural and inner city populations disproportionally lack access to technology,[31] including high speed Internet connectivity and mobile hardware platforms. Notably, this is the same population that stands to derive the most benefit from telemedicine.

Technical literacy becomes relevant in the discussion of telemedicine. At least 42% of patients older than 65 years are not online.[32] In an aging population, this becomes significant, as urology practices (and put more broadly, many medical practices) cater to this patient population. Even for those who are technically literate, many patients in this age group may find the telemedical encounter less satisfactory compared with the younger patients whose work schedule provides more incentive to avoid time spent traveling to and from health care appointments.

Reimbursement for telemedical encounters is an evolving topic and is considered a limitation to widespread adoption of telemedicine by urologists and other medical and surgical providers. Practitioners in states with fewer reimbursement mandates may be unmotivated to implement telemedicine into their practice given the expense and time associated with obtaining the hardware and software required for connectivity. Moreover, Health Insurance Portability and Accountability Act (HIPAA) compliance is a limiting factor for many connectivity and software platforms.

Physician satisfaction for urologists who were early adopters of telemedicine have indicated high satisfaction[21,23,24]; however, the logistics of telemedicine can be disruptive to the traditional clinic schedule. For those accustomed to the traditional schedule, eConsults that have accrued throughout the day may need to be performed after hours or technical difficulties during a video visit may delay a provider's clinic schedule. It is anticipated that the efficacy will offset some of the inconveniences like cost, need for technology, and disruption of the traditional schedule. Ideally, groups will customize their use of telemedicine in an effort to fit the needs of the practice group.

FUTURE CONSIDERATIONS/SUMMARY

With physician shortages and the push to do more with less, telemedicine has demonstrated a feasible solution to these barriers to health care. Telemedicine in urology has been met with favorable results. In this article, several examples of telemedicine in urology practice along with the associated benefits are reviewed. In particular, telemedicine has shown a benefit in addressing workforce shortages, increasing clinical and surgical productivity, broadening patient access to care, and improving data quality reporting. The benefits of telemedicine do not stop with the urology practice, as many of these telemedical modalities can be applied to the medical practice. As we overcome the limitations of telemedicine and as new technologies are developed, it is possible that telemedicine will become a standard practice in many medical and surgical practices.

REFERENCES

1. Bashshur RL, Shannon G, Krupinski EA, et al. Sustaining and realizing the promise of telemedicine. Telemed J E Health 2013;19(5):339–45.
2. Viers BR, Lightner DJ, Rivera ME, et al. Efficiency, satisfaction, and costs for remote video visits following radical prostatectomy: a randomized controlled trial. Eur Urol 2015;68(4):729–35.
3. Park ES, Boedeker BH, Hemstreet JL, et al. The initiation of a preoperative and postoperative telemedicine urology clinic. Stud Health Technol Inform 2011; 163:425–7.
4. Chu S, Boxer R, Madison P, et al. Veterans Affairs telemedicine: bringing urologic care to remote clinics. Urology 2015;86(2):255–60.
5. Yellowlees P, Burke MM, Marks SL, et al. Emergency telepsychiatry. J Telemed Telecare 2008;14(6):277–81.
6. Leong JR, Sirio CA, Rotondi AJ. eICU program favorably affects clinical and economic outcomes. Crit Care 2005;9(5):E22.
7. Miller GG, Levesque K. Telehealth provides effective pediatric surgery care to remote locations. J Pediatr Surg 2002;37(5):752–4.

8. Watson AJ, Bergman H, Williams CM, et al. A randomized trial to evaluate the efficacy of online follow-up visits in the management of acne. Arch Dermatol 2010;146(4):406–11.

9. Sathiyakumar V, Apfeld JC, Obremskey WT, et al. Prospective randomized controlled trial using telemedicine for follow-ups in an orthopedic trauma population: a pilot study. J Orthop Trauma 2015;29(3):e139–45.

10. Hwa K, Wren SM. Telehealth follow-up in lieu of postoperative clinic visit for ambulatory surgery: results of a pilot program. JAMA Surg 2013;148(9):823–7.

11. Matimba A, Woodward R, Tambo E, et al. Tele-ophthalmology: opportunities for improving diabetes eye care in resource- and specialist-limited sub-Saharan African countries. J Telemed Telecare 2016;22(5):311–6.

12. Brown EM. The Ontario telemedicine network: a case report. Telemed J E Health 2013;19(5):373–6.

13. Hawkins M. Physician appointment wait times and Medicaid and Medicare acceptance rates. 2014. Available at: http://www.merritthawkins.com/uploadedfiles/merritthawkings/surveys/mha2014waitsurvpdf.pdf. Accessed April 16, 2017.

14. McConnochie KM, Wood NE, Kitzman HJ, et al. Telemedicine reduces absence resulting from illness in urban child care: evaluation of an innovation. Pediatrics 2005;115(5):1273–82.

15. Cook J. There's my doctor from TV! 2015. Available at: http://healthier.stanfordchildrens.org/en/theres-doctor-tv. Accessed April 16, 2017.

16. Shivji S, Metcalfe P, Khan A, et al. Pediatric surgery telehealth: patient and clinician satisfaction. Pediatr Surg Int 2011;27(5):523–6.

17. Canon S, Shera A, Patel A, et al. A pilot study of telemedicine for post-operative urological care in children. J Telemed Telecare 2014;20(8):427–30.

18. Gettman M, Rhee E, Spitz A, et al. AUA Telemedicine Workgroup White paper on telemedicine in urology. Linthicum (MD): American Urological Association; 2016.

19. Nguyen B. New telemedicine pilot program merges robotics and urology in Boston. 2012. Available at: https://www.youtube.com/watch?v=pjqX0E8Kdal. Accessed April 16, 2017.

20. HealthIT.gov. Meaningful use definition & objectives. 2015. Available at: https://www.healthit.gov/providers-professionals/meaningful-us-definition-objectives. Accessed April 16, 2017.

21. Ellison LM, Nguyen M, Fabrizio MD, et al. Postoperative robotic telerounding: a multicenter randomized assessment of patient outcomes and satisfaction. Arch Surg 2007;142(12):1177–81 [discussion: 1181].

22. Daniel HE. 2015-16 MMS President Peter N. Bretan Jr., MD. Marin Medicine 2015; 61(2):21–8.

23. Kau EL, Baranda DT, Hain P, et al. Video rounding system: a pilot study in patient care. J Endourol 2008;22(6):1179–82.

24. Kaczmarek BF, Trinh QD, Menon M, et al. Tablet telerounding. Urology 2012; 80(6):1383–8.

25. Hinata N, Miyake H, Kurahashi T, et al. Novel telementoring system for robot-assisted radical prostatectomy: impact on the learning curve. Urology 2014; 83(5):1088–92.

26. Wang DS, Jani AB, Sesay M, et al. Video-based educational tool improves patient comprehension of common prostate health terminology. Cancer 2015;121(5): 733–40.

27. Brewin J, Ahmed K, Challacombe B. An update and review of simulation in urological training. Int J Surg 2014;12(2):103–8.

28. Affairs UDoV. VA telehealth services 2015. Available at: http://www.telehealth.va. gov/. Accessed April 16, 2017.
29. Ellimoottil C, Skolarus T, Gettman M, et al. Telemedicine in urology: state of the art. Urology 2016;94:10–6.
30. Painter R, Painter M. Telemedicine: reimbursement in fee-for-service, quality models. Urology Times 2017;17–8.
31. Viswanath K, Kreuter M. Health disparities, communication inequalities, and e-health: a commentary. Am J Prev Med 2007;32(5 Suppl):S131–3.
32. Perrin A, Duggan M. Americans' internet access: 2000-2015, vol. 2017. Washington, DC: Pew Research Center; 2015.

The Intersection of Medicine and Urology

An Emerging Paradigm of Sexual Function, Cardiometabolic Risk, Bone Health, and Men's Health Centers

Martin M. Miner, MD[a],*, Joel Heidelbaugh, MD[b],
Mark Paulos, MD[c], Allen D. Seftel, MD[d], Jason Jameson, MD[e],
Steven A. Kaplan, MD[f]

KEYWORDS

- Medicine and urology • Sexual function • Cardiometabolic risk • Bone health
- Men's health centers

KEY POINTS

- Men's mental health and how they think about their health are critical to the future of men's health. Poor health choice patterns are established during those years under the age of 50 when men are twice as likely to die compared with women.
- As the future of medicine focuses on quality and value, a better understanding of the social determinants of men's health will identify potential areas of improvement.
- The presentation of a man to a clinician's office with a sexual health complaint should present an opportunity for a more complete evaluation, notably the complaint of erectile dysfunction.
- The future of men's health will be well served by integrated men's health centers that focus on the entire man, with proper education and testing and careful shared decision making between patient and provider.

[a] Department of Family Medicine and Urology, The Men's Health Center, The Miriam Hospital, The Warren Alpert Medical School of Brown University, 164 Summitt Avenue, Providence, RI 02906, USA; [b] Departments of Family Medicine and Urology, University of Michigan Medical School, Ann Arbor, MI, USA; [c] Departments of Internal Medicine and Urology, Men's Health Center, The Miriam Hospital, The Warren Alpert School of Medicine, Brown University, Providence, RI, USA; [d] Division of Urology, Cooper University Hospital, Cooper Medical School of Rowan University, Camden, NJ, USA; [e] Division of Urology, Mayo Clinic, Scottsdale, AZ, USA; [f] Benign Urologic Diseases and The Men's Health Program, Icahn School of Medicine at Mount Sinai, Mount Sinai Health System, New York, NY, USA
* Corresponding author.
E-mail address: Martin_Miner@Brown.edu

Med Clin N Am 102 (2018) 399–415
https://doi.org/10.1016/j.mcna.2017.11.002
0025-7125/18/© 2017 Elsevier Inc. All rights reserved.

WHY MEN'S HEALTH?

Gender-based medicine, specifically recognizing the differences in the health of men and women, drew significant attention in the 1990s with regard to addressing disparities. The National Institutes of Health Office of Research on Women's Health was established in 1990, and in 1994 the US Food and Drug Administration (FDA) created an Office of Women's Health, resulting in a dramatic increase in the quantity and quality of research devoted to examining numerous aspects of women's health, rendering women's health in the mainstream today.[1]

Although decades of research have yielded many important findings about health disparities and disease burden in men, such knowledge has not resulted in the benefits expected. Men are still less likely than women to seek medical care and are nearly one-half as likely as women to pursue preventive health care visits or undergo evidence-based screening tests.[2] Recent data indicate that 68.6% of men aged 20 years and older are overweight,[3] and life expectancy of men continues to trail that of women by nearly 5 years in 2014 (76.4 years for men and 81.2 years for women).[4]

Men's health as a concept and discipline is in a nascent state compared with women's health. Most clinicians and the public consider men's health a field concerned only with diseases of the prostate and erectile dysfunction (ED). Men's health has recently become a hot topic in these specific areas, with millions of dollars spent on remedies for prostate health, improved urinary flow, and enhanced erections and by comparison a much smaller amount directed at improved preventive health.[5]

Adult men ages 18 years to 65 years do not use or react to health care services in the same ways as women[6] and are less likely to attend preventive health care visits.[7] Men are also less likely to follow medical regimens and are less likely to achieve control with long-term therapeutic treatments for chronic diseases, including hypertension, diabetes mellitus, and atherosclerotic heart disease.[8,9] The Commonwealth Fund did a mass survey in 2000 and found that "an alarming proportion of American men have only limited contact with physicians and the healthcare system in general. Many men fail to get routine check-ups, preventive care, or health counseling and they often ignore symptoms or delay seeking medical attention when sick or in pain."[10]

The presentation of a man to the clinician's office with a sexual health complaint should present an opportunity for a more complete evaluation, notably the complaint of ED. In a landmark article published in 2005, Thompson and colleagues[11] confirmed that ED is a sentinel marker and risk factor for future cardiovascular events. Incident ED occurring in the 4300 men without ED at study entry enrolled in the Prostate Cancer Prevention Trial was associated with a hazard ratio of 1.25 for subsequent cardiovascular events during the 9-year study follow-up. For men with either incident or prevalent ED, the hazard ratio was 1.45.

WHO IS THE MEN'S HEALTH DOCTOR: PRIMARY CARE PHYSICIAN, UROLOGIST, OR SUBSPECIALIST?

With the advent of the Patient Protection and Affordable Care Act in March 2010, millions of men ages 18 years through 45 years who previously did not have access to health care entered the marketplace to obtain health insurance. Although urologists are typically thought of as "men's doctors" and obstetrician-gynecologists are considered "women's doctors," the issue remains: Who is to shoulder the responsibility for men's health in the decades to come? Integrated men's health centers (MHCs) to deliver health care for years to come need to be created.

The appeal of an integrated MHC is of a single, highly personal medical or urologic issue home to address all of men's health needs, including sexual health.

The MHC paradigm at the Miriam Hospital Men's Health Center is admittedly challenging to replicate at the moment. The focus encompasses becoming a lifestyle coach as it deals with the parameters of cardiometabolic medicine: lifestyle, stress management, sleep, diet, and exercise.

The following sections provide a rationale for an integrated MHC in the primary care/urology intersection, focusing on ED, Testosterone (T) deficiency, osteoporosis, cardiovascular (CV) disease, and obesity. Although this includes a preventative focus, it does not include other relevant topics of men's health, such as affective and mood disorders, domestic and partner violence, and gender-specific issues. Disparities among multicultural differences in men's health, as it exists in a socioeconomic means, and disease prevalence among various multiethnic groups are beyond the scope of this article.

ERECTILE DYSFUNCTION AND SUBCLINICAL CARDIOVASCULAR DISEASE: AN INTERSECTION OF MEDICINE AND UROLOGY

The relationship between ED and clinical CV disease (CVD) was originally based on a shared clinical risk factor model (eg, hypertension, smoking, and diabetes mellitus) and the presumed overlap in pathophysiologic mechanisms, including endothelial dysfunction, inflammation, and atherosclerosis.[12] In the early 2000s, longitudinal studies on CVD and ED revealed a 2-way relationship, positing that patients with CVD are more likely to have ED and that patients with ED are more likely to develop future CVD, even when adjusted for risk factors.[13–16] The Princeton Consensus Conference identified ED as a substantial independent risk factor for CVD,[16] and the QRISK group published one of the first risk scores to incorporate ED as an independent risk factor into their updated 10-year CV risk model, calculating a 25% increased risk for average middle-aged men.[17]

The temporal relationship between ED and subclinical CVD progression is less clear. Is ED a precursor to CVD, or does underlying CVD first manifest as ED? Available data come from cross-sectional studies correlating symptoms of ED and overt CVD or highly limited prospective cohort studies correlating ED incidence or severity with incident CV events.[13–16,18–20] A few studies have revealed a 2-year to 3-year time interval between onset of ED symptoms and CVD symptoms,[14] whereas more recent studies have examined the interrelationships between subclinical CVD (ie, early atherosclerosis), ED, and overt CVD (myocardial infarction [MI] or major adverse cardiac events [MACE]).[18–20] The Multi-ethnic Study of Atherosclerosis (MESA)[21] showed subclinical CVD is a predictor of ED, which could predict MACE. This pivotal finding provided evidence that coronary artery calcium (CAC) score can serve as a "disease score" and surrogate for accelerated atherosclerosis process in arteries, including penile arteries and vascular ED.[22]

One-half of men with sudden CVD events have no previous symptoms of CAD and between 70% and 89% of sudden cardiac events occur in men.[23–28] ED may be the single warning of this risk of sudden CVD events.[28,29] ED severity has been correlated with atherosclerotic coronary disease burden, and the presence of ED has been independently associated with CVD events.[28,29]

THE TEMPORAL RELATIONSHIP OF ERECTILE DYSFUNCTION, SUBCLINICAL CARDIOVASCULAR DISEASE, AND CLINICAL CARDIOVASCULAR DISEASE

A systematic review demonstrating that men with ED at intermediate CVD risk had a higher relative risk of CVD events compared with those at low or high CVD risk: 0.93 for low risk, 1.51 for intermediate risk, and 1.30 for high risk.[1] Consistent with previous studies, they also showed an inverse relationship between prevalence and CV impact of age of onset on ED.[1,19,20] Relative risk of CVD events was higher among younger ED patients, with risk decreasing linearly as age in years increased.[1,19,20] This could indicate the potential usefulness of ED as a predictor in these young patients and the intermediate CVD risk score group, which commonly consists of middle-aged men, of the population who will benefit from a discussion about further testing, according to American College of Cardiology (ACC)/American Heart Association (AHA) 2013 preventive guideline.[30]

There is increasing interest in describing the burden of subclinical disease in patients with ED. The CAC score has been endorsed by recent ACC/AHA guidelines for further risk stratification of intermediate-risk patients and shown to be the single best predictor of CV risk.[21,31,32] To date, limited studies have examined CAC scores in patients with ED, showing that patients with ED have higher CAC scores compared with healthy subjects.[33] Consistent with this finding, Jackson[34] showed that among 65 ED patients aged 38 years to 73 years with no cardiac symptoms, 81% of patients had calcified plaque. Finally, Yaman and colleagues[35] categorized 60 patients with ED and 23 patients without ED according to the severity of ED measured by the International Index of Erectile Function (IIEF) and then compared CAC scores. An increasing IIEF score indicates decreasing ED severity. A significant negative correlation between IIEF scores with CAC scores was observed, implying a positive correlation between ED severity and CAC.[35]

The MESA study was the first study to explore temporal relationship between ED and subclinical CVD. Development of ED was found to occur sometime during the progression from baseline subclinical vascular disease to clinically overt CVD. A strong association was observed between baseline subclinical disease as assessed by CAC and carotid plaque and subsequent ED, highlighting the potential role of atherosclerosis testing—in particular, CAC scoring and carotid plaque—in predicting ED and overt CVD.[21] At the same time, given the strengths of ED as a predictor of future coronary and cerebrovascular events, there seem to be clear clinical implications and indications for the increased evaluation of subclinical CVD for at-risk patients before and once they develop ED.[36,37]

Few studies have examined the effect of CV risk factor modification on both ED and CVD, but much of the recent development of knowledge takes place in the men's health domain. Among the shared risk factors, modification of tobacco use, hyperlipidemia, and dietary change/weight loss/exercise in targeted patients has revealed symptomatic improvement in ED.[38–42] A randomized single-blind study of 110 obese men aged 35 years to 55 years, without diabetes, hypertension, or hyperlipidemia, who had an IIEF of 21 or less to determine the effect of weight loss and increased physical activity on erectile and endothelial function in obese men found that after 2 years, body mass index decreased more in the intervention group as did serum concentrations of interleukin 6 and C-reactive protein.[43] The mean IIEF score (Sexual Dysfuntion) in the intervention group improved from 13.9 to 17, with 17 men in the intervention group normalizing their sexual function.[43] These studies suggest that patients who are at high risk need aggressive risk factor modification, which then could delay or prevent the future onset of ED and perhaps overt CAD.

RECOMMENDATIONS FOR EVALUATION OF CARDIOVASCULAR RISK IN MEN WITH ERECTILE DYSFUNCTION

Given the relationship among ED, subclinical CVD, and clinical CVD, the authors recommend that all men with vascular ED should undergo CV risk assessment.[44,45]

In parallel, a sexual history assessment should be integrated into all CV risk assessments and may be of increased importance in populations with a lower burden of risk or predilection for more silent coronary disease as determined by the presence or absence of comorbidities or age.[44] All men should be questioned about their sexual history and functioning as part of the initial assessment of CV risk. Symptomatic men (eg, those with exertional chest pain, presyncope, or shortness of breath) with ED are presumed to have CAD and are, therefore, at high risk for CVD events and as such should undergo CV stress testing.[44,45]

The authors recommend evaluation of fasting plasma glucose, serum creatinine (estimated glomerular filtration rate), albumin/creatinine ratio, fasting lipids, and assessment of the cardiometabolic syndrome component, which may be used to further characterize CV risk.[44] The authors recommend measurement of total T levels, particularly for patients who have failed a trial of phosphodiesterase type 5 inhibitors.[44] Based on established guidelines, the authors recommend considering T supplementation for men with total T less than 300 ng/dL who are symptomatic (eg, decreased libido, decreased spontaneous erections, low energy, increased fatigue, or loss of muscle mass and strength).[46] The authors do not recommend T supplementation for total T greater than 350 ng/dL.[46]

The 2013 ACC/AHA risk assessment guidelines are an appropriate starting point for CAD risk stratification in younger, middle-aged men with ED or in diabetic men with ED.[45] Due to a reliance on a small number of traditional risk factors and the strong reliance of age in the risk estimates, the authors propose more advanced testing for all men aged 40 years to 60 years with vasculogenic ED because these patients normally do not score as high risk with the new ACC/AHA risk estimator and likely have significant unaccounted-for risk.[45]

Men who seem at high risk for CV events based on ASCVD score greater than 10% should be referred to a cardiologist.[47] The authors suggest that all other men with vasculogenic ED and no overt CVD symptoms undergo further noninvasive evaluation using CAC scoring as the primary diagnostic test to detect subclinical atherosclerosis for the purpose of advanced risk stratification.[47,48] Exercise stress testing with calculation of the FIT Treadmill Score may also have appropriate roles in the evaluation of men with vasculogenic ED.[49] In addition, imaging of CAC with the latest multidetector scans takes only a few seconds, and the cost of the test is currently less than $200 in many metropolitan areas in the United States.[50,51]

Given the limitations of other markers for CVD risk assessment and in light of the growing body of evidence supporting the use of CAC as a diagnostic and prognostic tool, the authors support the use of CAC scoring as the first diagnostic test for further risk assessment in all low-risk and intermediate-risk men 40 years to 60 year old with confirmed vasculogenic ED without overt CVD symptoms.[51,52]

This approach treats atherosclerosis as a continuum that can be impacted by many traditional and nontraditional risk factors that result in inflammation, subclinical atherosclerosis, and finally clinically apparent CVD.[53] In keeping with this theory, the presence of subclinical atherosclerosis has been shown to predict future CVD complications and death.[54] The growth of technology over the past 2 decades has allowed for direct measurement of subclinical atherosclerosis and, therefore, further stratifying individual risk for a CVD event.[51] The authors propose the use of CAC score to guide initiation of pharmacotherapy in low-risk and intermediate-risk patients and to guide intensity of therapy in high-risk patients.[47,51,54]

AN UPDATE ON TESTOSTERONE REPLACEMENT THERAPY AS ANOTHER EXAMPLE OF THE POTENTIAL OF THE MEN'S HEALTH CENTER

In March 2015, all US commercial T products underwent an FDA-mandated label change that restricted the indicated population and warned against the possible risk of MI and stroke.[55] Investigators from the responsible FDA team subsequently published their rationale and perspective in a leading medical journal in 2015.[56]

The actions by the FDA were extensively covered by the lay and medical media, and contributed to concerns that T therapy (TTh) is associated with previously underrecognized risks and is overprescribed. The label change regarding indicated populations created an unusual situation in which TTh prescriptions for a large majority of men with well-recognized condition of T deficiency, also known as adult-onset hypogonadism, suddenly became off-label literally overnight, adding to the concern that physicians are prescribing T for no reason other than "normal aging."[57] These changes may have reduced the willingness of many professionals to consider treatment of affected men with T deficiency. In addition, health insurers have created policies based on these changes to justify reduced coverage for T products.

CHANGES TO THE FOOD AND DRUG ADMINISTRATION LABEL

Although the addition of a CVD warning to the label for TTh products received considerable attention, warnings of this type are not uncommon. It states, "Long term clinical safety trials have not been conducted to assess the cardiovascular outcomes of testosterone replacement therapy in men. To date, epidemiologic studies and randomized controlled trials have been inconclusive for determining the risk of major adverse cardiovascular events (MACE), such as nonfatal myocardial infarction (MI), nonfatal stroke, and cardiovascular (CV) death, with the use of testosterone compared to nonuse. Some studies, but not all, have reported an increased risk of MACE in association with use of testosterone replacement therapy in men."

In addition, the language for indications was changed by the FDA to provide an inclusive list of conditions causing hypogonadism, termed *classical hypogonadism*, and removing the term *idiopathic*, which accounted for a large majority of treated cases prior to the issuing of the warning. Finally, a statement was added as follows: "Safety and efficacy of AndroGel 1.62% in men with 'age-related hypogonadism' (also referred to as 'late-onset hypogonadism') have not been established.[55]

STATUS OF PUBLISHED STUDIES LEADING TO ADDITION OF CARDIOVASCULAR RISK WARNING

The FDA pharmacovigilance team identified only 4 studies suggesting increased CV risks with T therapy. The first, in 2010, was a 6-month placebo-controlled T gel study in frail men, with limited mobility, in which more CV events were noted in the T arm compared with the placebo arm.[58] A majority of these events, however, were not clinically significant and included nonspecific changes on electrocardiogram, palpitations, and pedal edema not associated with heart failure. The FDA's own written assessment indicated they dismissed these results as concerning because the numbers of MACEs were too few for evaluation.[59]

The second study, by Vigen and colleagues,[60] reported that men who subsequently received TTh had an absolute rate of MI, stroke, or death of 25.7% at 3 years after angiography compared with 19.9% in untreated men. Soon after publication it was discovered the investigators had reversed their results, because the absolute rate of events was only 10.1% among men who received TTh and 21.2% in untreated men.

Later, the investigators revealed they had miscategorized more than 1000 individuals in the original publication, and nearly 10% of the all-male population was discovered to be women.[61]

A third study by Finkle and colleagues[62] reported increased rates of nonfatal MI in the 90 days after a T prescription compared with the prior 12 months. Apart from serious methodological concerns (the period prior to the prescription represents physician prescribing behavior rather than a natural rate of MI), there was no control group of hypogonadal men who did not receive a T prescription, so it is unknown whether rates of MI were higher, lower, or unchanged in this population. Finally, a meta-analysis of placebo-controlled Testosterone Trials reported increased CV events for men who received T.[63] As the FDA noted, however, this study's results were confounded by incorrect data culled from the component studies and an overly broad definition of what constituted a CV event.[59] The FDA's own analysis indicated that the number of important CV events were similar in the T-treated and placebo-treated groups.[59] At least 6 other meta-analyses found contradictory results, with no increased T-associated CV risks.[64–70] The largest of these suggested decreased risks for men at high CV risk due to cardiometabolic disorders.[64]

Substantial literature indicates that low T levels are associated with increased mortality, coronary artery disease (severity and incidence), increased fat mass, and decreased lean mass. Two observational studies reported reduced mortality, by half, in men with low T who received TTh compared with untreated men.[71,72] Several small to moderate-sized placebo-controlled trials showed CV benefits with T administration in men with known CV disease, specifically angina and heart failure.[73–77]

Although the new FDA warning is accurate in that some studies did report increased CV risks with T administration whereas others did not, the strength of the few studies suggesting any increased risk was remarkably weak. The European Medicines Agency performed its own review and declined to add a new CV warning.[78]

REVIEW OF NEW CARDIOVASCULAR STUDIES

Since the FDA advisory committee meeting in 2014, 22 new studies were published addressing CV risks of TTh, including 11 clinical trials and 11 observational data analyses. Five of these studies comprise the Testosterone Trials. None has proved that T is associated with an increased risk of CV events.

In 2016, the primary results of the Testosterone Trials were published.[79] This was arguably the most important Testosterone Trial to date, representing the first large, government-funded, multicenter, placebo-controlled trial involving 790 men 65 years or greater assigned to either T gel or placebo for 1 year. The trial included a second year to monitor for safety outcomes. The Testosterone Trials confirmed that T therapy improved sexual function, sexual desire (increase in T levels was associated with significantly increased sexual activity, as assessed by the Psychosexual Daily Questionnaire as well as significantly increased sexual desire and erectile function), physical activity, and mood. Rates of MACE were identical in the first year for the T arm and placebo arms, with N = 7. In the second year, however, there were only 2 MACEs in the T arm compared with 9 in the placebo arm, albeit not statistically significant.

Subsequently, Budoff and colleagues[80] presented results of CT angiography in subset of 138 men from the Testosterone Trials. Compared with placebo, T treatment was associated with a significantly greater increase in noncalcified and total plaque volume but not in calcified plaque. No major CV events occurred in either treatment group. First, the volume of noncalcified plaque has not been associated with CV outcomes, so the significance of this finding is unknown. Second, CAC scores do have a well-established association with CV outcomes, and this measure did not change with T administration. Finally, there were no adverse CV events in this subgroup, and as discussed previously, for the entire study population of 790 men in the Testosterone Trials there were a greater number of MACEs in the placebo arm than the T arm (16 vs 9, respectively).[80]

Testosterone's Effects on Atherosclerosis Progression in Aging Men was a 3-year placebo-controlled, double-blind, parallel-group randomized trial involving 308 men 60 years or older with low or low-normal T levels[81]; 156 participants were randomized to receive 7.5 g of 1% T and 152 were randomized to receive placebo gel packets daily for 3 years, with dose adjustment targeted to achieve T levels between 500 ng/dL and 900 ng/dL. Results were that T administration for 3 years versus placebo did not result in a significant difference in the rates of change in either common carotid artery intima-media thickness or CAC. No MACEs were reported because this trial was only powered to evaluate atherosclerosis progression and, therefore, these findings should not be interpreted as establishing CV safety of T use in older men.

SUMMARY OF CARDIOVASCULAR STUDIES BECAUSE FOOD AND DRUG ADMINISTRATION LABEL CHANGE

Although the newly added CV warning to T products mandated by the FDA is technically accurate, in that some studies have reported increased CV risks and others have not, it is incomplete to note the few observational studies reporting an increased CV risk that are weak with regard to scientific evidence and quality and omit studies that provide evidence to the contrary. Specifically, the overall safety results from the Testosterone Trials revealed fewer MACEs for men who received T compared with placebo by 9 to 16, respectively. Two observational studies showed reduced hazard ratio of MACEs for men whose T levels normalized with treatment compared with those whose T levels failed to normalize, indicating suboptimal treatment may increase CV risk. The attention raised by the FDA investigation into CV risk seems to have prompted additional studies, together with published results from the Testosterone Trials, yet not a single study has emerged to provide evidence to support concerns that T therapy increases CV risk. On the contrary, the totality of evidence of these studies strongly suggests either a neutral or a protective CV effect for T therapy.

Thus, the MHC provides the infrastructure to affect change as seen in this comprehensive review of T replacement therapy. The MHC provides for a comprehensive and thoughtful evaluation and treatment plan to ensure that T replacement therapy is given in accordance with both the FDA guidelines and the latest CV contributions.

FINAL EXAMPLE OF THE POTENTIAL OF THE MEN'S HEALTH CENTER: OSTEOPOROSIS IS A MEN'S HEALTH CONCERN: INCIDENCE AND GENDER DISPARITIES

Osteoporosis is the most common metabolic bone disease in the United States and worldwide. The National Osteoporosis Foundation estimates that there are 10 million Americans with osteoporosis and an additional 43 million with low bone mineral density (BMD).[82] In 2005, more than 2 million incident fractures were reported in the United States alone.[83] Worldwide, osteoporosis causes more than 8.9 million fractures annually, resulting in an osteoporotic fracture every 3 seconds.[84] The economic burden of incident osteoporosis related fractures is staggering and the direct medical cost of osteoporosis related fractures in the United States is estimated to be more than $13.8 billion.[85]

With the US population 50 years of age or older predicted to increase by 60% from 2000 to 2025, the economic burden of osteoporosis related fractures is estimated to increase to 23.5 billion dollars, and at least 25% of this cost will be attributed to treating osteoporosis related fractures in men.[86] In 2010 the National Osteoporosis Foundation estimated that there were 2.8 million men with osteoporosis and another 14.4 million men with low bone mass.[86] Worldwide, men account for 25% of hip fractures,[87] and in the United States men account for nearly 30% of all hip fractures.[88] By 2050, the worldwide incidence of hip fracture in men is projected to increase by 310% compared with 240% in women.[86] In 2025, the estimated number of hip fractures occurring worldwide in men will be similar to that observed in women in 1990.[86]

The estimated lifetime risk of an osteoporosis-related fracture in US men is at least 1 in 5.[86] This is in contrast to the 1 in 7 lifetime risk of prostate cancer. Studies of older men's knowledge about osteoporosis demonstrated that 83% of men did not believe that they were susceptible to osteoporosis, and 43% could not correctly define osteoporosis. Osteoporosis-related fractures in men lead to significant disability, diminished quality of life, and increased mortality.[87] One in 6 men will sustain a hip fracture by age 90, and a man's risk of death from complications of a hip fracture is 34%.[88] After a hip fracture 15% of men are unable to walk at 2 years, and only 34% are able to walk without an assisting device.[88]

Despite these remarkable statistics, significant gaps still remain in the management of osteoporosis in men. A study of 51,000 adults admitted with a hip fracture in the state of North Carolina showed that only 2.2% of men admitted with a fracture received treatment of osteoporosis, and men were 75% less likely than women to be treated.[89] Of those men who did receive treatment, two-thirds received calcium and vitamin D only.[90]

GAPS IN TREATMENT IN MALE OSTEOPOROSIS ARE SIGNIFICANT

Although the health and economic impact of osteoporosis on men is well described, there remains a paucity of research on osteoporosis therapies in men. A systematic review and meta-analysis of osteoporosis treatment efficacy in men could identify only 22 randomized clinical trials that evaluated the efficacy of a treatment of osteoporosis or low BMD for adult men that reported fracture outcomes.[91] A prior systematic review and meta-analysis completed in 2011 included only 5 studies reporting fracture outcomes and concluded that "the evidence of the efficacy of osteoporosis treatment to reduce fracture risk in men was inconclusive."[92]

Vertebral fractures are a marker of bone fragility and indicate a higher risk of fractures. The presence of 1 or more prevalent vertebral fractures on lateral spine radiographs is a strong predictor of future incident vertebral fractures and a moderate predictor of nonvertebral fractures independent of BMD.[93] The National Osteoporosis Foundation recommends routine DXA screening for all men over 70 and for men over 50 based on risk factor profile.[94]

Treatment includes making healthy lifestyle changes, including getting 1000 mg to 1200 mg of calcium daily through dietary sources and using supplements if dietary sources are insufficient.[95] Vitamin D supplementation to achieve blood 24-hydroxyvitamin D levels of at least 30 ng/mL is also recommended as is 30 minutes to 40 minutes of weightbearing exercises 3 times to 4 times per week, limiting alcohol to fewer than 3 drinks per day, and smoking cessation, recommended for all men.[95]

Treatment with a specific bone-forming medication is indicated in any man with a low impact fracture, a T score−2.5 SD below mean for normal young white men, or T score from −1 to −2.5 with high 10-year risk of fracture greater than or equal to 20% overall or 3% at the hip using FRAX or long-term glucocorticoid therapy greater than 7.5 mg daily. Currently there are 5 FDA-approved drugs for treatment of osteo-porosis in men, including alendronate, risedronate, zoledronic acid, teriparatide, and denosumab. Response to treatment should be monitored by serial BMD at the hip and spine every 1 year to 2 years, and markers of bone turnover or bone formation may be considered.[95]

Recently updated guidelines from the American College of Physicians for treatment of low BMD and osteoporosis to prevent fractures in men and women reiterate that low BMD as measured by dual-energy x-ray absorptiometry is an imperfect predictor of fracture risk, identifying less than one-half of the people who go on to have an oste-oporotic fracture.[96] There is low-quality evidence showing the appropriate duration of treatment is uncertain, although high-risk patients may benefit from more than 5 years of treatment.[96] Newer imaging modalities to improve on fracture risk estimation include quantitative CT and trabecular bone score. Quantitative CT improves quanti-fication of tissue density within a region of interest and trabecular bone score can pro-vide information regarding bone architecture and quality rather than bone quantity.[97]

THE COMPONENTS OF A MEN'S HEALTH CURRICULUM: AN OUTGROWTH OF THE MEN'S HEALTH CENTER

A dedicated men's health curriculum is long overdue and would be a natural outgrowth of an MHC. Such a curriculum would begin with a deep understanding of the social determinants of men's health, why men do or do not seek health care, and, most importantly, how they view and address their acute and chronic health con-ditions. Teaching men's health should not be limited to conditions solely focused on urologic or CV conditions but should focus on the interaction between the 2 and the implications for morbidity and mortality. Common conditions that are often overlooked in men's health include the impact and burden of mental health, gastrointestinal, rheu-matologic, and renal diseases. More men than ever are considering complementary and alternative solutions toward addressing health care issues. Health care providers need to be adequately trained to care for men who have sex with men, transgendered patients, and complex geriatric men. The future will see fellowships based on such curricular platforms to train men's health specialists.

Men's health should be categorized into 4 general categories:

1. Conditions that are unique to men (eg, prostate cancer, prostate disease, and ED)
2. Diseases or illnesses that are more prevalent in men compared with women (eg, CV disease, stroke, and renal disease)
3. Health issues for which risk factors and adverse outcomes are different in men (eg, obesity)
4. Health issues for which different interventions to achieve improvements in health and well-being at the individual or population level are required for men (eg, access to care)

A men's health curriculum must be rooted in the deep understanding of the impact of masculinity factors on health care engagement and outcomes. Hegemonic mascu-linity is the idealized cultural standard that sets the ideal of "how to be a man" and sets the standards by which men are judged in society. As various psychosocial stressors directly and indirectly contribute to high rates of unhealthy behaviors, chronic disease diagnoses, and premature mortality among men, these factors help explain men's self-representation and internalization of notions of masculine social norms that drive or avoid the receipt of appropriate health care services. Understanding poor health status and literacy in men includes considering how masculinity and gendered social determinants of health (eg, social norms and expectations of biological males at a certain age and setting) shape men's lives and experiences through their economic and environmental factors.

Special populations of men also deserve attention in a broad-based men's health curriculum. Education should include caring for men who have sex with men, incarcerated men, men with significant mental health concerns, athletes, male executives, veterans, immigrants, and transgendered patients. Each population has unique needs, social determinants, biases, and outcomes. Teaching of a men's health curriculum for these and other populations should be comprised of primary care providers, urologists, advanced practice providers, mental health providers and social workers, medical experts across all specialty fields, and allied health professionals with expertise in the aforementioned arenas.

BUILDING A MEN'S HEALTH CENTER

Before developing a business plan for a MHC, it has to be decided what and whom it will encompass, organization, revenue versus expenses, sustainability, and opportunities for growth. To build a successful enterprise, there must be a buy-in from leadership (in either an academic or private practice setting) as well as a cadre of specialties, including partnerships with various subspecialists in cardiology, endocrinology, psychiatry, orthopedics, and dermatology, who are truly vested in the need for integration of thought, goals, and vision. In the past, most MHCs have focused on sexual health and administration of T.

This is a time of great stress on the medical system and health care providers. The adaptation of the patient-centered medical home model, electronic medical records, and increasing scrutiny of testing and outcomes all add to the burden of clinical management of male patients. Men tend to present to health care providers later with symptoms and far more advanced along the disease spectrum than their female counterparts. A men's health program and concentration can allow those symptoms men see as vital to a healthy life (eg, sexual function) and propel them to a softer landing for a greater preventative focus and risk factor analysis. This effort requires an astute urologist who acknowledges and seeks evaluation of appropriate medical comorbidities coupled with a productive partnership with primary care clinicians or focused within the context of a men's health program or MHC established to address these needs.

THE FUTURE OF MEN'S HEALTH

Men's health has received both praise and skepticism over the past decade, with some bona fide controversy. The importance of men focusing on their health with regular preventive care is highlighted by numerous awareness events throughout the year, including Men's Health Month in June, and November, which highlights prostate cancer, testicular cancer, and mental health in men during that month. Because women make up to 80% of the health care decisions for their families, including men, the future of men's health can be positively affected by a better understanding of men's health issues by women. Many MHCs have notoriously treated thousands of men with T or injections for ED without progressing through the proper guidelines of national organizations, often charging patients hundreds of dollars for proprietary treatments that could be offered for much less with standard prescriptions. The future of men's health will be well served by integrated MHCs that focus on the entire man, with proper education and testing and careful shared decision making between patient and provider.

The latest annual statistics from the Centers for Disease Control and Prevention (www.CDC.gov) show for the first time in decades the life expectancy in 2015 for US men decreased by 0.2 years to 76.3 years.[98] Age-adjusted cancer deaths was the only area of improvement because 9 of the 10 top causes of death increased, including heart disease, chronic lower respiratory disease, unintentional injuries, stroke, Alzheimer disease, diabetes, kidney disease, and suicide. Despite improvement in most other age groups and races over the past decade, middle-aged (ages 45–54 years) white Americans have slowly been experiencing an increase in all-cause mortality due to significant increases in poisonings (including opioids), suicide, and chronic liver disease. The largest gap in life expectancy between men and women occurred in 1979 (7.8 years favoring women) and decreased to 4.8 years in 2010 and has remained fairly stable since. As men's health specialists hope to continue to decrease the life expectancy gap between men and women, addressing these concerning trends will be critical, especially dealing with the opioid crisis in America.

Men's mental health and how they think about their health are critical to the future of men's health. Poor health choice patterns are established during those years under the age of 50 where men are twice as likely to die compared with women. Being male is the single largest demographic factor for early death.[99]

Addressing these important men's health issues will not be easy. As the future of medicine focuses on quality and value, a better understanding of the social determinants of men's health will identify potential areas of improvement. Advocating for men's health will become more important in the years to come because access to care and costs of care are limiting factors in a population that has not typically focused on their own health. Reaching boys and men at all stages of life with important health behavior education will allow them to live their lives to the fullest. The American Urological Association Men's Health Checklist is a comprehensive outline of health topics for providers to address for various ages of men. Women and other social support systems can have a positive impact on male health, which ultimately improves the lives of men, women, and children. Men's health is family health!

REFERENCES

1. Fontanarosa PB, Cole HM. Theme issue on men's health: call for papers. JAMA 2006;295:440–4.
2. Agency for healthcare research and quality. Evidence Based Report. December, 2005.
3. National Center for Health Statistics Fact Sheets. December, 2005.
4. National Center for Health Statistics. Health, United States, 2015: with special feature on racial and ethnic health disparities. Hyattsville (MD). 2016.
5. Penson D, Kreiger JN. Men's health. Are we missing the big picture? JGIM 2001; 16:717–71.
6. Schlichthorst M, Sanci LA, Pirkis J, et al. Why do men go to the doctor? Sociodemographic and lifestyle factors associated with healthcare utilisation among a cohort of Australian men. BMC Public Health 2016;16(Suppl 3):1028.
7. Courtenay WH. Constructions of masculinity and their influence on men's well being: a theory of gender and health. Soc Sci Med 2000;50:1385–401.
8. Rose I, Kim MT, Dennison CR, et al. The contexts of adherence for African Americans with high blood pressure. J Adv Nurs 2000;32:587–94.
9. Plascencia A, Ostfield AM, Gruber SB. Effects of sex on differences in awareness, treatment, and control of blood pressure. Am J Prev Med 1988;4:315–26.

10. Sandman D, Simantov E, An C. Out of Touch: American Men and the Health Care System. The Commonwealth Fund. March 2000.
11. Thompson IM, Tangen CM, Goodman PJ, et al. Erectile dysfunction and subsequent cardiovascular disease. JAMA 2005;294(23):2996–3002.
12. Vlachopoulos CV, Terentes-Printzios DG, Ioakeimidis NK, et al. Prediction of cardiovascular events and all-cause mortality with erectile dysfunction: a systematic review and meta-analysis of cohort studies. Circ Cardiovasc Qual Outcomes 2013;6:99–109.
13. Fung MM, Bettencourt R, Barrett-Connor E. Heart disease risk factors predict erectile dysfunction 25 years later: the Rancho Bernardo Study. J Am Coll Cardiol 2004;43:1405–11.
14. Montorsi P, Ravagnani PM, Galli S, et al. Association between erectile dysfunction and coronary artery disease. Role of coronary clinical presentation and extent of coronary vessels involvement: the COBRA trial. Eur Heart J 2006;27:2632–9.
15. Hotaling JM, Walsh TJ, Macleod LC, et al. Erectile dysfunction is not independently associated with cardiovascular death: data from the Vitamins and Lifestyle (VITAL) study. J Sex Med 2012;9:2104–10.
16. Nehra A, Jackson G, Miner M, et al. The Princeton III consensus recommendations for the management of erectile dysfunction and cardiovascular disease. Mayo Clin Proc 2012;87:766–78.
17. Hippisley-Cox J, Coupland C, Brindle P. Development and validation of QRISK3 risk prediction algorithms to estimate future risk of cardiovascular disease: prospective cohort study. BMJ 2017;357:j2099.
18. Banks E, Joshy G, Abhayaratna WP, et al. Erectile dysfunction severity as a risk marker for cardiovascular disease hospitalisation and all-cause mortality: a prospective cohort study. PLoS Med 2013;10:e1001372.
19. Inman BA, Sauver JL, Jacobson DJ, et al. A population-based, longitudinal study of erectile dysfunction and future coronary artery disease. Mayo Clin Proc 2009; 84:108–13.
20. Chew KK, Finn J, Stuckey B, et al. Erectile dysfunction as a predictor for subsequent atherosclerotic cardiovascular events: findings from a linked-data study. J Sex Med 2010;7:192–202.
21. Feldman DI, Cainzos-Achirica M, Billups KL, et al. Subclinical vascular disease and subsequent erectile dysfunction: the Multiethnic Study of Atherosclerosis (MESA). Clin Cardiol 2016;39:291–8.
22. Jackson G, Boon N, Eardley I, et al. Erectile dysfunction and coronary artery disease prediction: evidence-based guidance and consensus. Int J Clin Pract 2010; 64:848–57.
23. Go AS, Mozaffarian D, Roger VL, et al. Heart disease and stroke statistics—2013 update: a report from the American Heart Association. Circulation 2013;127(1):6–245.
24. Fox CS, Evans JC, Larson MG, et al. Temporal trends in coronary heart disease mortality and sudden cardiac death from 1950 to 1999: the Framingham Heart Study. Circulation 2004;110:522–7.
25. Kuller L, Cooper M, Perper J. Epidemiology of sudden death. Arch Intern Med 1972;129:714–9.
26. Podrid PJ, Myerburg RJ. Epidemiology and stratification of risk for sudden cardiac death. Clin Cardiol 2005;28:I3–11.
27. Ni H, Coady S, Rosamond W, et al. Trends from 1987 to 2004 in sudden death due to coronary heart disease: the Atherosclerosis Risk in Communities (ARIC) study. Am Heart J 2009;157:46.

28. Shin D, Pregenzer G, Gardin JM. Erectile dysfunction: a disease marker for cardiovascular disease. Cardiol Rev 2011;19:5–11.

29. Gandaglia G, Briganti A, Jackson G, et al. A systematic review of the association between erectile dysfunction and cardiovascular disease. Eur Urol 2014;65:968–78.

30. Goff DC Jr, Lloyd-Jones DM, Bennett G, et al. 2013 ACC/AHA guideline on the assessment of cardiovascular risk: a report of the American College of Cardiology/American Heart Association Task Force on Practice Guidelines. J Am Coll Cardiol 2014;63:2935–59.

31. Greenland P, Alpert JS, Beller GA, et al. 2010 ACCF/AHA guideline for assessment of cardiovascular risk in asymptomatic adults: executive summary. J Am Coll Cardiol 2010;56:2182–99.

32. Blaha MJ, Yeboah J, Al Rifai M, et al. Providing evidence for subclinical CVD in risk assessment. Glob Heart 2016;11(3):275–85.

33. Chiurlia E, D'Amico R, Ratti C, et al. Subclinical coronary artery atherosclerosis in patients with erectile dysfunction. J Am Coll Cardiol 2005;46:1503–6.

34. Jackson G. Erectile dysfunction and asymptomatic coronary artery disease: frequently detected by computed tomography coronary angiography but not by exercise electrocardiography. Int J Clin Pract 2013;67:1159–62.

35. Yaman O, Gulpinar O, Hasan T, et al. Erectile dysfunction may predict coronary artery disease: relationship between coronary artery calcium scoring and erectile dysfunction severity. Int Urol Nephrol 2008;40:117–23.

36. Gibson AO, Blaha MJ, Arnan MK, et al. Coronary artery calcium and incident cerebrovascular events in an asymptomatic cohort. JACC Cardiovasc Imaging 2014;7:1108–15.

37. Detrano R, Guerci AD, Carr JJ, et al. Coronary calcium as a predictor of coronary events in four racial or ethnic groups. N Engl J Med 2008;358:1336–45.

38. Kostis JB, Dobrzynski JM. The effect of statins on erectile dysfunction: a meta-analysis of randomized trials. J Sex Med 2014;11:1626–35.

39. Cui Y, Zong H, Yan H, et al. The effect of statins on erectile dysfunction: a systematic review and meta-analysis. J Sex Med 2014;11:1367–75.

40. Kałka D, Domagała Z, Dworak J, et al. Association between physical exercise and quality of erection in men with ischaemic heart disease and erectile dysfunction subjected to physical training. Kardiol Pol 2013;71:573–80.

41. Gupta BP, Murad MH, Clifton MM, et al. The effect of lifestyle modification and cardiovascular risk factor reduction on erectile dysfunction. Arch Intern Med 2011;171:1797.

42. DeLay KJ, Haney N, Hellstrom WJ. Modifying risk factors in the management of erectile dysfunction: a review. World J Mens Health 2016;34:89–100.

43. Esposito K, Giugliano F, Di Palo CD, et al. Effect of lifestyle changes on erectile dysfunction in obese men: a randomized controlled trial. JAMA 2004;291:2978–84.

44. Miner M, Nehra A, Jackson G, et al. All men with vasculogenic erectile dysfunction require a cardiovascular workup. Am J Med 2014;127:174–82.

45. Shah NP, Cainzos-Achirica M, Feldman DI, et al. Cardiovascular disease prevention in men with vascular erectile dysfunction: the view of the preventive cardiologist. Am J Med 2016;129:251–9.

46. Bhasin S, Cunningham GR, Hayes FJ, et al. Testosterone therapy in men with Androgen deficiency syndromes: an endocrine society clinical practice guideline. J Clin Endocrinol Metab 2010;95:2536–59.

47. Same R, Miner M, Blaha M, et al. Erectile dysfunction: an early sign of cardiovascular disease. Curr Cardiovasc Risk Rep 2015;9:49–57.

48. Blaha MJ, Silverman MG, Budoff MJ. Is there a role for coronary artery calcium scoring for management of asymptomatic patients at risk for coronary artery disease? Clinical risk scores are not sufficient to define primary prevention treatment strategies among asymptomatic patients. Circ Cardiovasc Imaging 2014;7(2): 398–408.

49. Ahmed HM, Al-Mallah MH, McEvoy JW, et al. Maximal exercise testing variables and 10- year survival: fitness risk score derivation from the FIT Project. Mayo Clin Proc 2015;90(3):346–55.

50. Yeboah J, McClelland RL, Polonsky TS, et al. Comparison of novel risk markers for improvement in cardiovascular risk assessment in intermediate-risk individuals. JAMA 2012;308(8):788–95.

51. Hecht H, Blaha M, Berman D, et al. Clinical indications for coronary artery calcium scoring in asymtomatic patients: expert consensus statement from the society of cardiovascular computed tomography. J Cardiovasc Comput Tomogr 2017;11:157–68.

52. Blaha MJ, Dardari ZA, Blumenthal RS, et al. The new intermediate risk group: a comparative analysis of the new 2013 ACC/AHA risk assessment guidelines versus prior guidelines in men. Atherosclerosis 2014;237(1):1–4.

53. Gofman JW. The quantitative nature of the relationship of coronary artery atherosclerosis and coronary heart disease risk. Cardiol Dig 1969;4:28–38.

54. Pastuszak AW, Hyman DA, Yadav N, et al. Erectile dysfunction as a marker for cardiovascular disease diagnosis and intervention: a cost analysis. J Sex Med 2015;12:975–84.

55. FDA Drug Safety Communication: FDA cautions about using testosterone products for low testosterone due to aging; requires labeling change to inform of possible increased risk of heart attack and stroke with use 2015. Available at: http://www.fda.gov/Drugs/DrugSafety/ucm436259.htm. Accessed December 14, 2017.

56. Corona G, Isidori AM, Buvat J, et al. Testosterone supplementation and sexual function: a meta- analysis study. J Sex Med 2014;11(6):1577–92.

57. Nguyen CP, Hirsch MS, Moeny D, et al. Testosterone and "Age Related Hypogonadism"–FDA concerns. N Engl J Med 2015;373(8):689–91.

58. Basaria S, Coviello AD, Travison TG, et al. Adverse events associated with testosterone administration. N Engl J Med 2010;363:109–22.

59. US Food and Drug Administration. Citizen petition denial response From FDA CDER to Public Citizen. Published July 16, 2014. Accessed August 31, 2014. Available at: http://www.citizen.org/documents/2184_FDA%20Denial%20of% 20Petition_July%2016, %202014.pdf. Accessed April 28, 2016.

60. Vigen R, O'Donnell CI, Baron AE, et al. Association of testosterone therapy with mortality, myocardial infarction, and stroke in men with low testosterone levels. JAMA 2013;310(17):1829–36.

61. Morgentaler A, Lunenfeld B. Testosterone and cardiovascular risk: world's experts take unprecedented action to correct misinformation. Aging Male 2014; 17(2):63–5.

62. Finkle WD, Greenland S, Ridgeway GK, et al. Increased risk of non-fatal myocardial infarction following testosterone therapy prescription in men. PLoS One 2014; 9(1):e85805.

63. Xu L, Freeman G, Cowling BJ, et al. Testosterone therapy and cardiovascular events among men: a systematic review and meta-analysis of placebo-controlled randomized trials. BMC Med 2013;11:108.

64. Corona G, Maseroli E, Rastrelli G, et al. Cardiovascular risk associated with testosterone-boosting medications: a systematic review and meta-analysis. Expert Opin Drug Saf 2014;13(10):1327–51.

65. Borst SE, Shuster JJ, Zou B, et al. Cardiovascular risks and elevation of serum DHT vary by route of testosterone administration: a systematic review and meta-analysis. BMC Med 2014;12:211.

66. Calof OM, Singh AB, Lee ML, et al. Adverse events associated with testosterone replacement in middle-aged and older men: a meta-analysis of randomized, placebo-controlled trials. J Gerontol A Biol Sci Med Sci 2005;60(11):1451–7.

67. Fernández-Balsells MM, Murad MH, Lane M, Lampropulos JF. Clinical review 1: adverse effects of testosterone therapy in adult men: a systematic review and meta-analysis. J Clin Endocrinol Metab 2010;95(6):2560–75.

68. Haddad RM, Kennedy CC, Caples SM, et al. Testosterone and cardiovascular risk in men: a systematic review and meta-analysis of randomized placebo-controlled trials. Mayo Clin Proc 2007;82(1):29–39.

69. Isidori AM, Giannetta E, Gianfrilli D, et al. Effects of testosterone on sexual function in men: results of a meta-analysis. Clin Endocrinol (oxf) 2005;63(4):381–94.

70. Shores MM, Smith NL, Forsberg CW, et al. Testosterone treatment and mortality in men with low testosterone levels. J Clin Endocrinol Metab 2012;97(6):2050–8.

71. Muraleedharan V, Marsh H, Kapoor D, et al. Testosterone deficiency is associated with increased risk of mortality and testosterone replacement improves survival in men with type 2 diabetes. Eur J Endocrinol 2013;169(6):725–33.

72. English KM, Steeds RP, Jones TH, et al. Low-dose transdermal testosterone therapy improves angina threshold in men with chronic stable angina: a randomized, double- blind, placebo-controlled study. Circulation 2000;102(16):1906–11.

73. Caminiti G, Volterrani M, Iellamo F, et al. Effect of long-acting testosterone treatment on functional exercise capacity, skeletal muscle performance, insulin resistance, and baroreflex sensitivity in elderly patients with chronic heart failure a double-blind, placebo-controlled, randomized study. J Am Coll Cardiol 2009; 54(10):919–27.

74. Malkin CJ, Pugh PJ, West JN, et al. Testosterone therapy in men with moderate severity heart failure: a double-blind randomized placebo controlled trial. Eur Heart J 2006;27(1):57–64.

75. Pugh PJ, Jones RD, West JN, et al. Testosterone treatment for men with chronic heart failure. Heart 2004;90(4):446–7.

76. Iellamo F, Volterrani M, Caminiti G, et al. Testosterone therapy in women with chronic heart failure: a pilot double-blind, randomized, placebo-controlled study. J Am Coll Cardiol 2010;56(16):1310–6.

77. Available at: http://www.ema.europa.eu/ema/index.jsp?curl=pages/medicines/human/referrals/Testosteronecontaining_medicines/human_referral_prac_000037.jsp&mid=WC0b01ac05805c516f. Accessed December 14, 2017.

78. Snyder PJ, Bhasin S, Cunningham GR, et al. Testosterone trials investigators. Effects of testosterone treatment in older men. N Engl J Med 2016;374(7): 611–24.

79. Budoff MJ, Ellenberg SS, Lewis CE, et al. Testosterone treatment and coronary artery plaque volume in older men with low testosterone. JAMA 2017;317(7): 708–16.

80. Basaria S, Harman SM, Travison TG, et al. Effects of testosterone administration for 3 years on subclinical atherosclerosis progression in older men with low or low-normal testosterone levels: a randomized clinical trial. JAMA 2015;314: 570–81.

81. Campion JM, Maricic MJ. Osteoporosis in men. Am Fam Physician 2003;67(7): 1521–6.
82. Gullberg B, Johnell O, Kanis JA. World-wide projections for hip fracture. Osteoporos Int 1997;7(5):407–13.
83. Cooper C, Campion G, Melton LJ 3rd. Hip fractures in the elderly: a world-wide projection. Osteoporos Int 1992;2(6):285–9.
84. Stevens JA, Rudd RA. The impact of decreasing U.S. hip fracture rates on future hip fracture estimates. Osteoporos Int 2013;24:2725–8.
85. Day, Cheeseman J. Population projections of the United States by age, sex, race, and hispanic origin: 1995 to 2050, U.S. bureau of the census, current population reports. Washington, DC: U.S. Government Printing Office; 1996. p. 25–1130.
86. Schnell S, Friedman SM, Mendelson DA, et al. The 1-year mortality of patients treated in a hip fracture program for elders. Geriatr Orthop Surg Rehabil 2010; 1(1):6–14.
87. Pande I, Scott DL, O'Neill TW, et al. Quality of life, morbidity, and mortality after low trauma hip fracture in men. Ann Rheu Dis 2006;65(1):87–92.
88. Ip TP, Leung J, Kung AWC. Management of osteoporosis in patients hospitalized for hip fractures. Osteoporos Int 2010;21(Suppl 4):605–14.
89. Kiebzak GM, Beinart GA, Perser K, et al. Undertreatment of osteoporosis in men with hip fracture. Arch Intern Med 2002;162(19):2217–22.
90. Nayak S, Greenspan S. Osteoporosis treatment efficacy for men: a systematic review and meta-analysis. J Am Geriatr Soc 2017;65(3):490–5.
91. Schwarz P, Jorgensen NR, Mosekilde L, et al. The evidence for efficacy of osteoporosis treatment in men with primary osteoporosis: a systematic review and meta-analysis of antiresorptive and anabolic treatment in men. J Osteoporos 2011;2011:2598–618.
92. Kim SH, Choi HS, Rhee Y, et al. Prevalent vertebral fractures predict subsequent radiographic vertebral fractures in postmenopausal Korean women receiving antiresorptive agent. Osteoporos Int 2011;22:781.
93. Schousboe JT, Vokes T, Broy SB, et al. Vertebral fracture assessment: the 2007 ISCD official positions. J Clin Densitom 2008;11(1):92–108.
94. Watts NB, Adler RA, Bilezikian JP, et al. Osteoporosis in men: an endocrine society clinical practice guideline. J Clin Endocrinol Metab 2012;97(6):1802–22.
95. Qaseem A, Forciea MA, McLean RM, et al, For the Clinical Guidelines Committee of the American College of Physicians. Treatment of low bone density or osteoporosis to prevent fractures in men and women: a clinical practice guideline update from the American College of Physicians. Ann Intern Med 2017;166:818–39.
96. Expert Panel on Musculoskeletal Imaging, Ward RJ, Roberts CC, et al. ACR appropriateness criteria osteoporosis and bone mineral density. J Am Coll Radiol 2017;14(5S):S189–202.
97. Kochanek KD, Murphy SL, Xu J, et al. Deaths: final data for 2014. Natl Vital Stat Rep 2016;65(4):1–122.
98. Neese R, Kruger DJ, Nesse RM. Economic transition, male competition, and sex differences in mortality rates. Evol Psychol 2007;5:358–74. Available at: www.CDC.gov.
99. AUA Men's Health Checklist: Am Urological Assn Publication 2014.